MANUAL

OF

HOMŒOPATHIC

THEORY AND PRACTICE.

DESIGNED FOR THE USE OF

Physicians and Families.

BY ARTHUR LUTZE, M. D.

Man can what he wills,
But he must have faith and trust!

TRANSLATED FROM THE GERMAN, WITH ADDITIONS,

BY CHARLES J. HEMPEL, M. D.

FROM THE SIXTIETH THOUSAND OF THE GERMAN EDITION.

NEW YORK:
WILLIAM RADDE, 300 BROADWAY.
PHILADELPHIA:
WILLIAM RADDE, No. 635 ARCH STREET.
1862.

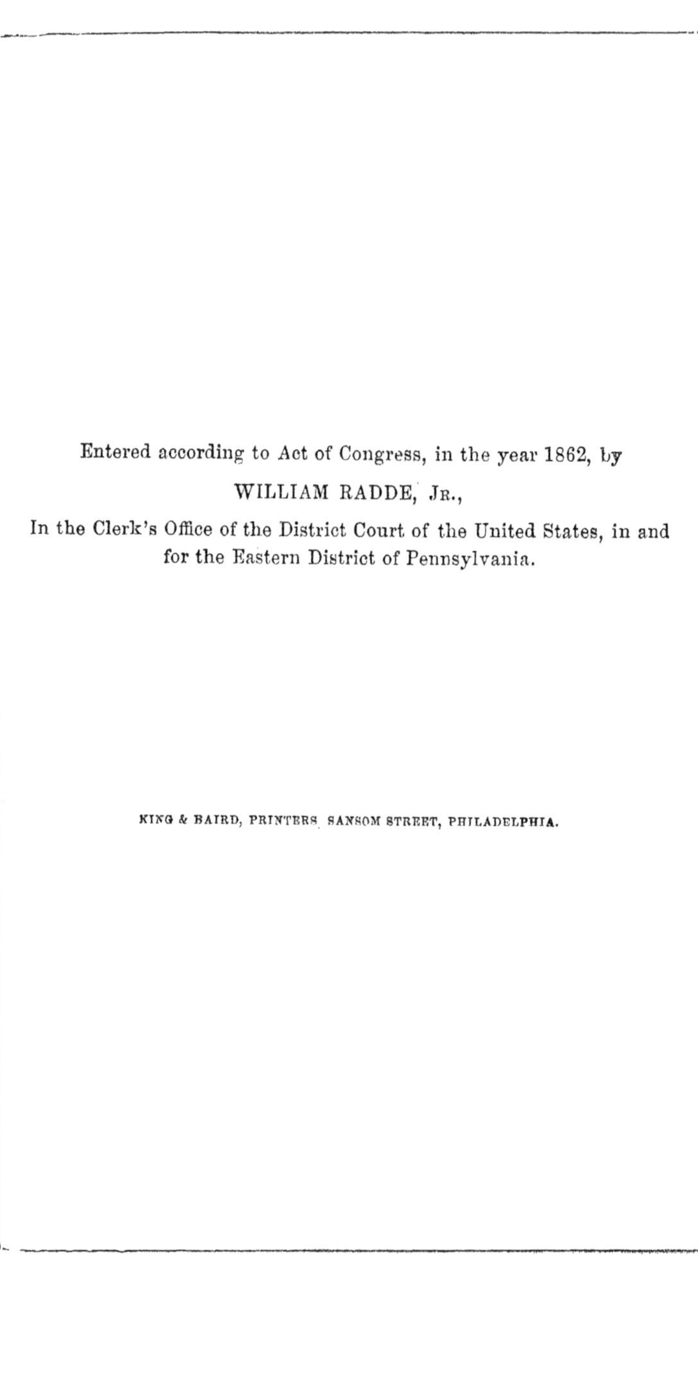

KING & BAIRD, PRINTERS, SANSOM STREET, PHILADELPHIA.

TO

His Highness

THE

REIGNING DUKE BERNHARD,

OF

SAXE-MEININGEN.

Although I have not the honor to be one of your Highness' subjects, yet you are so generally known and admired as a promoter of the Homœopathic Healing Art, and you occupy such an eminent position in the history of Homœopathy that it affords me the highest honor and delight to be permitted to dedicate to your Highness my Manual of Homœopathy.

Would that many reigning Princes might follow your Highness' example, and protect and promote the new Healing Art fraught with blessings.

With deep respect, I am your Highness'

Faithful and obedient servant,

ARTHUR LUTZE.

CŒTHEN, August 10th, 1860.

TABLE OF CONTENTS.

THE PUBLISHER'S ANNOUNCEMENT.

DR. LUTZE'S work on the Theory and Practice of Homœopathy is the most popular treatise on this science which has yet been published in Europe. No less than sixty thousand copies of this work have been sold at the present moment. No physician in Europe can boast of a larger and more lucrative practice, or of a larger number of patients of the highest social standing and education than Dr. Lutze. He adheres with the utmost rigidity to Hahnemann's original doctrines, and his practice is crowned with undeniable and, in many respects, unparalleled success. In one particular Dr. Lutze deviates in the treatment of inveterate chronic diseases from the established rule of homœopathic practitioners; we allude to a combination of remedies. This proceeding is, however, applied only to a few remedies, and then only in chronic maladies.

The section where the use of combined drugs is explained, does not form an integral part of this work; but, in order not to omit any thing of the original text, the publisher has deemed it advisable to insert this section of Lutze's work in this Announcement, together with the letters to and from Hahnemann where the discovery of a combination of drugs is sanctioned by the author of Homœopathy as a legitimate development of the homœopathic healing art. This innovation, however, need not shock the orthodox reader; it is never alluded to in the body of the work; all that need be said in reference to this matter is that in chronic cases, Dr. Lutze, instead of alternating drugs, frequently gives the two remedies, each of which is supposed to be homœopathic to the case, in combination. The reasons which have prompted him to innovate thus far upon the general practice of homœopathic physicians, are fully stated in Section VII. of his work, which is here transcribed for the benefit of the American reader.

SECTION VII.

"An important subject is the combination of remedies. As in acute cases we often have to give two remedies in alternation, because the symptoms of the case are not always covered by one, so in chronic cases two remedies may be given not in alternation, *but in combination,* three to four globules of each remedy being dissolved in the same tumbler of water, and a spoonful of this solution being taken morning and night for several days in succession. In a case of tetter, for instance, or debility from loss of blood, *Sulphur* and *China* may be given in combination. Sulphur for the psora, China for the debility, and the result shows that this combination cures much more effectually than either of these drugs, if given singly. In cardialgia the symptoms of which are covered by *Nux,* I give Nux and Sulphur in combination, if an eruption had existed previously. In tetter which breaks out after suppressed itch or syphilis, I give *Mercurius* and *Sulphur* in combination.

In making such a combination I have to warn against using drugs each of which is not homœopathic to the existing case. This, however, is a matter of course, for no cure can be expected of a remedy which is not homœopathic to the case.

Any two remedies may be combined, if highly potentized, even antidotes. Experience shows that, if two antidotes are indicated in a case, they produce striking effects, *if given in combination.* The explanation of this phenomenon is not difficult. I suppose that the process of mixing does not apply to higher potencies, but that the two may assist each other in their mutual effects; but even this fact does not extend to antidotes which repel each other, and each of which pursues its own action to the end of the cure.

This important discovery of the combination of drugs was first announced twenty-four years ago, by Doctor Julius Aegidi, at that time physician to the Princess Frederica of Prussia, and now medical counsellor. This discovery was communicated to Hahnemann in the year 1833, corroborated by two hundred and thirty-three cures with combined remedies, and was joyfully received by Hahnemann, but kept secret from the public by the imbecility of the foes of truth, whereas the worthy discoverer was insulted and derided by those who were unworthy of unloosening his shoe-strings.

Read Hahnemann's reply to Aegidi's letter where he announces his discovery, and relates the history of two hundred and thirty-three cures with remedies administered in combination. The letter bears date May 15th, 1833.

"DEAR FRIEND AND COLLEAGUE:

"Do not suppose that I reject any thing good from mere prejudice, or because it might lead to modifications in my doctrine. All I desire is the truth, and I know that this is all you care for. I am rejoiced that you should have had such a happy thought, at the same time confining its execution to proper limits. Two remedies should only be given in combination, in a highly potentized form, provided each is, in its own way, homœopathic to the case. In such a case, this proceeding is an advantage to our art which should not be repudiated. I shall take the first opportunity of making a trial, and I doubt not that it will be successful. I am likewise glad to hear that Bœnninghausen approves of this plan. I believe that two remedies may be given in combination, which we do even now when *Sulphur* and *Calcarea* are given in combination in the form of *Hepar sulphuris;* or *Sulphur* and *Mercurius,* when Cinnabaris is administered. Permit me to communicate your discovery to the world, in the fifth edition of the Organon which is soon to appear. Until then please keep this discovery to yourself, and request Dr. Jahr, whom I esteem very highly, to do the same. At the same time I shall protest and earnestly warn against the arbitrary combination of any two drugs indiscriminately.

"Truly yours,
"S. HAHNEMANN."

In another letter to Dr. Aegidi, Hahnemann writes, under date of June 19th, 1833:

"——— I have devoted a special paragraph to your discovery of a combination of drugs, in the fifth edition of my Organon, the manuscript copy of which was sent last night to Arnold, with a request that the work should be printed very speedily and that my likeness should be placed in front of the title-page. The rivalry for priority is a most anxious chase. Thirty years ago I, too, had the weakness of wooing it. But for a long time past I have not felt any other desire than that the world should know the best and most useful truth, whether through me or any body else."

These are the words of the master, and we now ask, What has become of this paragraph? We search the Organon from the first page to the last, *without finding it!*

Here is the explanation. Hahnemann laid the new discovery which he had kept secret heretofore, before the meeting of homœopathic physicians on the 10th of August, 1833. Their number was as yet small, but instead of meeting with open hearts, he found stubborn minds that were incrusted with old prejudices, and, instead of accepting the blissful truth, assailed it with all sorts of persecutions, comparing it to the mixtures of allœopathic practitioners, and persuading Hahnemann to abandon the publication of this discovery and even to allow one of his friends, while passing through Dresden, to suppress the paragraph which had already been printed.

Thus it is that the world has been robbed of a most important discovery these twenty-one years; for Aegidi's publication of his discovery in the 14th volume of the Archive, 1834, was assailed in such a shameless manner by a number of enemies, that it was soon forgotten by those who only heed the cry of the multitude, and that the worthy discoverer preferred remaining silent to exposing himself to abuse and to the assaults of an imbecile crowd.

I do not know the persons who have perpetrated this robbery against humanity, nor do I care to hear their names mentioned; most of them may be in their graves, and the balance are already judged; therefore we will not condemn them any further, but pray for them: Father, forgive them, for they knew not what they were doing.

The time of requital has come; the hitherto suppressed discovery rises like a phenix from its ashes, and the name of its author, *Julius Aegidi*, shall be snatched from oblivion. I am thankful for the privilege I enjoy of wresting the new truth from its slumber, not like a feeble infant, but grown up to manhood and armed with the sword of intelligence and power, which will enable it to resist the persecutions of darkness.

In comparing the use of *combined remedies* to the mixtures of allœopaths, the opponents of this discovery showed most conclusively that they have neither apprehended the essence of homœopathy nor the meaning of potentization. If a medicine is selected *homœopathically*, or in conformity with the law of similarity, every arbitrary proceeding which prevails in allœopathic practice, ceases; an arbitrary compounding of drugs cannot be compared with a combination of remedies based upon law. In the next place, the term mixture only applies to coarse materials, but not to high dynamisations which are deprived of their material constituents, and have been converted into purely spiritual powers by means of which the most astonishing effects can be produced, such as the instantaneous cure of a violent toothache, by simply smelling of the appropriately-selected agent; thousands of cases illustrate these marvellous effects. Spiritual forces can be mixed no more than mental productions received into the storehouse of the mind; a proof of this is our memory in which thousands of objects, whether acquired or invented, are ranged side by side without being mixed; if this should take place, it shows mental disease, derangement, insanity.

Mesmerism exhibits a form of *combined medicines.* If a person has a headache in both sides of the forehead or in both temples, and I first make a pass over the right side of the forehead, the pain disappears in this region; if, then, I make a similar pass over the left side, the pain there disappears likewise; we know this from experience. In making simultaneous passes with both hands down both sides of the forehead, the pain disappears in both sides at the same time. Who will assert that this is not in strict accord with the requirements of art? On the contrary, any one who is acquainted with mesmerism, will proceed in this very manner, and will obtain striking results. This is the case with *combined remedies.*

I do not mention this by way of an explanation, but my intention has only been to illustrate my position by analogous facts; for no fundamental or elementary phenomenon can be explained.

Hahnemann commits a slight mistake by ranging Hepar sulphuris and Cinnabaris with combined remedies; the difference is, that the former are mixed in their crude elements, and then potentized and proved as identical units; whereas combined remedies consist of two high dynamizations acting side by side with each other, *each in its specific manner.*

Three or four years ago the discoverer first acquainted me with the combination of remedies; having had thousands of opportunities of trying them in my clinic, it is useless to deny their efficacy. But I must request my colleagues who are anxious to institute similar experiments, to do so with carefully prepared potencies. Our excellent Bœnninghausen has informed me orally, that he has obtained equally fortunate results with the high potencies, and every honest experimenter will be able to achieve a similar success.

I made my first experiments in Berlin, on the very day when the discovery of a combination of remedies was first made known to me. It was in the case of a lady who had been operated on for cataract by Jûngken nine months ago, and who had been suffering since then with such a violent ophthalmia and such intense pains in the eyes that she prayed for death, since Jûngken was unable to order any thing for her relief except leeches to the temples, a stupid remedy which had the effect of determining the blood to the head more and more. As soon as she heard my steps, she exclaimed: Oh, relieve me of my boundless misery, else I shall prefer death! I at once mixed 3 globules of *Aconite* and 3 of *Belladonna* in a small tumblerful of water, and ordered a dessertspoonful every hour. Half an hour after the first dose she felt relieved; in two hours the pains had left her, and in twenty-four hours pains and inflammation had disappeared. Now she was for the first time able to enjoy the benefit of the operation which had otherwise been performed with perfect success. Homœopathy has converted ophthalmic surgery into a true blessing; I can show numbers of cases where I have operated without the least inflammation supervening; for immediately after the operation I give *Aconite* 30 in water every two hours, and if the patient complains of pains in or over the eyes, I give *Belladonna* 30 in alternation or combination with Aconite.

I will now relate a few cases which I have treated in my clinic :

2. Antonia D., aged 25 months, was thrown down by a cat jumping against her, with such violence that her head was knocked against a chair, and she trembled with fright. Half an hour after she commenced to stutter, which grew worse from day to day. I gave a solution of *Arnica* 30, and *Opium* 30 *in combination*, a dessertspoonful every morning and night, for four days in succession (Arnica for the concussion, and Opium for the effects of the fright). After a trifling aggravation the child improved, and, in a fortnight, talked with her usual ease.

3. Mrs K. had pulmonary phthisis for some time past. Cough with expectoration of yellow mucus, having a saltish and sometimes a bitter taste. Hoarseness, faint sound of the voice. Slight fever without thirst, oppression of the chest, palpitation of the heart, whining mood. Complete suppression of the menses for the last three months, they had been scanty and watery for a long time previous. Great debility, constant night-sweats. Every other day all the symptoms were worse. Gave *Pulsatilla* 30 and *China* 30 in water, in combination, for four days as above. Eight days after commencing the treatment the menses became regular and a general improvement set in. Cough and expectoration likewise disappeared. She was cured in four months.

4. Mrs. K., 40 years old, had been affected for many years with violent pains in the abdomen, especially when the menses happened to be suppressed, which took

place very irregularly in consequence of severe confinements. The menses had been suppressed for six months. The pain in the abdomen set in with so much chilliness that the limbs trembled, and the pain affected the whole body. In the right side of the abdomen a hardness was sometimes perceived, which disappeared again. Stool generally hard, attended with great pain. In consequence of great weakness the patient had almost always to keep her bed; when she attempted to rise, the pain grew worse. It lasted from three in the morning until evening. When a child, she had the itch which was removed by means of an ointment. I gave *Nux* and *Sulphur* 30 in combination. Six weeks after, I received the following report: "After the first dose the pains ceased, the menses returned in a fortnight, and I feel quite well except a little weak."

5. Augusta F., 12 years old, had been afflicted with vomiting of the ingesta since her birth, except bread. She could not even retain her mother's milk, so that she had to be brought up on bread; afterwards she was unable to keep any thing on her stomach except dry bread. After having employed several physicians, among whom some homœopaths, she applied to me. I ascertained that she was occasionally troubled with an eruption in the face, and that her fingers were covered with small warts. I gave *Sulphur* and *Ipecac.* 30 in combination, dissolved in water, morning and evening, for four days, Sulphur for psora, Ipecac. for the vomiting. Three days after taking this medicine she was seized with such violent vomiting for three days, that even the dry bread was rejected; after this she was able to keep every thing on her stomach, even water, and any kind of nourishment. The vomiting ceased en-

tirely, the warts diminished in size from week to week, disappeared first on the left hand, in eight weeks after likewise on the right (because Sulphur first acts upon the left side), so that a single dose of this combined remedy effected a cure.

6. Mr. W., 29 years old, after every slight cold was attacked with chilliness, followed by pains in the head, chest and back which continued for some time. The pain then extended throughout the whole head and was most violent on the top. During the attack the bowels remained costive for three or four days, he had no appetite, his sleep was restless and disturbed by anxious dreams. In his 17th year he had spitting of blood and pains in the chest; he had occasional attacks of congestion of blood to the chest, so that he had to tear his clothes open. In his youth he had a tetter on the legs which was removed by an ointment. This was followed by swelling of the knee-joints, sour, nauseous taste in the mouth on waking in the morning, frequent itching of the hands. Gave *Nux* and *Sulphur* in combination. A fortnight after, he had another attack, and another in four weeks which only lasted one day, after which the attacks ceased entirely, even when he took a violent cold.

7. Mr. F., 32 years old, had a fall six years ago, which caused a contusion of the testicles, in consequence of which *hydrocele* developed itself which increased continually. He complained of constant pain in the testes, especially in stormy weather. I gave *Arnica* and *Rhod.* 30 in combination (Arnica for the contusion, Rhod. on account of the influence of stormy weather). The pains abated after the first dose, and disappeared entirely in four days, without ever returning. The hydrocele was cured in six weeks.

8. Mrs. L., 35 years old, was afflicted with spasmodic attacks which recurred several times a day. They were attended with distortion of the mouth, trembling of the hands and feet, paralysis of the tongue, flow of mucus from the mouth, sweat on the whole body. The paroxysms lasted half an hour, and were worse in the evening than in the morning. Delirium after the paroxysms. Suppression of the menses for the last three months, pains in the small of the back, stinging in the rectum. Gave *Bellad.* and *Pulsat.* 30 in combination. On the second day after taking the medicine, the menses reappeared normally, but the spasms grew worse, especially on the third day; they were much less on the fourth and fifth day, ceased on the sixth, and on the seventeenth the patient only complained of a feeling of dullness in the head, which disappeared very speedily.

9. Miss S., 19 years old, took a violent cold, in consequence of which she had almost lost her voice for eight days past. She felt a dryness and heat in the throat, sensation as of a foreign body having lodged in the throat, which cannot be raised. Painful feeling when moving the throat. Menses scanty, but occurring every three weeks. Gave *Chamom.* and *Sepia* 30 in combination (Chamomilla for the hoarseness, Sepia for the scanty menses). The patient took her first dose in the evening, slept well, and was able, after taking her second dose in the morning, to answer a question with a clear and ringing voice; every painful feeling in the throat had disappeared, and she was cured. Afterwards the menses appeared every four weeks and a little later.

10. Frederick, aged 18 years, had been troubled with ulcers for two years past, one of which at least broke out on the arms, legs or back, and caused violent pain.

The patient was so feeble that he sometimes was scarcely able to stand. This weakness was the result of masturbation which he had practiced for four years. I gave *Hepar* and *China* 30 in combination. Eight days after taking the medicine a large ulcer broke out on the thigh; this was the last that ever troubled him; the weakness likewise disappeared, and he soon felt better than he had ever done.

11. Julius, aged three years, had had several attacks of tertian fever, for which nothing had been taken. The child had not much chilliness or sweat, but a good deal of dry heat, and some breaking out around the mouth. He took *Aconite* and *Sulphur* 30 in combination. He had another violent attack, which was the last.

12. Mrs. H., 24 years old, was attacked with violent stitches in both breasts after weaning her infant, dry heat and vertigo so that she had to hold on to something to prevent her falling. I gave *Acon.* and *Bell.* in combination. A few minutes after the first dose, pain, stitches, etc., disappeared completely.

13. Mr. S., 75 years old, had been hard of hearing of the right ear since his infancy. The ear discharged a yellow, fetid pus, as is sometimes the case after scarlet-fever. For four weeks past he did not hear well of the left ear where I observed a good deal of indurated, dark-brown cerumen. The itch had been suppressed on him in his youth. I gave *Bell.* and *Sulphur* 30, in combination. On the twelfth day, on waking, he heard the ticking of the watch: he had recovered the hearing of both ears.

14. Mr. W., aged 23 years, had been affected with figwarts for some years past; they were cauterised, cut, tied, but they invariably broke out again. Three weeks ago, syphilis had supervened. He took *Thuja* and

Mercurius 30, in combination; in a fortnight the fig-warts fell off, and the syphilitic symptoms disappeared in a month; several years after, he assured me that he never enjoyed such good health as after my treatment.

15. The most remarkable case is that of the stocking-manufacturer Harnisch, of Hoheneck in Saxony. This case is so remarkable that the prime-minister von Gossler, examined the patient, and Drs. Moldenhawer and Loewenstein, who attend my clinic, were instructed to relate the case officially. The patient sent me the following report: Is 44 years old, has had caries of the left leg for thirteen years and a-half, which had six suppurating sores. The leg was one and a-half inches shorter than the other, so that he had been limping for fourteen years. The many physicians whom he had consulted, had never been able to heal the sores which had discharged four pieces of bone. Owing to his exertions in walking, the right thigh had likewise become affected, so that he frequently complained of tearing pains and stiffness in the hip-joint. Every year he had been bled two or three times for a rush of blood to the head; he hadbeen practising this for twenty-five years past, and had been much weakened by it. I gave him *Sulphur* and *China* 30, in combination, the former for the psora, the latter for the weakness from loss of blood. Six weeks after the treatment he sent me the following report: "After the first dose I had ease in my leg, so that I was able to sleep for three nights, which I had not been able to do for the four weeks past in consequence of the tearing pain, and the anxiety. After that, I was again attacked with burning, especially in the right hip, and colicky pains, with distention of the abdomen. On the twelfth day I experienced a stretching in the legs, which, however,

made me feel stronger, so that I desired to stretch all the time. In the night from the 13th to the 14th, this desire was very strong, and when I arose, behold! *both legs had the same length.* Those who did not see me, would not believe it, nor could the physicians account for this change, for they had seen me limp on a stick for fourteen years, whereas I was now able to walk erect like a soldier. The weakness in the hip-joint has likewise left me, so that I am now able to walk for ten hours on a stretch, whereas, formerly, I was hardly able to walk a mile."

This case created quite a sensation in Saxony, and brought daily from fifty to sixty people to my clinic who expected to be cured in the same striking manner. Harnisch who visited me every few weeks, brought me some thirty or forty reports of cases at each visit, and this case has converted many persons to homœopathy who did not believe in it previously. It is interesting to every friend of homœopathy that a single dose of a combined remedy effected this cure in a fortnight. Every physician will want to know how it happened that the shortened limb acquired its natural length back again. Upon examination I found that the bones of the left leg were not shortened, and that only single splinters had been detached by the ulcerative process; the pus had become healthy, and the pain had disappeared. The inequality could not, therefore, be owing to any defect in the left leg, but must depend upon the right leg being abnormally elongated. The patient indeed recollected that, fourteen years ago, previous to the breaking out of the sores, he experienced a violent pain in the right hip. I infer from this that he was then affected with coxitis or coxarthrocace (hip-disease,) which was arrested in the first stage of elongation of the limb, in consequence of the morbid process developing itself in the left limb, and terminating in ulceration. My deeply-penetrating combined remedy re-excited the former ailment and cured it. I have several cases of inveterate coxarthrocace, where a cure was effected and where both limbs were restored to the normal size and length. The difference is that in some cases it takes years to effect a cure, whereas twelve days were sufficient in Harnisch's case.

These cases point out the method I pursue, with sufficient clearness to any one who chooses to understand it. To him who does not choose, a thousand additional cases would afford no light.

The following is my formula for prescribing two remedies in combination. I unite them by means of this sign &, and moreover by the sign + placed underneath the former, and a ◡ thus: *Acon.* & *Bell.*"
+
◡

The reader will see at a glance that this work is an eminently practical treatise, and that both laymen and beginning practitioners may derive great benefit from its use. Dr. Lutze uses throughout the 30th potency of Hahnemann. The publisher has deemed it sufficient to make this general statement in his Announcement, instead of repeating it on every page. The translation has been carefully prepared by competent hands, and all that now remains for the publisher to do is to plead in justification of his undertaking his firm conviction that Lutze's work will prove a most useful and interesting addition to the popular literature of our School.

WM. RADDE, Jr.

1861, *Philadelphia.*

PREFACE.

THERE are still many who have not the remotest idea of Hahnemann's true greatness and of his doctrine. Some only know him as a great physician and discoverer of a new system of cure, others as a medical reformer whom they range side by side with other reformers of the sciences and believe to have sufficiently honored by comparing him to Newton, Galiläi, Copernicus, etc. But what have all these discoverers accomplished in comparison with Hahnemann?

They have indeed discovered new laws, conquered old prejudices, removed abuses, and announced unknown truths; but they were enabled to continue that which had been begun by their predecessors, and to improve existing knowledge.

Hahnemann, on the contrary, had to overthrow the present and was not even able to make use of the ruins of the past; he had to create every thing anew, and, like a phœnix above the ashes, his new doctrine hovers over the ancient chaos of errors, prejudices and fatal abuses which have tortured poor humanity for nearly two thousand years, and have prepared premature graves for thousands of victims.

Finally Hahnemann's doctrine affects the very life of the whole human race. It not only blesses a few, a certain class, the learned, but *all men;* learned and unlearned, rich and poor, kings and beggars, even animals, enjoy the fruits of Hahnemann's discovery. Hahnemann nurses and promotes the belief in God, and in his inscrutable Providence by showing that even the smallest and almost imperceptible quantity of a medicine may produce great and astonishing results.

Samuel Hahnemann has discovered the irrefutable law, which proves true without exception, in every science and in all our relations of life. *Like* can only act upon and promote *like*, in speech, act or medicine. This law pervades all nature like a shining meteor.

We see how only animals and plants that are alike, support and fecondate each other, how only like forces and passions combat each other: a teacher can only teach with effect, if he accommodates his instruction to the capacities of his pupils; a preacher can only exercise a powerful effect upon the minds of his hearers, if his discourse is adapted to the nature and comprehension of his hearers; even the mechanician and the naturalist can only act with forces that are alike; only similar poles can attract each other, only like hearts can realize a happy union.

That which is entirely dissimilar, opposite, like the same poles of a magnet, repels its contrary, and may even produce disaster and ruin like the allœopathic practice of medicine which ignores or denies the universal law of homœopathy.

But what would avail all theory in medicine; of what use would it be to the world and to the human race, if the theory were not confirmed by the brilliant achievements of experience.

Our practice and theory go hand in hand, and it is because our accumulated and brilliant cures furnish the most indubitable evidence of the truth of Hahnemann's discovery: that it becomes our sacred duty not to be idle spectators of this new order of things, but to institute active inquiries until we too are favored with a knowledge of the truth which remains hidden from no one who earnestly seeks it.

To many minds it is both a problem and a stumbling-block that the infinitesimal, imponderable and imperceptible, but highly refined doses should act more *powerfully*, more *intensely* and more *penetratingly* than the crude material of these same drugs; but let us consider that the nervous system likewise is refined and enfeebled; that a sound, a blow, even the ticking of a clock may cause one to start, and may excite a feeling of fright and anxiety; how much more powerful are the most refined homœopathic doses than these vibrations of the air, true *nothings to the healthy organism, but the causes of considerable aggravations, and even of death in severe diseases.*

By curing a number of otherwise incurable sufferings, homœopathy furnishes the proof that every disease has its main seat and origin in the nervous system; a medicine is to act upon the nerves, this exceedingly subtile fluid which has never yet been perceived by the senses. Should we not, then, operate with the most refined medicinal preparations which are most adapted to the nerves, and has not the discoverer of homœopathy realized these preparations?

It is only such exceedingly minute doses that are assimilable to the affected nerves; a cure can only take place where such an assimilation exists; in the same way nutrition can only take place by the food being assimilated to the digestive organs. The digestive process is to food what potentization is to drugs.

ARTHUR LUTZE.

INTRODUCTION.

The law of Homœopathy, "*similia similibus*," or "*like by like*," has been verified since its discovery by Samuel Hahnemann in the year 1790, in all the departments of life, as an irrefutable *law of nature*, one of those laws which enable us to look into the internal economy of nature, and to observe the connection between cause and effect. It is a sad thing that this great law which should not only govern the treatment of diseases but social life, and more particularly the education of children, is still comprehended and acknowledged by such a small number. But since the homœopathic healing art is spreading so rapidly, it may be supposed that the law of homœopathy will likewise become more and more deeply-rooted in life, although the progress of the law has so far been comparatively slow and is still retarded by imbecility, indolence and arrogance until, like the sun piercing the mist, it shall conquer all obstacles and illumine the horizon like a shining star. Lichtenberg says: "When Pythagoras had discovered his theorem, a hundred oxen were sacrificed to the gods; since then all oxen tremble at every new discovery."

Section II.

Any one who is still unacquainted with the meaning of homœopathy, may read my "*Hahnemann's Todtenfeier*," (Hahnemann's funeral solemnities,) where the homœopathic doctrine is explained in a popular manner. After that, *Hahnemann's Organon* may be studied, which is instructive to physicians and teaches the science of homœopathy.

Section III.

After having mastered the principle of homœopathy and comprehending the truth that a disease can only be cured by a remedy which is capable of producing a similar disease in healthy organisms, it then becomes a matter of importance to learn the symptoms of the different remedies.

The first provings of our drugs are found in Hahnemann's "Materia Medica Pura," and in his "Chronic Diseases." But inasmuch as the student of homœopathy is fairly inundated with symptoms in these works, and the symptoms of the various drugs are so frequently alike, that it is almost impossible to find out the characteristic action of each drug, it has frequently happened that these difficulties have caused physicians to abandon the study of homœopathy which they had commenced.

For this reason I have extracted the characteristic symptoms of every drug, so that they can be studied and remembered without difficulty. Any one who has mastered this knowledge, will find it easy to study further; but it is only in this way that these studies can be continued with success and advantage.

SECTION IV.

If I have not arranged the symptoms of the most approved remedies according to the parts of the body, it is because it was my design to premise the most important particulars in the case of each drug; in the case of ACONITE, for instance; "*vascular erethism, dry heat,* alternate chilliness and heat (fever), *restlessness, anxiety, palpitation of the heart, irritable mood.*" If these few symptoms were all that we know of Aconite, they would be of the utmost importance, since no remedy has been found more adapted to vascular erethism and inflammation than Aconite. NUX VOMICA commences with "*cardialgia, oppression of the stomach with sour eructations, sour vomiting,* water in the mouth, *distension of the abdomen, backache,* costiveness," etc. For among one hundred cases of cardialgia, eighty are cured with Nux, because this agent acts principally upon the nerves of the stomach, back and abdomen, and this simple knowledge is sufficient to cure numbers with Nux. In the case of PULSATILLA we read first: "*Menses retarded and scanty; suppression of the menses, especially in consequence of taking cold; chlorosis; irregular menstruation,* pains and cramps in the abdomen, previous to or during the appearance of the menses;" for most uterine derangements are cured with Pulsatilla, and these few symptoms make it one of our most important remedies. SULPHUR commences with these words: "*Principal remedy for psora; herpes and eruptions of every kind; itch;*" these few statements contain the gist of the remaining 1079 symptoms; for Sulphur is required in all diseases depending upon or connected with psora, and it alone secures their radical and comprehensive cure.

These are the reasons of my arrangement, and which could not operate in the case of new drugs, such as mancinella, pyrocarbon, etc., with which I myself am but imperfectly acquainted.

The "*Characteristic Symptoms*" owe their existence to the fact that a physician who studied homœopathy under my direction, requested me to make him acquainted with the most thoroughly tested effects of drugs, and which I dictated to him in my leisure hours from memory. The polychrests have been marked with an *.

Section V.

If the beginner has mastered these particulars, and should desire to have a more detailed knowledge of each drug, he may obtain it by studying Bœnninghausen's "Affinities of Homœopathic Medicines," and the more comprehensive treatise: Possart's "Characteristics of Homœopathic Medicines." After this work has been studied, "Jahr's Symptomen-codex"† may then be consulted, and "Bœnninghausen's Therapeutic Manual;" these works will enable one to get along in the most complicated cases.

For the treatment of *acute diseases* the beginner is in need of a treatise like the present one, where the course of every disease is described and the appropriate remedies are fully indicated, previous to using which the whole image of the disease has to be fully considered and the most strictly corresponding drug to be chosen with great care.

† Both works may be had in English, with considerable additions, of W. Radde, 635 Arch St., Philadelphia.

My first resource was Hering's Domestic Physician, first edition, and I am thankful to Providence that such a genuine homœopath has been my first teacher, for to him I am indebted for my first reputation as physician. What I then missed so keenly, I have endeavored to add in the present work, I mean the size and repetition of doses, concerning which I offer the following general remarks:

SECTION VI.

We have to distinguish *acute* and *chronic* diseases.

1. *Acute* diseases, violent, breaking out suddenly, and frequently endangering life, running a rapid course, such as inflammations, croup, cholera, acute fevers, etc. In all such cases I give the medicine in water, which has been found advantageous even at Hahnemann's time. I fill a clean tumbler with one or two cupfuls of well-water, into which I drop from three to five pellets of the appropriate remedy. I stir the mixture with a horny spatula or a silver spoon which should be carefully wiped after being used; the tumbler is covered with a clean saucer or plate. The solution should be kept in a cool place.

The repetition of the dose is regulated by the violence of the disease. In acute fevers I give a teaspoonful or a swallow every hour or two hours; in croup every ten or fifteen minutes; in cholera every five minutes; in erysipelas every two to four hours; if an improvement takes place, the repetition is less frequent. In fever-and ague I give the remedy morning and evening, during the apyrexia, for four or five days, after which I discontinue the medicine, for, if the remedy is properly chosen, the disease will either be arrested at once, or will disappear in the course of eight or twelve days.

I may mention that violent pains are sometimes very speedily relieved by *simply smelling* at a vial containing a few pellets of the appropriate remedy. In this way toothache for instance, is cured in a very speedy manner, also headache, or violent pains caused by contusions or wounds. If smelling should only produce temporary relief, the same medicine may then be given in water.

If it should be inconvenient to take the medicine in water, when traveling, for instance, the pellets may be taken dry on the tongue, placing no more than one pellet on the tongue and allowing it to dissolve.

In all diseases beginning with *dry heat, glowing cheeks, hurried respiration, full pulse,* restlessness and anxiety, we first give Aconite in water, as stated above, one teaspoonful every hour or even more frequently. If another remedy is indicated whose symptoms are not covered by Aconite, the two may be given in alternation.

This alternation of drugs in acute diseases is very convenient, provided both drugs are indicated at the same time; in typhus, for instance, Byronia and Rhus; in pneumonia, Aconite and Bryonia; in meningitis, Acon. and Belladonna, or Acon. and Hyoscyamus; in cholera, Cuprum and Veratrum, or Veratrum and Arsen.; in croup, Acon. and Hepar, Hepar and Spongia, Brom. and Iodine, or Acon., Hepar and Bromine; as the stages of a disease can never be sharply circumscribed, but lap over into each other, so the remedies which are administered in alternation, form the transition from one stage into another, even to a cure.

2. It is different in the cases of *chronic diseases*, or diseases which run a long course, have existed for years, and deeply taint the organism; for instance: deafness, blindness, gout, paralysis, old eruptions, open sores and old ulcers, fistulæ, herpes, curvatures of the back and bones, caries of bones.

In such chronic affections the medicine should never be frequently repeated, nor should the same medicine be given twice in succession. Each dose should be allowed sufficient time to develop its full effect, since it is the subsequent action of the drug that achieves a cure.

Formerly I gave a pellet of the indicated remedy, and in two or five months thereafter a pellet of some other remedy; but it seemed that also in chronic cases the medicine acted more penetratingly, if given in water, which may be accounted for by the fact that the medicinal water presents a more extensive surface of contact to the absorbent mucous membranes, and the torpid nerves are more frequently and hence more permanently touched by the repeated administration of the drug.

On this account I have adopted the practice of dissolving three to five pellets of the thirtieth potency in a cupful of fresh water, of which I give a swallow morning and evening for four or five days, after which I allow the medicine to act for three or four months, sometimes even for five or six months, or even longer, if the improvement continues; if it should cease, and three months should have elapsed, I then give another remedy.

The reason why I do not give another remedy under three months (except in case acute symptoms supervene,) is because I have noticed that the primary action of the drug is sometimes not developed under two or three months, after which a cure takes place, which could not have been accomplished, if I had not waited a sufficient length of time to allow the medicine to manifest its full action, or if I had interfered with it by the untimely repetition of the dose.

The curative process should not be viewed as materially as it is very frequently done. The *properly selected remedy starts the cure, the natural curative power finishes it.*

If the pendulum of a clock is once set in motion, it keeps moving as long as the clock is wound up; if we kept starting the pendulum every now and then, its vibrations would soon become disordered, and would finally be arrested. If I hide an apple-seed in the ground, it will germinate and sprout in due time, will penetrate to the light of day, and slowly but surely will grow up to the tree, according to Nature's behest. If man, becoming impatient, should undertake to lay one seed above the other, the former would become choked, no tree would grow, because Nature had been interfered with by short-sighted man.

This remark applies to chronic diseases which generally arise from some acrid matter, from some hereditary or externally inòculated *dyscrasia.* In order to expel this, the natural curative power of the organism only requires *to be started,* after which this power achieves the cure as certainly as earth and sun accomplish the unfolding of the tree from the seed. If we unwisely interfere with these mysterious rulings of Nature, a cure can no more take place than a tree can be developed from the seed.

Although Hahnemann has taught these truths most satisfactorily, yet we only become fully conscious of them, if we have experienced them in our own practice.

Years ago I had adopted the practice of not giving another dose in chronic affections under several months; but the following case taught me a different lesson.

Louise B., of H., 16½ years old, of a scrofulous habit, became so distorted after a fall which she had in her seventh year, that the cervical vertebræ stood out in an almost horizontal direction, and the sternum had assumed a similar direction in front, the head was twisted backwards. She had continual pain in the spine, sternum, and in both thighs. The latter had become weaker and weaker ever since her eighth year. At first she was only able to drag her lower extremities, but gradually she lost the use of her limbs entirely and had to be carried like a child. In this condition she was brought to my clinique where the treatment was commenced with a pellet of *Sulphur* 30. The mother returned in two months and a-half, stating that the pains had considerably increased. I gave a pellet of *Silica* 30. In three months and a-half I was informed that the sufferings of the patient had gone on increasingly. On Dec. 30th, 1847, I gave a pellet of *Calcarea* 30. No change having occurred in three months, I began to suspect that I had given my remedies too soon one after another, thus destroying the primary effect of each. I now gave powders of sugar of milk, and a favorable change took place, and continued from month to month. The pains abated more and more, the spine became straighter, the limbs more vigorous, so that, six months after taking the Calc., she was able to be led a few steps. Eight months after the cure, the father wrote: "Last Friday my daughter Louise walked a few steps alone, without being supported." A few months afterwards a tumor formed under the right scapula which terminated in an abscess and discharged after *Hepar* 30. The pus being thin and fetid, I gave *Asafetida* 30, after which it soon became yellow and thick. The suppuration weakened the patient so much that she again lost the use of her limbs; but the psoric poison having been removed from her organism, she was enabled to go to church with her parents in the spring of the same year, and to take short walks. At the end of May she took a pellet of *Lycopodium* 30, after which she improved so rapidly that she was able to walk for miles in the summer, and to do the housework; she considered herself cured. A cure would probably have been effected more rapidly, if I had allowed the former remedies to act more fully. I trust that this case will prove a warning to my colleagues, and that every one who only gives low doses, will ask himself whether he has ever performed such a cure by means of them.

Another case. Mr. H., from Holstein, had been suffering for years. He sought my advice in writing. Age 40 years. Almost constant pains in the left side of the chest; frequent yawning, sneezing and eructations. Occasional pain and swelling in the pit of the stomach, empty eructations when pressing upon this region. Deaf of the left ear from his infancy. Swelling at times of the left cheek, at other times of the mouth, nose and eye. Stiffness in the nape of the neck. Drawing pains in the left thigh. Weakness of the stomach and nerves. In former years, inflammation of the glands and lungs. He had the itch when young, which had been removed with an ointment. I sent him four powders, to be taken in eight weeks, No. 1 containing four pellets of *Sulphur* 30, which were to be dissolved in a cupful of water, a swallow to be taken morning and night for four days. After eight weeks the following report was sent to me: A few weeks after taking the medicine, all the symptoms grew worse, but in three weeks a general improvement set in. The left ear began to discharge again, which had not been the case for years, and the flatulence and pains in the chest have abated, so that the patient feels much better. I sent four powders of sugar of milk, for the effect of Sulphur now first began to show itself. The next report being still more favorable, I continued the non-medicinal powders. Twelve months after the commencement of the treatment I received the following report: The hearing of the left ear which had been deaf these thirty-two years, is restored, and I am cured except a small swelling near the left eye, and some stiffness of the nape of the neck. Another non-medicinal dose completed the cure. One dose of *Sulphur* 30, did all this in the space of four months.

Another case is Lady H., 67 years old. For forty years this patient had attacks of hemicrania which deprived her of her senses for three and more days every two or three weeks. She felt as if her brain were torn and sore. She constantly complained of nausea, rush of blood to the head, throbbing and shooting pain in the temples, towards the ear, worse on one side. Roaring and whizzing in the head and ears, so that she was not able to hear during the attack, and was unable to open her eyes in consequence of the extreme sensitiveness of her eyes. She was, moreover, affected with backache, and pains in the limbs, hæmorrhoidal tumours and such an obstinate constipation that very frequently she had only a hard and painful stool every fortnight in spite of all injections.

After a careful examination I considered *Sulphur* 30 the best remedy, and gave her one pellet, informing her at the same time that the medicine would probably excite former ailments, the first of which was an obstinate constipation which lasted a fortnight, and was followed by regular stool. This, however, may have been promoted by the magnetized water which is very apt to remove such difficulties. In the fourth week she had an attack of hemicrania, where every symptom was most intense, but I gave no medicine, confident that I must allow the Sulphur full time to act. Every two or three weeks some former ailment made its appearance. Ten years ago the patient had had violent pains in the left side; these set in for two days, after which they disappeared. Four weeks later the patient was troubled with asthmatic complaints which she had had fifteen years ago; these, too, disappeared again in a few days. Now an inflammation of the liver showed itself which had troubled the patient twenty years ago for eight weeks, and had brought her to the brink of the grave. The inflammation increased to such an extent that I had to give her two pellets of *Aconite* in water, after which the inflammation disappeared in two days. Two months after this time she was attacked for two days with coxagra, an attack of which she had twenty years ago. Soon after she had a pain at the left elbow which had preceded the former complaint during the first attack. In the mean while the attacks of hemicrania became less frequent and violent, until during the sixth month, she had an eruption about the head and on other parts of the body, after the removal of which, she was perfectly cured seven months after the beginning of the cure.

What is interesting to know in this case is that this patient had had nothing but homœopathic treatment for twenty years past; but her physicians had not cured her because they did not allow the medicine to develop its full effect. At a consultation of homœopathic physicians it had been agreed that Sulphur was the right remedy, and Dr. Rau had ordered her to take one pellet every fourth evening. This had no effect for the simple reason that one dose destroyed the other, and the frequent repetition of the same medicine prevented the natural remedial power of the organism from improving the start imparted by the appropriate remedy for the purpose of achieving the cure.

This precaution being duly observed, Sulphur not only developed its full curative power, but likewise excited all her previous ailments which had only been suppressed heretofore, and gradually effected a perfect cure in the space of seven months.

It seems as though every physician of intelligence and good-will should feel disposed to follow this example.

These cases show that no second dose of a remedy should be given as long as the first dose has not exhausted its action, and in cases where no effect is observed, as in the case of deaf and dumb patients, to allow a dose to act at least for three to five months, since it is impossible to know what is going on in the interior of the organism, and it is so easy to injure the salutary action of a drug by the untimely exhibition of another remedy, of which we have had repeated instances in the case of externally perceptible ailments.

Section VIII.

In answer to the question, how such a small dose can produce such wonderful effects, I repeat what I wrote in 1849, for I have nothing better or clearer to offer:

Explanation

Of the efficacy of homœopathic potencies by means of animal magnetism.

Nobody has known heretofore how it happens that homœopathic potencies act so powerfully, and the most diversified theories have been offered in explanation. Some years ago I made the discovery, and have since verified it by repeated observations, that animal magnetism is the vivifying, efficient power of our potencies.

Every one who frequents my clinic, has seen that the most violent pains often yield to a pass with my hand, to a breath, to a mere word, hence to the *power of the will;* that even ailments which had lasted for years, frequently cease suddenly and even permanently.

This is a gift of God which cannot be acquired by study or comprehended by the reason, but which has a real existence although depending upon faith and the will. We have to believe that man is capable of such a power, and that it is bestowed upon him by God's omnipotence. If this faith is accompanied by the firm will of relieving an afflicted brother, I may then either impose my hand or make a pass, or simply extend the hand, or breathe upon him, or only speak a word, and the pain will cease.

If relief is not procured, it must be because the magnetiser was deficient in faith or will-power, or he must have felt that he ought not to have afforded any help in this case; powerfully-magnetic individuals are conscious of this, as though it were whispered to them by an invisible power.

The zoo-magnetic power may likewise be transmitted to natural objects, pure water, pulverised sugar, wood, etc. I have the most striking proofs showing that a powder of sugar upon which I had breathed, or a glass of water which I had touched *purposely*, has produced the most marvelous effects.

A most striking example is afforded by Mr. Moses Philipps, of Dessau, aged 72 years. For the last six months he had vomited whatever food he swallowed, first after the lapse of twenty-four, then after twelve, and finally after six hours, and for the last eight days immediately after swallowing food, so that he was unable to walk in consequence of his debility, and the most distinguished physicians gave up the thought of saving his life. He was brought to me in this condition, and said: "I am a dead man unless you help me; I know you can help me!"

I took a glass of water in my left hand, magnetised it with my right by placing it upon the tumbler, and told him to drink it. To his astonishment he kept the water on his stomach, whereas he had rejected even fluids heretofore; soon after he experienced hunger, and I had him eat a plate of soup with some wheat bread; this, too, was retained, and he was able to eat more solid food and never vomited after this. The violent cardialgia with which he had been constantly afflicted, had likewise disappeared; and in a fortnight he returned to Dessau quite well. A few years after his return he wrote me that he continued in excellent health, that he was able to digest the heaviest aliments and that he had grown quite stout.

This and many other similar cures induced me to draw the following inference: If mere water, by a mere imposition of hands, is rendered so medicinal that it will cure at once a severe affection of years' standing, how much more must this medicinal power be imparted to a properly attenuated agent whose peculiar effects we have become acquainted with by experience and provings upon the healthy, by continued shaking with the hand!

This inference seems quite plain, but it would have remained problematical, if daily experience had not demonstrated its correctness.

The thing happens in this wise:

The noxious constituents of the drug, for instance of poisons, is removed by attenuation; but the peculiarly specific principle which constitutes, so to say, the soul of the drug, remains, and is wonderfully excited during the shaking by the magnetic influence, and by it is rendered capable of curatively affecting the disordered nerves, which would have been overwhelmed by the coarse material.

The selection of the appropriate remedy in a given case depends upon the law that the drug must be capable of producing in its coarser form, on healthy individuals, the very symptoms which the potentized agent is expected to cure. This is the law of similarity which Hahnemann has discovered, and which has given rise to the name homœopathy. Even Paracelsus makes mention of this law, and Hippocrates alludes to it in this proposition: Fevers are sometimes most readily cured by remedies which induce fever.

This affords an explanation why the improperly-selected remedy has no injurious effect upon the body. By virtue of the law of similarity the remedy can only act upon a condition of the nervous system analogous to the drug; where this analogy is wanting, the highly potentized remedy can hurt no more than a magnetic pass hurts a person in health, which will sometimes cure a diseased individual in an instant.

Many persons may have rejected homœopathy because they were unable to comprehend its law. We have furnished an explanation and support it with undeniable facts.

Although the phenomena of animal magnetism cannot be accounted for, yet its effects are seen, and are only denied by a small number.

Every body possesses it more or less;* for what else is it but the vital power which is extinguished only by death. It is undermined by irregular and licentious living, by excesses of the body or mind. It is preserved and fortified by a careful observance of the laws of health, by self-control, and by an increasing consciousness that the body is only the envelope of an immortal spirit.

---

* Hence any body may prepare homœopathic medicines; but their power will depend upon the degree of magnetic power which he possesses. This is probably the reason why some who use my preparations, assert that the medicines prepared by me, act more powerfully than those prepared by other persons. This seems to have been verified by a number of experiments. The experiments which I have instituted with Jenichen's high potencies in chronic affections, have satisfied me that they act less intensely than my own preparations, without accomplishing any more; and that in the case of all potencies the main point is to *allow each dose to act to the end.* I use throughout the 30th potency which I prepare with 60 strokes of the arm.

It is in us that the divine spark slumbers which enables us to attain by faith and will to whatever is not beyond the boundaries of Nature.

He who believes and wills this, and steps to his sick brother's bedside with a loving heart, will behold, not without amazement, the wonder of fulfilment.

Section IX.

I have shown that in *acute* diseases the dose may be repeated quite frequently, and in chronic diseases much less frequently; and that a change in the symptoms, in the case of acute diseases, necessitates a change of remedy, or the alternate use of two remedies. In acute cases it is generally more expedient to alternate than to combine remedies, because one may be withdrawn and another substituted in its stead. In meningitis, for instance, with dry and burning heat, I give *Acon.* and *Bell.* 30 in alternation, every hour or half hour; but as soon as the heat is over, and sweat sets in, I discontinue the *Acon.*, and give *Bell.* alone, or alternate this remedy with *Bryon.*, in case the patient should move the jaws as when chewing; if the sweat should cease, and the burning heat should return, I have again recourse to *Acon.* In this way the dangerous symptoms of a violent disease may be controlled speedily and safely; but care must be had not to give too much of a remedy, and not to continue it after it has removed the symptoms for which it was selected.

I have likewise shown that an entirely different method has to be pursued in chronic cases; that the trifling incidental symptoms of an acute character need not be considered, and that the totality of all the symptoms has constantly to be kept in view, if a cure is to be effected. This proceeding is followed by many of my colleagues who admit that they had failed in obstinate cases until they pursued the course indicated by me. A homœopath of 20 years' standing who had been in the habit of repeating the dose, or changing the remedies in four or eight days, writes as follows: "I am more and more confirmed in the conviction that remedies should be allowed full time in all chronic affections to exhaust their action. I am now curing a case of salt-rheum where the pains under the former rash change of remedies inflicted the most excruciating sufferings upon the patient. After returning from your clinic I again besought the patient to accept my help. I gave her 5 pellets of *Sulphur* 30 in water, and this dose has already been acting for four months. At first the pains disappeared entirely; an itch-like eruption has made its appearance (she had the itch in former times), and the sores are healing perceptibly, so that this affection which has lasted for years, will yield to one dose."

I have likewise given a chapter on the combination of remedies, which is so important in chronic cases, and I have endeavored to account for the action of high potencies by means of the influence of animal magnetism.

Although this may enable the beginner to determine the size and repetition of the dose in a given case, yet he is not yet acquainted with the best method of selecting the appropriate remedy.

Much, and in many cases every thing, depends upon the similarity of the morbid symptoms to those of the drug, but it is likewise important to find out the more immediately-existing cause of the disease, and to keep in view the constitution, the age, temperament and disposition of the patient.

A young girl, for instance, had bilious vomiting for several months past, with violent pains in the stomach, which were moderated by gentle exercise. The menses were scanty and retarded; stool normal, sometimes papescent, slimy; little appetite; no thirst, gloomy mood. Feeble frame, face pale. Gentle disposition.—The first cause of the vomiting was a violent attack of anger.

The symptoms as far as the first dash correspond with *Pulsatilla;* frame, disposition and age indicate this drug; but the cause points to *Chamom.* which likewise cures vomiting of bile. *Puls.* and *Cham.* 30 would therefore have to be given in alternation, and such a case would speedily and radically yield to such alternate remedies.

It is therefore important that a physician should first be acquainted with the characteristic symptoms of drugs, and that he should gradually obtain a knowledge of all our remedies, because in many cases we neither know the cause of the disease, nor the other points upon which the selection of a remedy depends.

In the next place, a physician should have a ready knowledge of the remedies which correspond with the most common exciting causes of diseases, such as Opium for fright; Coffee for a joyful surprise; Aconite for fright and anger; Cham. for anger; Nux vomica for violent indignation; Ignatia and Phosph. ac. for silent grief, unfortunate love, suppressed mortification; Hyoscyamus for jealousy and homesickness; for a violent cold: Acon., Nux vom., Dulc., Bell., Cham.; for exposure in water or dampness: Calc. carb. or Rhus tox.; for the consequences of a blow, shock or concussion generally: Arnica or Rhus tox.; for loss of animal fluids, China.

If the physician knows the exciting cause, which should always be inquired into, the remedy which is in relation with this cause, should always be given first; or else, if it does not cover the totality of the symptoms, the remedy which is indicated next, or the two in alternation.

In the third place, in selecting a remedy the physician should have regard to the patient's constitution. He has to observe whether the patient is scrofulous, distorted, in which case Sulphur should never be omitted; likewise, whether the patient is now or has been afflicted with eruptions, tetter, ulcers, itch, caries, in which case Sulphur has always to be given alone, or in alternation with some other remedy. If the patient is bloated, inquiry has to be made whether the bloat is the result of dropsy (*China, Arsen.,*) or of an excessive deposit of fat (*Calc. carb.*) In a case of emaciation *Ars.* and *China* have to be given; heat in the head requires Bell.; pregnancy points to *Sepia, Ipecac., Bell., China.*

In the fourth place the patient's age has to be considered, and in the case of infants the experienced physician will first think of *Acon.* and *Cham.;* in the case young girls between the ages of 13 and 17, *Puls.* and *China* are very frequently required; in the critical age, between the years of 46 and 52, *Sepia* and *Lachesis* are required; old age is benefited by *Bar. carb.* and *Opium.* Of course, age is no criterium for the selection of a remedy; in comparing remedies, these remedies should not be overlooked, if they are otherwise indicated by the symptoms.

Fifthly, the temperaments and disposition have to be

considered. In the case of gentle and quiet, and generally also in the case of pale, blond, blue-eyed persons, we generally think of *Puls.*, *Chin.*, *Lach.*; in the case of violent, irascible, and dark-complexioned persons, with red and full faces, we think of *Nux. vom.*, or *Bell.*; in the case of persons who are disposed to weep, of *Ignat.*, *Puls.*, etc.; these indications, however, are not binding, but may suggest a remedy; they are only to be followed, if other marked symptoms are wanting, and a choice is to be made between two remedies of an opposite character.

A lady of a sanguine temperament, for instance, who had been full of life and of a vehement disposition, lapsed into a derangement of the mind which induced a constant disposition to weep; all the other bodily functions were carried on with regularity, and no precise exciting cause could be discovered. I gave *Nux vom.* because it was indicated by the temperament (and Nux. has "weeping" among its symptoms); if the patient had been of a quiet or gentle disposition, I should have given *Puls.* or *Ignat.*; she was speedily restored.

Every patient should furnish his physician an exact description of his symptoms, either orally or in writing. The latter should not content himself with a superficial statement of the case, for in our practice the most trifling accessory symptoms are sometimes of the utmost importance. In a case of *hemiplegia*, for instance, without any more precise indications, I should be unable to prescribe, unless I knew whether the left or right side is affected; for if the right side is affected, I give *Causticum*, *Crotalus* or *Rhus tox.*; if the left side, *Lachesis* or *China.*

It is likewise of importance to know when and by what

cause a symptom is made worse or better; *aggravation*, for instance: in the evening (Puls.) or in the morning (Nux), at night (Sulph., Merc.), or in the day-time after a meal (Nux vom.), in the open air (Nux vom.), or in a warm room (Puls.), during rest (Rhus tox.), or during motion (Bry.), in the warmth of the bed (Sulph., Rhus tox., Merc., Lyc.), by dampness and wet (Calc. carb., Rhus tox., Chin.); *improvement*, in the warmth of the bed (Caust., Nux vom., Bry.), in the open air (Puls.), etc.; again, improvement or aggravation by certain kinds of food, work, exertions, mental exertions, (Nux vom.), or bodily (Arn., Rhus tox.), and other similar indications which are of the utmost importance to the genuine homœopath.

Next to the history of the disease and all the accessory symptoms, the ordinary bodily functions have to be considered, such as stool and urine, appetite and thirst, sleep, respiration, cutaneous exhalations, catamenia; the absence or presence of one of these functions frequently determines the selection of the remedy. The catamenia constitute in most cases the characteristic symptom. Deafness or hardness of hearing, for instance, if no other accessory symptoms are known, or the exciting cause cannot be ascertained, can only be cured in the case of females by ascertaining all irregularities in the sexual sphere and selecting the remedies which are indicated by them. In general, this point should never be overlooked in selecting a remedy, otherwise we might be unable to effect any satisfactory result.

In order to facilitate the examination of a case, I have established the following seven points which I send to all patients at a distance who have sent me an imperfect report, and who are desirous of obtaining my advice.

A FEW HINTS TO PHYSICIANS AT A DISTANCE REGARDING THE MANNER OF TAKING DOWN THE TOTALITY OF THE SYMPTOMS OF A DISEASE.

1. *Name, age, condition, residence, street, number of the house;* if the patient resides in a village, the mail-station has to be indicated from which letters are sent to the village.

2. *Correct description of the disease,* duration and probable exciting cause of the same. If pains exist, the seat of the pains should be correctly indicated, indication of the period when the pains are either less or worse, whether in the day-time or at night, in the morning or evening, by cold or warmth, during rest or motion, etc.

3. *Temperament* and disposition, whether cheerful or gloomy, gentle or vehement, disposed to weep, etc., whether this has always been the case, or has set in with the disease.

4. *Frame of body,* whether tall or small, stout or thin, robust or delicate, with red cheeks or pale and sickly.

5. *Bodily defects:* hernia, prolapsus, defects of hearing or sight, whether distorted, lame, etc. Causes thereof.

6. *Stool* and *Urine,* appetite and thirst, sleep, respiration, cutaneous secretions; chilliness, heat, sweat (fever); in a case of fever and ague, whether and when thirst is present; whether the menses appear regularly; duration of the same, color, consistence (pale, red or dark); coagulated, tenacious; profuse or scanty, with or without pain; leucorrhœa, its character

7. Whether *an eruption* has ever existed, even in infancy, glandular swellings, herpes, ulcers, itch or any

other acrid humors; whether the patient has been guilty of self-abuse or other excesses.

It should be ascertained whether the patient had been bled frequently, had taken much calomel or china, etc., or had indulged in coffee, wine, brandy, etc.

In examining a patient, this order of questions should never be departed from.

The patient should first be allowed to relate his case without interruption; cross-questions are very apt to cause patients who have not much power of concentration, to forget various points which may be of great importance to a physician, and which would have to be ascertained at the next visit. Let the patient speak slowly so that every thing can be noted down. After he has said every thing, he may then be questioned more specifically, but in such a manner that the answers are not suggested to him; for instance: he should never be asked, have you headache? but, have you any other painful sensations? If he should say: Yes, I suffer with headache, we should not ask: in the temples or forehead, stinging or boring? but we should say: describe the headache more minutely. After this, we do not ask: is it worse in the evening or morning? but: at what time of the day or night is it worse? Again, we do not ask: is it made worse by cold or heat, by sitting or moving about, by loud talking, etc., but: by what influences or changes in the temperature is the headache made better or worse?

We should never omit inquiring into the condition of the sexual sphere; this can be done without any difficulty by a physician who knows how to win his patient's confidence by an earnest and sympathising manner. The physician should know most positively whether the patient had been guilty of masturbation. Every apparently trifling symptom is important to the proper selection of a drug; the statements of hypochondriac and hysteric patients, however, should be subjected to a careful criticism.

Every thing bearing upon the case is to be carefully noted in this manner, and to be transferred to the clinical journal which every physician should keep with conscientious care. Any one who applies for it, can obtain such a paper from me, containing seven divisions: 1. The number of the journal; 2. Date; 3. Name, condition, residence, age; 4. Symptoms of the disease; 5. Remedy, potency and prescription; 6. Result; 7. Particular remarks. I have kept such a journal for six to eight years; but my practice increasing so much that I had to employ several assistant physicians and secretaries for my foreign correspondence, I arranged a so-called flying journal. I had sheets, of the size of a third part of a common sheet of letter paper, printed as follows:

To be avoided during the treatment.

Coffee, tea, strong beer, wine, gin, rum, acids, spices, herbs and roots, fat pork, fat meat and vapors of sulphur. All other ordinary aliments are permitted.

Dissolve a powder in a cupful of fresh water, and keep it well covered. First. No. 1.	Take every day, morning and evening, a dessertspoonful, so as to finish the whole in four days; then wait seven days.	In dissolving the powder, stir the mixture with a horny spatula, or a goose-quill, but no metal-spoon.

This paper has to be preserved, and brought or sent to me at every consultation.

Cœthen. DR. ARTHUR LUTZE.

My clinic is open every day, except Sunday, from 8 to 1 o'clock and from 4 to 7 in the afternoon.

In the middle space I write the date, name, condition and residence of the patient. On the reverse blank page are found the symptoms of the patient, his age, the duration of the malady, a general description of the same, and finally the most particular symptoms. The symptoms of the disease of which, if sent in writing, the assistant physicians make an extract, are followed by my prescription, which is inclosed in the paper, after which the whole is sent off by mail, or handed to the patient if present.

Example: Mrs. F., 31 years. Cardialgia for seven years past, caused by a cold. A spasmodic pain commences in the stomach, extends to the small of the back, and upwards between the shoulder-blades. These symptoms are accompanied by sour eructations, gulping-up of sour water, sometimes vomiting. Worse in the morning and after eating. Violent temperament, irascible; slender and looking well. Stool hard, every two or three days. Little appetite, restless sleep. Menses regular, profuse and dark. Had never any eruption. *Nux vom.* 30., $\dot{4}\,\overline{\text{P.}}$

This last expression signifies that only the first powder contains five pellets, and that the other powders are non-medicinal. If the two first powders contained medicine, I should express it thus: Nux vom. $\ddot{4}\,\overline{\text{P.}}$

When sending off medicine, I wrap these four powders in the printed envelop, so that they fill exactly the middle space, and in six weeks the report and the envelop are sent back to me; the case is continued in the same paper; as soon as this paper is filled, a second paper is attached to it, and the flying journal is composed of these papers, which every patient takes good care of, for he knows that they are important.

This arrangement has enabled me to make in the year 1853 eighty thousand prescriptions by mail, and twenty thousand to thirty thousand in my clinic. This fact has been doubted, until physicians came to my clinic and convinced themselves by ocular demonstration of the truth.

Let no beginner neglect to read Hahnemann's Organon, §§ 84–99, where the investigation and description of the symptoms of a case are more particularly explained.

Section X.

One of the most important chapters is that of *diet;* for a cure may not only be promoted, but also prevented by it.

As a general rule, the following articles should be absolutely forbidden, both during and some time after a homœopathic cure: coffee, vinegar, lemon-juice, pungent and aromatic condiments in food or drink, wine, spirituous beverages, strong and stupefying perfumes or odors, such as the smell of sulphur and phosphorus in lighting matches.

As regards *coffee,* it is generally known that it excites the nerves, but few are acquainted with the fact that coffee is the cause of most of the ruling ailments, especially among females. All sorts of cardialgia and abdominal complaints, hæmorrhages, headache and toothache, sur-excitation of the senses and nerves, owe their existence to the abuse of coffee. This beverage should never be used by children and women, more particularly if they are affected with rush of blood to the head and chest.

Every homœopathic physician should prohibit coffee

from the following three reasons: First, because it is more or less hurtful in every case; second, because it antidotes most of our homœopathic preparations; third, because the patient who is anxious to recover his health should be willing to suffer a trifling privation, in order to be placed in possession of this precious gift of God. Such a privation will induce him to be very particular in following the directions of his physician; he ought to be carefully reminded of the fact that he is sick, for an ever-present consciousness of this fact will keep the desire of recovering his health keenly alive in his heart, and will facilitate the operations of the medical adviser. These are the moral reasons, imposed by common sense and duty, why coffee should be avoided.

As regards *tea*, I do not prohibit the absolute use of it, but I allow the so-called black tea, which is not injurious to homœopathic preparations, except *China* and *Pulsatilla*.

But even black tea should be strictly forbidden, if patients are not accustomed to its use; for it excites the nerves, especially those of females; whence it may be inferred that the use of tea has a deleterious effect upon the nerves of those who experience the least stimulating influence from it; such persons should abstain from the use of tea altogether.

Instead of coffee and tea, fresh milk should be used, immediately after it is drawn; this is a most wholesome and natural beverage, more particularly for children.

A beverage prepared from roast-corn and sweet carrots may likewise prove a good substitute for coffee. Pure chocolate or ground cocoa may likewise be resorted to, but not the so called prepared chocolate without the oil, which is recommended by ignorant traders, but is of difficult digestion. Cocoa-shells likewise afford a wholesome and pleasant beverage, or a plain soup, such as our ancestors were in the habit of eating at breakfast or supper, and is still used in many parts of Germany and France.

Vinegar and *lemon-juice* are forbidden because they interfere with the action of most homœopathic preparations. If not under treatment, mild acids may now and then be used with the food by persons in health; such acids should be used very sparingly by children, but should be rigorously avoided by chlorotic girls, or by girls of a chlorotic habit of body, who have frequently a strong desire for acids, which should not be gratified, inasmuch as such gratifications may be followed by disastrous results.

Sourkrout, without vinegar, may be eaten by chronic patients whose digestive organs are in good condition; curd may likewise be eaten by those who are not incommoded by it.

Sharp and *aromatic spices* heat the blood, on which account both healthy and sick persons should abstain from them, but especially the latter. The custom of spicing the food so as to cause the mouth to burn for hours has been very generally abandoned; it is a most unwholesome practice.

Cinnamon causes a tendency to hæmorrhage, and should be prohibited; *parsley* excites the urinary organs, and *celery* the sexual organs; for this reason these two articles should be avoided in affections of these organs respectively; on the other hand, in chronic affections of other organs, a cure is not interfered with if patients should now and then eat a little parsley or celery, or some other simple herb, in the soup or vegetables.

Wine should be prohibited during homœopathic treatment; it interferes with the operation of many drugs, stimulates the circulation, and is more especially prejudicial to *rheumatic* and *arthritic* individuals.

Healthy persons should use wine in moderate quantities, if they do not wish to be injured by it. This is particularly advisable in the case of young persons. The proper way would be to drink wine only on extraordinary occasions of rejoicing, when it may contribute to promote hilarity; it should not be used as a common beverage.

It may do good when drank after eating heavy or fat food, on journeys, more particularly when the weather is cold and damp; at such times a little wine is craved by the natural instinct, which should always be obeyed by persons in health.

Wine proves *true medicine* after debilitating diseases, such as typhus. In such cases a teaspoonful of it should be taken at a meal. Wine, taken at dinner, proves invigorating to old people.

On the other hand, wine will prove injurious to health if used immoderately, without due regard to hygienic laws.

Spirituous beverages, such as brandy, rum, grog, punch, liquors, etc., should not only be rigorously abstained from by patients, but likewise by persons in health, for such things destroy life and peace.

It has been ascertained by recent investigations that all fermented liquors contain alcohol, which does not act as a sudden poison, but slowly and very gradually undermines health and weakens the vital power. Most drunkards die of delirium tremens, and some are even said to have perished by spontaneous combustion. This termination of a drunkard's fate occurs so rarely that its occurrence is doubted by many. The Prince E. Gagarin, of Odessa, has assured me that he has witnessed several such casualties with his own eyes.

An examination of the stomachs of recently-deceased drunkards has shown that the inner coat of these organs has a reddish color, arising from the congested condition of the capillaries. The stomach of a drunkard who gets intoxicated several times a week has a blueish appearance, and the blood-vessels are very much distended with blood. The stomach of a drunkard is intensely inflamed, and scarcely able to retain food; the stomach of one who died of delirium tremens, or of schirrus of the stomach induced by drinking, has an offensive look. He who considers these things must be aware that even the moderate use of brandy is not innocuous, as is supposed by many ignorant persons, who fancy that brandy is necessary to those who are exhausted by hard labor. All that brandy accomplishes is to excite the nervous system, and inasmuch as these artificial stimulations lead to excessive waste, every drop of brandy is destructive to health and life. Instead of spending money for the deleterious brandy, even poor people might procure for themselves strength and comfort, if they would buy meat instead of liquor.

Sensible people should constantly endeavor to impress these teachings upon the minds of the uneducated masses, who could easily be made to understand such a simple and important matter.

Look at a drunkard: not only his physical strength is ruined, but likewise his moral energies. All his finer feelings are blunted; the sense of honor and shame, the love of that which is great and good, have disappeared; the only desire that is not extinguished in his soul is the desire for brandy. Hufeland says: "I do not know anything that is more capable of begetting a character of beastly brutality, and of destroying the divine features in man's nature, than the abuse of brandy. Other vices still leave the hope of improvement, but the vice of drunkenness ruins man throughout, for the reason that it destroys his sensibility. It seems to me that these considerations should engage the attention of the public authorities, and should induce them to devise measures to diminish the consumption of brandy, instead of allowing gin-shops and brandy-distilleries to be multiplied. A country where this vice becomes universal must perish, for industry, virtue, humanity, sobriety, moral sentiment, and all the other qualities without which no country can preserve its existence and growth, are banished by this horrid vice. History shows that the introduction of brandy among savage tribes is the beginning of their physical weakness and degradation, and that this disastrous gift by the white man secures their subjugation much more readily than gunpowder and artillery."

The best evidence of the correctness of these statements is furnished by the following words addressed years ago by a delegate of many Indian tribes to the President of the United States: "We pray thee to grant us ploughs and other tools, and to send us blacksmiths who can teach us to mend them. But, my father, whatever we undertake will prove without avail, unless the assembled Congress of the sixteen States forbids the sale of brandy and other spirituous beverages to the red man. Father, the sale of this poison has been forbidden in our fields, but not in our cities where many of our hunters not only sell their furs for this poison, but likewise their rifles and blankets, and return to their families in a state of nudity. Father, thy children are willing to labor, but the introduction of this deleterious poison keeps them poor. Thy children have not yet learnt to govern themselves as thy people have. When our white brethren first came to our country, our ancestors were numerous and happy; but since the arrival of the white man, and since the introduction of this deleterious poison they are less numerous, and less happy."

What a joyful message it must be to the unfortunate victims of the vice of drunkenness, that the new healing art offers means of salvation even to them, not by secret remedies, but by enabling man to mend his ways by his own free will; for man's feeble strength can only be supported and his ruin can only be prevented, if he is willing to accept help. I have frequently succeeded in saving a poor unfortunate from the consequences of drinking; even two years ago I rescued the father of a family whom the vice of drunkenness had well nigh led to the brink of ruin; since then he has not touched a drop of brandy, and the members of this family now form a happy and comfortable group.

In regard to *ale*, I have been in the habit of forbidding it, because it is most generally mixed with a little alcohol, especially when brought from a distance, for a little alcohol is then added by the brewer in order to secure its better preservation; but pure beer made from malt and hop may be drank in moderate quantities without injuring the medicine.

A Bavarian brewer once informed me that he had been in the habit of mixing his beer with quassia, lolium temolentum, centaury, and even nux vomica; although these poisonous ingredients are only added in small quantity, yet their continued use must necessarily have a deleterious influence upon the human body. In more than one case of insanity, it has been traced to the constant use of this adulterated ale.

The public authorities in every country should see to it that such adulterations do not take place.

Although fresh water is undoubtedly the most wholesome beverage, yet a glass of pure beer need not be interdicted; more particularly in the case of an industrious laborer who uses beer as a substitute for brandy. Children, however, should abstain from beer, or should drink it only exceptionally.

Cider had better be avoided by persons under treatment; if perfectly pure and not acid, it may be drank occasionally by chronic patients whose digestive organs are not affected by it.

All strong and stupefying odors should be carefully avoided. Nevertheless it is unnecessary to follow this rule with pedantic anxiety. Nobody, for instance, need be afraid of the perfume of flowers in the open air; fragrant flowers, however, should not be kept in a close room, much less in a bed-room, because the exhalations emitted by such flowers may cause death. The perfuming of rooms and linen, which fashionable persons were formerly in the habit of resorting to, is likewise injurious to the nerves which are weakened by such influences. Fumigations in rooms for the purpose of dispelling bad odors, are likewise condemnable; they only tend to increase the bad air. The only proper mode of purifying the air in rooms, is to ventilate them, more especially sick-rooms the windows of which should be opened several times a day, if such a thing is feasible, and currents of air should be induced by large fans.

In lighting matches, care must be taken to avoid the vapors of sulphur and phosphorus which are even injurious to persons in health. The best place to light matches is in the stove or fire-place, where the vapors can ascend into the chimney without affecting the atmosphere in the rooms. In public rooms, bar-rooms, etc., a little flame should be kept burning with paper-matches; the common phosphor-matches are especially to be avoided when lighting cigars or pipes.

Tobacco injures the health on account of its narcotic power. Persons with weak nerves are even affected by the smell of tobacco; they, as well as those who are suffering with sore throat, pulmonary and ophthalmic complaints, should avoid the use of tobacco as much as possible.

Chewing tobacco is a bad practice which should never be permitted.

Smoking not only induces a waste of saliva, but spoils it, and deranges the natural process of digestion. Hence tobacco will prove injurious to persons affected with abdominal and nervous complaints.

Nicotine, the active principle of tobacco, when prepared from fresh leaves, destroys life almost as speedily as prussic acid; yet the vapors of such a poison are inhaled by the mouth and nose.

The action of homœopathic medicines is impaired by smoking and taking snuff; hence tobacco should be strictly avoided during treatment.

Patients whose physician permits them to smoke,

should not smoke cigars, which are always injurious, but should use pipes with long stems, and smoke light tobacco, but never immediately before or after a meal.

Smoking is very much abused now-a-days by young persons. Even boys are seen walking about the streets with cigars in their mouths. Parents and guardians should put a stop to this reprehensible practice which enfeebles the rising generation, and gives rise to the diminutive stature, and to the many pulmonary affections of young people, that were never so frequent in former times.

Hufeland who was as humane as he was experienced, writes: "Smoking spoils the teeth, dries up and emaciates the body, causes paleness of the face, weakens the sight and the memory, causes determinations of the blood to the head and lungs, predisposes to head and chest-affections, and may cause hæmoptysis and pulmonary phthisis in those who have a hectic habit of body. Moreover the habit of smoking is an additional want, and the more wants a man has, the more his freedom and happiness are limited. For this reason, I warn every body of the vile practice of smoking, and shall deem myself happy, if my remarks should contribute ever so little to its decrease.

Taking snuff is not much better, and much worse in point of uncleanliness. Moreover it irritates the nerves, weakens them in the end, and gives rise to headache and sore eyes.

What increases the injury caused by smoking and taking snuff, are the acrid and often poisonous ingredients which are mixed up with the tobacco by the venders of this weed, for the purpose of increasing the desire for it by artificial means. I am unable to comprehend why life-insurance companies which institute such rigorous inquiries into all other things that may prove injurious to health, are not more particular in regard to the use of tobacco, for in the end it is the same whether a person is poisoned by swallowing or by smoking and snuffing up poison. Let me instance a single fact, the occurrence of which is well known to me. It was the custom in a snuff-factory to mix up the tobacco leaves with vermillion, in order to impart to them a beautiful red color, and an increased weight. In this case the persons who used this snuff, snuffed up every day a quantity of the most deleterious, but slowly-acting poison. Is it to be wondered, if many kinds of snuff induce incurable blindness, nervous disorders, (instances of which have occurred to me,) and is it not time to expose these dangerous adulterations, and not to permit the sale of snuff or smoking tobacco until it has undergone a chemical examination, and has been declared pure and innocuous by the public authorities?"

Symptoms of lead-poisoning have occurred from snuff being packed in lead-foil (staniole).

So far I have only mentioned the articles which should be forbidden during treatment; these constitute the smaller number, for as a general, rule, patients may be guided by this proposition:

During homœopathic treatment patients may use all ordinary articles of diet, both solid and liquid, not mixed up with forbidden spices, condiments, acids.

I shall afterwards allude more especially to particular articles of food.

As a matter of course every body should pay attention to that which agrees or disagrees with him, since different organisms, especially when sick, are differently affected by different aliments.

In all dietetic regulations it is a supreme law:

Never eat unless thou art hungry, and stop eating as soon as the hungry stomach ceases to crave food.

Never eat from habit, or from fear of offending by refusing the proffered food. This is foolish politeness; so is the custom of drinking with each other at table, which is only kept up among uneducated people.

We should endeavor, by obeying the laws of Nature, to re-awaken the instinct which man seems to have lost, and which should be obeyed whenever it prompts us to abstain from any kind of food or beverage.

The stomach is not only deranged by mixing up quantities of food, but such a derangement may even be caused by eating a single morsel which is repulsive to the stomach. It should not be touched, nor should the least effort be made to eat it.

This rule should likewise be followed in the education of children. They should be accustomed to regularity, but should never be compelled to eat if they are not hungry; for this might make them sick. All eating between meals, especially cakes, candies, etc., should be prohibited.

It is well known that meat is more nourishing and heating than vegetables. For this reason meat should be eaten sparingly by persons of a plethoric, bilious habit, and irascible temperament; and is especially adapted to chlorotic, cold, lax, phlegmatic and nervous individuals.

The best method is to eat a proper admixture of meat and vegetables; however it is easier to live exclusively on vegetables than meat, an excess of which deteriorates the fluids. In the war against Spain, after the vegetables, bread, etc., had all been eaten, and the army had to live on meat alone, the first consequence was that the soldiers were attacked with diarrhœa, after which a most devastating putrid fever set in, which continued until vegetables and bread were procured.

Full-grown chickens, and all kinds of flying fowl, if not too old and tough, or too young, are comparatively of easy digestion; young pigeons, for instance, are not advisable.

Rabbit and *deer-meat*, if tender, is very digestible and nourishing.

Likewise tender and young *beef*.

Mutton is not quite as digestible, but wholesome, and is especially useful when a disposition to diarrhœa prevails.

Veal should only be used if the calves are large and not too young; but it is neither as digestible nor as nourishing as mutton; if too young, it frequently causes diarrhœa and cardialgia.

Pork is more difficult to digest than any other kind of meat; if eaten in too large a quantity, it causes impurities; hence it should be strictly avoided by all those who are affected with phlegm, acridities, eruptions, ulcers, etc. Persons of a nervous temperament, and those who take much active exercise in the open air, such as day-laborers, digest it more readily than others.

These remarks likewise apply to goose-flesh, whereas duck is rather more digestible.

Eggs contain the nutriment matter in a concentrated form. A fresh and soft-boiled egg is equivalent to one-third of a pound of common boiled beef. Hard-boiled eggs are hard to digest, constipating, and less nourishing;

baked in butter, they are the most indigestible. Bad eggs may cause a good deal of mischief.

Milk, especially when fresh from the cow, is a most wholesome beverage, and exceedingly nourishing and easily digested. It may be said to occupy a mean rank between meat and vegetables. It is particularly useful to children, enfeebled persons, consumptive individuals, and persons who are inclined to cough and other chest affections. It is less suitable to hypochondriacs and to persons with acid stomachs, unless such individuals take much exercise in the open air. Trifling ailments which may be caused by the use of milk, may be removed by homœopathic medicines.

Cheese is nourishing when fresh, but old cheese is indigestible, and irritates rather than nourishes. If eaten in quantity, it causes much phlegm, constipation, acrid humors, diseases of the skin and kidneys. Old cheese has often caused symptoms of poisoning; in overload ing the stomach, it may act as a medicine; hence it may prove useful after a copious dinner.

Fresh butter is the mildest of all kinds of fat, but is easily digested only if a thin layer of it is spread on bread. Old or fried butter is hard to digest, acrid, and should be avoided by all persons under homœopathic treatment.

Cold-blooded animals, such as fish and conchylia, are less nourishing and generally harder to digest than the meat of warm-blooded animals. The most wholesome kind of fish is that which lives in flowing water, with a bottom of sand or gravel; fish from stagnant water is less wholesome. Sea-fish is more nourishing than fresh-water fish.

The more easily the flesh of fish is crumbled between

the fingers the more easily it is digested; the fatter and more tallowy the flesh, the harder it is to digest. The most wholesome kinds of fish are trout, young pike, cod-fish, haddock, perch, shad, black-fish, white-fish from Lake Michigan, carp, flounders, etc. Halibut and salmon are not adapted to delicate stomachs.

The flesh of fish being easily decomposed, it should always be eaten fresh, and sufficiently salted, especially by persons under homœopathic treatment. Boiled fish should be eaten with fresh butter and potatoes. Otherwise it might prove very indigestible, and cause fever and ague, especially in those whose stomachs are turned by eating this kind of food. For this reason it is not well to make a meal exclusively of fish.

Fresh oysters are easily digested and nourishing, and may be eaten by patients, but without lemon-juice. Fried or baked oysters are hard to digest.

Vegetables, being less nourishing and heating than meat, they should be recommended to all robust, plethoric individuals of sanguine temperament and irascible disposition.

Vegetable-diet favors a mild disposition, meat-diet a vehement and irascible temper.

Vegetable-diet is less favorable to putridity, and should be chiefly resorted to by all who are inclined to scurvy, carcinoma, etc. On the other hand, vegetables are more flatulent, and give rise to acidity more readily than meat and eggs; for this reason vegetable diet has to be used cautiously by hypochondriacs and by persons who are disposed to acidity.

In summer, and in hot climates, people should live chiefly on vegetables and fruit, whereas the people of the North require meat, especially during winter. These facts are even taught by an unsophisticated instinct.

SECTION XI.

The duty of a physician not only consists in prescribing the necessary medicines, but likewise in regulating the diet adapted to each case. This includes not only the diet, but the whole mode of life, clothing,* distribution of the day's work, rest, etc.

But even this does not limit the functions of a true physician; on the contrary, after all this has been attended to, the most important matter still remains to be done—watching the state of the mind. If all these various duties are properly attended to, the physician will be able to fulfill the highest object of his calling, which is *to prevent diseases.*

All truly humane physicians seek to accomplish this noble task. In this respect physicians should go hand in hand with teachers and ministers. Among the ancients the priests were likewise physicians; it was only at a later period when medicine ceased to be limited to a knowledge of a few popular remedies, and became a vast reservoir of nauseous decoctions and health-perverting poisons, that physicians became a distinct class. Homœopathy, which is destined to upset the whole allœopathic plunder, will likewise restore the union between medicine and theology, for a physician should attend to the welfare of the soul as well as the body, both of which are inseparable.

---

* How often has too tight lacing laid the foundation of incurable diseases, affections of the heart, etc.!

Even if physicians and ministers still constitute two distinct classes, yet every true physician is anxious to ascertain whether the soul is in any manner involved in the production of the bodily disease; this knowledge may be the first indispensable stepping-stone to a cure.

How often do both mental and physical derangements arise from a want of faith and love!*

It is the duty of the physician as well as of the minister to kindle these living fires in the patient's soul, the extinction of which may cause diseases and death.

To be a true physician, one must understand and do these things.

As love is the alpha and omega of Christianity, which induces the apostle Paul to say: "If I had faith, and could remove mountains, and had not love, I should be nothing;" so love should be the main motive of a physician's doings. It is only when the patient knows and feels this that he will follow his physician's instructions with perfect confidence; he will even listen to kindly-meant censure, and the physician will become both the helper and the friend of his patient.

Physicians whose hearts are full of love, are honored with a confidence which is alone capable of restoring health.

I must not omit to mention an instance which has frequently incited me, at a time when I was not yet accustomed to physical fatigue, to make renewed efforts in behalf of poor sufferers; for the poor are more in need of advice than those who are more fortunately endowed.

---

* Insanity, for instance, is very frequently caused by anxious care, grief, religious scruples, pride, greediness, etc.

One evening when old Dr. Heim had retired to rest before his accustomed hour, the bell rang; his wife who was anxious not to disturb the doctor's rest, sought to send the inquiring invalid away; but the old doctor who had heard the sound of the bell, called out: "Who is there?" His wife replied: "Never mind, the old watchman is sick, and his wife may call in some other physician." "No," said Heim, "nobody will visit this poor man at night, he is an old patient of mine, I must get up and see him." He rose from his bed, and visited his poor patient. In return for his many acts of kindness Heaven has blessed him with a long life and a happy age.

This example should be an admonition to every physician to go and do likewise.

If this truly Christian feeling which is not manifested by turning up the eyes, by praying and fasting, but by deeds of love, and by a firm and unshakeable faith that nothing can happen to us which is not ordained by the Providence of God, shall have penetrated the hearts of men; then these two important offices of the ministry and medicine, will be again filled by the same person, *for every pastor should be a physician, and every physician a pastor.*

CHARACTERISTIC SYMPTOMS.

***Aconitum Napellus.** (Monk's-hood, wolf's-bane.)

A remedy for the blood. *Vascular* excitement, dry and burning heat, alternate chills and heat (fever). Restlessness, anxiety, palpitation of the heart, excitement; consequences of sudden chagrin and fright, such as: trembling, inflammations of every organ, where the treatment is always commenced with Aconite, such as: pneumonia, pleurisy, etc.; *croup;* measles, purple-rash, jaundice, stye; violent *rheumatic pains* in the limbs, with sensations in the whole body as if bruised, after taking cold, with heat and chilliness, or only heat (stiffness of the limbs); gout, with feverish symptoms. Arthritic, rheumatic and nervous *toothache,* with restlessness and anxiety, vertigo and fainting fits. Short and hurried breathing. Paroxysms of anxiety and suffocation. *Asthma; apoplexy; pulmonary hæmorrhage,* with frequent pulse, anxiety, expectoration of fluid blood when hawking, the blood comes up with a sensation of scraping or burning in the chest. Short and dry, or hollow and hoarse cough, especially in the case of children after taking cold, also with fever. Vomiting, especially of drinks, cardialgia, constipation, colorless stools. *Anxious urging to urinate.* Suppression of the urinary secretions. Brown, dark, burning, scanty urine.

Uterine hæmorrhage, miscarriage with fever; typhoid fever, with dry skin and burning heat (together with Bell., Bry. and Rhus.); burning swelling of injured parts; unquenchable thirst; intermittent fever with heat and thirst prevailing (in the case of scrofulous individuals give Silicea); *sleeplessness*, owing to mental anxiety, also with wandering of the mind. Anxiety and restlessness, even until the patient is beside himself. Apprehensive mood.

If fever is present, Aconite should be given in every case, and should invariably initiate the treatment.

Agaricus muscarius. (Bug-agaric.)

Rheumatic tearing pains in the limbs, worse during rest, less during motion (in conjunction with Rhus); ailments which break out cross-wise, for example; in the right arm and left leg; epilepsy; aversion to work; feeling of icy-coldness on top of the head (together with Calc. carb. and Sepia); contraction of the eye-lids which seem less widely apart; twitching of the eyelids; short-sightedness, also with dimness of both eyes, as through a gauze; *muscæ volitantes;* cold urine; many symptoms are worse after singing.

Agnus castus. (Chaste-tree.)

Deficiency of milk, in the case of lying-in women (in conjunction with Pulsat.); chronic distortions of the joints (after Arn. and Rhus); arthritic nodes; sadness, apprehension of near death; swelling and induration of the spleen; chronic gonorrhœa, with suppression of the sexual instinct and deficient erections; swelling and induration of the testes, also after suppression of gonorrhœa; sterility.

Alumina. (Argilla, oxide of alumen.)

Trembling of the extremities; involuntary motions and twitching of the limbs; humid scurfs and spreading herpes; inability to think coherently; falling and dryness of the hair; cold feeling in the eyes; squinting of the eyes; vibrations and sparkling before the eyes; purulent discharge from the right ear; swelling and redness of the nose; sore and scurfy nostrils, with discharge of a thick, yellowish mucus; ulceration of the Schneiderian membrane; tubercular blotches in the face; swelling and cracking of the lips, also with blisters and crusts on the same; painfulness of the teeth when chewing, the teeth feel loose and elongated; swelling and bleeding of the gums; sore throat when swallowing, and pressure under the sternum when swallowing, as if the œsophagus were contracted; potatoes cause unpleasant symptoms; protrusion and incarceration of existing hernia; constipation of pregnant females and infants; fluent piles; premature, scanty and short-lasting menses; acrid leucorrhœa during and after the menses. The skin on the hands is rough, chapped, bleeds readily. Whitlow. At night the legs go to sleep.

Ambra grisea.

Ailments of old people (in conjunction with Baryta and Opium); tearing or crampy pains in the muscles, also in the joints, often on one side of the body only.

In the evening, when lying down, or in the warmth the pains are worse; they abate during a walk in the open air or by lying on the affected part; talking fatigues. The skin feels numb all over; *itching and burning of the skin,* as from the itch; *brings the suppressed itch and tetter out again*; burning herpes; disconsolate loathing of life; aversion to talking and laughing; embarrassed manners in company; rush of blood to the head when listening to music; the hair feels sore when touched, it falls out; roaring, whizzing in the ears; drawing pains in the teeth, especially in *hollow* teeth, worse by eating warm food, abating when touched by cold things, disappearing after eating; fetid breath; sore throat; sour mouth after eating milk, hiccough after smoking; sour or suppressed eructations; tasting of the ingesta; nausea and vomiting; burning pressure and spasm in the stomach; pressure in the region of the liver; pressure, crampy or cutting pains, cold feeling in the bowels; urging to urinate, inability to retain the urine, secretes three times as much urine as the quantity of liquid taken followed by dull pains in the region of the kidneys; sour odor of the urine; premature menses; discharge of blood between the catamenia; lucorrhœa; spasmodic cough, especially in the case of thin persons; nightly trembling in the chest; stiffness of the small of the back, after sitting; the arms incline to go to sleep, especially when lying upon them; tearing and drawing in the arms, trembling of the arms; continual coldness of the hands; tearing in the legs: unpleasant coldness of the legs; cramp in the legs, almost every night; swelling or coldness of the feet burning of the soles.

Ammonium carbonicum. (Carbonate of Ammonia.)

Stinging and tearing, abating in bed (with Causticum); pains in the joints as if sprained; glandular swellings; chronic rash; the skin is scarlet-red; scarlet-fever (after Bell.); warts; nightmare when about to fall asleep; dreams of death and dead bodies; anxiety every afternoon as if one had committed a crime; loathing of life; fearful disposition; forgetfulness, inability to collect one's ideas; throbbing headache; falling off of the hair; ophthalmia, nightly agglutination of the lids; diplopia at a distance, shortsightedness, catarrh; hardness of hearing; nosebleed, especially when washing in the morning; chronic dryness of the nose; itching eruption in the face; ulcerated corners of the mouth; chapped lips; dullness or long-lasting looseness of the teeth; even sound teeth fall out; blisters on the tongue; swelling of the tonsils, rendering deglutition difficult; aversion to milk; excessive desire for sugar; cardialgia; burning, boring stitches, pressure and soreness in the region of the liver; when stepping, pain in the abdomen as from shaking; excoriating and sore hæmorrhoidal tumors; discharge of blood from the anus during and between stool; flowing piles; wetting the bed at night, especially when occurring towards morning; frequent emissions, almost every night; menses premature and profuse, the discharge taking place principally at night, in lumps; toothache during the menses; acrid leucorrhœa; dry cough, excited by titillation in the windpipe; cough with expectoration of mucus, especially in the morning in bed; shortness of breath, especially when going up stairs; numbness of the arms and finger; the legs go to sleep; swelling of the feet.

Anacardium. (Malacca-bean.)

Pressure in various parts of the body, as from a plug; sensitive to cold and to currents of air; the skin is insensible to external stimuli; deep and long sleep, finds it hard to wake in the morning; dreams of fire; apprehensive for the future, dread of men; the moral sense seems blunted; sensation as if mind and body were disconnected; pain in the back part of the head, when making a wrong step; dimness of sight, as from cobwebs and spots before the eyes; hardness of hearing, roaring in the ears; discharge of brown pus from the ears; pale complexion, sickly look; fetid breath; excited sexual instinct; cough, with vomiting of the ingesta; hæmoptysis; trembling of the hands; burning of the soles.

Antimonium crudum. (Crude antimony.)

Lienteria; eructations tasting of the ingesta; nausea, vomiting of bile and mucus (together with Ipec and Puls.,) cardialgia, derangements caused by overloading the stomach; mucous hæmorrhoids; fungus articularis; intermittent fever with mucous diarrhœa and gastric ailments, especially in the morning; twitching pain in decayed teeth; indurated, horny skin; adiposis (after Calc.); spongy swelling of the knee.

Apis mellifica. (Honey-bee.)

Consequences of suppressed, repelled or imperfectly developed acute eruptions, such as measles, scarlatina, urticaria, etc. Consequences of stings of insects especially of bees ; ophthalmia ; obscuration and cicatrices of the cornea; staphyloma; styes; fistula lachrymalis; œdematous swelling of the face ; erysipelas of the face, especially of a pale, livid color; inflammation and swelling of the tongue; ulcers on the tongue; carcinoma of the tongue ; inflammation of the palate, mouth, fauces ; inflammation of the abdominal organs; diabetes ; gonorrhœa ; affections of the ovaries and uterus, especially dropsy of these organs, without thirst ; menstrual difficulties, swellings of the labia ; miscarriage ; metrorrhagia; induration of the mammæ; hydrothorax; pericardia; rheumatism, nodous gout; œdema of the extremities; swelling of the knees; furuncles, etc.

Vertigo when standing, sitting, lying, closing one's eyes, with obscuration of sight, nausea, headache, sneezing; fullness, heaviness; pressure in the head, especially when rising from a sitting or lying position, worse in a warm room, less when compressing the head; sharp, stinging pains in the temples; headache, with sensitiveness to the light or redness of the eyes; weakness of the eyes, with dread of straining them ; twitching of the eye-ball, especially at night; heaviness, fullness and pressure in the eyes and lids; cutting, burning and redness of the eyes. Weeping of the eyes, and sensation as if they were full of mucus; agglutination and swelling of the lids; dropsical, erysipelatous swelling around the eyes; itching, redness and swelling of the nose; burning stinging in the face, with sensation of fullness, heat and redness, desire for cold water; livid, blueish-red color of the face; swelling of the lips; tongue as if scalded, especially along the edges, where it is blistered; the blisters burn and sting ; dryness, fiery redness, burning stinging and swelling of the tongue;

dry mouth, fauces and throat, with pain as if scalded; ptyalism ; difficult deglutition, with burning, excoriating and stinging sensation; inflamed, swollen and painful tonsils; no appetite; absence of thirst in dropsy, with dryness of the throat, and heat; eructations tasting of the ingesta, worse after drinking water; nausea, vomiting, with dizziness, fainting, prostration, when these symptoms accompany other ailments; pressure, stinging, soreness and burning in the stomach; contused feeling under the ribs; colic, in the morning, with urging to stool; burning and soreness in the abdomen which is sensitive to the least pressure; greenish-yellow, watery or mucous diarrhœa, without pain, especially in the morning; scanty or suppressed secretion of urine, very painful; increased urination, day and night; burning and smarting in the urethra as if scalded; pains in the ovaries as if strained, or cutting, drawing, stinging pains, with pressure downwards; pressing downwards in the uterine region, as if the menses would appear; swelling of the labia; metrorrhagia, with expulsion of the fetus; hoarseness, with sensitiveness in the larynx, roughness in the throat, dryness; slow and difficult respiration, with constriction of the throat; fullness in the chest, obliging one to sit up; pressure in the chest, especially in the upper part; stitches, especially in the left side of the chest; coldness and heat in the chest; stitching pains in the region of the heart, impeding respiration; pulse hurried, full and strong, or hard, small and quick; pains under the scapulæ, worse during motion; stiffness in the small of the back; pains from the shoulders through the arms, drawing pains to the tips of the fingers; the arms go to sleep; burning and stinging of the hands, with redness, heat and swelling; itching, burning and chapping of the hands; the nails seem loose; falling off of the finger and toe nails; lupus; pains in the knee, or swelling of the knee, with burning and stinging; burning of the feet and toes; swelling of the feet; itching blotches in the joints; excessive sensitiveness of the flesh to pressure; the symptoms are made worse by warmth; cold water diminishes the pains in the inflamed parts; this agent chiefly affects the left side.

Argentum foliatum. (Silver-foil.)

Tearing and drawing in the bones, with pressure; profuse nose-bleed, especially after blowing the nose, or preceded by tickling and creeping in the nose; mercurial sore throat; nocturnal emissions; affections of the larynx, in the case of preachers, teachers, actors, singers; the pains are worse every day at noon.

Argentum nitricum. (Nitrate of silver.)

Aching or stinging, semi-lateral pains; epilepsy with dullness of mind; semi-lateral paralysis; dropsy depending upon affections of the liver; itch-like eruptions; catarrhal and syphilitic ophthalmia; fiery bodies and flashes before the eyes; black, carious teeth; the sound teeth are exceedingly sensitive to cold water; loose, readily bleeding gums; colicky pains in the case of hypochondriac or hysteric persons; thin brown stools having a foul smell; bloody and mucous diarrhœa; inflammation and stricture of the urethra; hæmaturia; deficient sexual desire, with shrinking of the parts; chancrous ulcers on the prepuce; cough induced by violent titillation in the larynx; nightly palpitation of the heart.

*Arnica montana. (Leopard's bane.)

Hæmorrhage and injuries of internal and external organs, by blows, a fall, strain, sprain, contusion; ecchymosis, boils, varices, (in alternation with Puls.,) arnica may be used externally as a lotion; bed-sores, (externally and internally;) nose-bleed; cough after every exertion, after crying; paroxysms of whooping-cough, commencing with crying; violent coughing fit ceasing after eating; sensation of tenesmus in the rectum, after stool; anasarca and ascites (after Acon.;) cardialgia, pleuritis after a strain or an effort; intermittent fever after abuse of cinchona, with rheumatic pains in the limbs, aggravation by motion, talking or noise; aggravation or supervention of the pains when exposed to the vapor of coal.

*Arsenicum album. (Arsenious acid.)

Burning pains in internal and external parts; *sudden prostration of strength;* watery diarrhœa, painless or else with burning in the bowels and anus; fetid diarrhœa, with constant coldness; white diarrhœic stools, bloody, also with tenesmus, brown and black; violent vomiting of the ingesta and of liquids, also of brown and black substances; aversion to farinaceous food; *Burning pains in the stomach,* relieved for a short time by warm drinks; gastritis, carcinoma of the stomach; Asiatic cholera, last stage, with cold breath or pains in the region of the spleen (after Cuprum or Veratrum;) anasarca, ascites, hydrothorax, especially after abuse of cinchona; constriction of the chest during motion, with dyspnœa; dry titillating cough during a walk in the open air, as if caused by the vapors of sulphur; spasmodic asthma; nocturnal palpitation of the heart, with great anguish; *Ichorous ulcers,* with burning pains, or with everted margins, having a foul smell, (carcinoma;) warts, surrounded by an ulcerated circle with hard, everted border; anthrax; gray tetter; greenish complexion; spontaneous limping; intermittent fever, with absence of thirst during the chill, great prostration, trembling or also paralysis of the extremities, or dropsical bloat of the body, especially after abuse of cinchona; with intense thirst and burning heat, *frequent drinking,* though little at a time; typhus; extreme *emaciation;* atrophy of childdren with large abdomens and glandular swellings; affections of the spleen and liver, after abuse of cinchona; phthisis laryngea (in connection with Carbo veg., Hep., Phosph., Spong;) mucous phthisis (in connection with Stannum;) illusions of smell, as if one smelled pitch; the pains are made worse by smoking, relieved by eating a copious meal; consequences of animal poisons that have been introduced into the stomach or have become absorbed into the blood.

*Asafœtida.

Ulcers and caries, with thin, fetid ichor; hysteric complaints; intermittent, pulsative, stinging, tearing pains, they are felt from within outwards and are changed to other pains by contact; bone-pains after suppression of syphilis, aggravated by the warmth of the bed; cough with expectoration tasting of onion.

Asarum europæum. (Common asarabacca.)

Headache with nausea, even unto vomiting, made worse by thinking; hemicrania on the left side, every afternoon at five o'clock; burning in the eyes, in the evening, with continual lachrymation; inflamed, weeping eyes; constant nausea; unsuccessful efforts to vomit, causing all the pains to be worse; vomiting, with great anxiety, or accompanied by diarrhœa, or vomiting of mere water; soreness in the region of the spleen; lienteria, potatoes are passed undigested; discharge of thick, black blood at stool; protrusion of the rectum; Menses premature and long lasting, with black blood; stitches in the lungs, especially when drawing breath; some symptoms abate while washing one's face.

***Aurum foliatum.** (Leaf-gold.)

Hernia, prolapsus of the uterus (after Nux v., in connection with Bell., Kreas., Lyc., Plat., Sep., Sil.;) *nightly bone-pains;* caries; syphilitic and mercurial affections of bones; ulcerated nose, with fetid discharge; swelling and suppuration of the inguinal glands; induration or swelling of the testes; melancholy, longing for death, oppressive anxiety, especially in the præcordia, as if one should die; mania of suicide; jumping of the heart, palpitation during motion; feels better in the open air.

Baryta carbonica. (Carbonate of baryta.)

Affections of old people (in connection with Ambra and Opium;) scrofulous ailments; atrophy of children, with large bowels and glandular swellings; paralysis after apoplexy; nocturnal twitching of the muscles; swelling and induration of glands; warts; steatoma, sarcoma; tearing, stinging, twitching, throbbing in the head, especially in the forehead, over the eyes (in connection with Bell.;) falling off of the hair; baldness (with Graph. and Lyc.;) humid and dry scaldhead; inflammation of the eyes and lids, especially in the case of scrofulous persons, with photophobia; muscæ volitantes; eruption on and behind the ears; scurfs under the nose; eruption in the face; inflamed throat, with suppuration of tonsils, especially when frequently recurring after the use of the other remedies; weak digestion; violent singultus; pressure in the stomach as from a stone, even after eating the least quantity of food; *weakness of the male organs;* aversion to sexual intercourse (in females, with Caust.;) painful stiffness of the back and nape of the neck; rheumatic tearing in the limbs; ulcers on the legs; fetid sweat on the feet; the pains are chiefly felt in the left side of the body, when sitting, they pass off during exercise in the open air.

*Belladonna. (Deadly night-shade.)

A medicine acting chiefly on the brain Vertigo, meningitis, hydrocephalus (after Acon.;) delirium; screaming of children, without any apparent cause, all the time, when carried or lying; headache, over the eyes, stitches in the temples; headache, with sensation as if the brain were balancing to and fro; hemicrania, especially on the right side; prosopalgia, toothache, with heat and swelling of the cheek, or gums, the pains are lancinating or tearing, affecting the whole side, sometimes it is impossible to point out the affected tooth, the pains extend to the temples, cold air, contact, chewing or hot drinks aggravate the pains, the teeth feel elongated; *hot, red, shining swelling,* erysipelas, especially of fleshy parts; *scarlatina* and sequelæ, such as hardness of hearing, otorrhœa, difficulty of speech, stuttering; *glandular swelling,* especially with heat and stinging, also stiffness of the neck and nape of neck, glandular indurations; chilblains, with bright-red, erysipelatous appearance; ophthalmia (after Acon.;) swelling of the eyelids, aversion or bleeding of the lids, thickening of the conjunctiva, spots, obscuration of the cornea; *weak sight;* dilated pupils; *diplopia;* hemeralopia; amaurosis; rush of blood to the head and chest; apoplexy; paralysis; *palpitation of the heart;* oppression of the chest, angina pectoris; convulsions, spasms, epilepsy with screams, delirium, laughter, worse by the least contact; tetanus; *chorea;* mental derangement after a fright or chagrin, illusions of the fancy, insanity; spasmodic cough as if the head would burst; paralysis of single parts; stitches and lameness of the hip-joint (with Caust.;) wetting the bed; intermittent fever, with delirium, headache over the eyes, or setting in in the afternoon, with violent chilliness and thirst, aversion to drink; discharge of blood between the menses; fetid metrorrhagia; prolapsus and induration of the uterus; the pains improve while the patient is lying on a hard couch, or when looking out in a straight line; this remedy is particularly adapted to stout, plethoric individuals.

Borax.

Ailments in consequence of taking cold during damp

and chilly weather; unhealthy skin; tetter; twisting of the hair as in plica polonica; inflammation of the eyes, and especially of the lids, with inversion of the lids; the eyes are sensitive to the light of lamps or candles; otorrhœa; tearing pains in decayed teeth, in cold and damp weather; the gums are swollen and bleed readily; aphthæ, as in stomatitis; hiccough, especially of infants; vomiting of sour phlegm; menses premature and profuse; chronic, corrosive leucorrhœa; sterility; galactirrhœa; cough, with musty expectoration; the pains are worse during a dance or when swinging.

Bovista. (Puff-ball)

Humid, scurfy tetter; objects seen nearer than they are; chronic fetid diarrhœa; scurfy nostrils; eruption in the corners of the mouth; scrofulous swelling of the lips; drawing, digging, boring pains in decayed teeth; chronic backache, with stiffness after stooping; the pains are made worse by the vapors of coal.

Bromine.

Very drowsy in the day-time; starting during sleep; violent chill, with stretching of the arms, as during an attack of fever and ague; sensation of burning in the whole body, as if surrounded by hot vapor; small, accelerated pulse; cool and damp hands; sweaty palms; small, moveable glandular swellings on the neck and nape of the neck; goïtre; vertigo when crossing a stream; hemicrania on the left side; headache after drinking milk; lachrymation, also with sensitiveness of the eyes to the light; photophobia, with pressure in the eyes when moving them; stitches in the ears, with heat in the same; soreness and scurfs in the nose; pains in decayed teeth, they are sensitive to cold water; inflammation of the fauces and uvula; sore throat, with swelling of the tonsils, difficult deglutition, pains when swallowing a drink; pains in the stomach, made worse by pressing upon the part; pains in the region of the liver, especially when pressing upon the same, also when riding in a carriage; slimy or papescent, diarrhœic stool; menses premature and too copious, preceded by frontal headache and accompanied by pain in the small of the back; *stitching constriction in the larynx; inflammation of the larynx and trachea; hoarseness, feeble low voice; rough, hollow, dry cough, with weariness, or with paroxysms of suffocation, or with wheezing sound and rattling breathing; or with croupy sound; croup,* even in the last stage; swelling of the mammæ; stitches in the chest, especially on the right side, during a rapid walk, worse during an inspiration; violent palpitation of the heart, especially in the evening, not permitting one to lie on the left side; the pains are worse in the evening until midnight, they abate during a walk in the open air.

*Bryonia alba. (White bryony.)

Acts chiefly upon the joints. Erysipelas of joints; rheumatic and arthritic pains in the joints, especially with redness of the affected parts, aggravated by motion, relieved by rest; stitches and rigidity of joints; rash, especially of lying-in females and infants, also miliaria alba (with Arsen.;) purpura hæmorrhagica; *intermittent fever,* especially quotidian and tertian, with chilliness prevailing, thirst during the chilly and hot stage, and *dry cough with stitches in the chest;* typhus with burning heat and thirst, dryness of the skin (after Acon.;) delirium, especially on waking; throbbing headache, worse during motion; meningitis (after Acon. and Bell.; *cough,* with *pleuritic stitches,* worse when entering a warm room and drawing a long breath; *pneumonia, pleurisy* (after Acon., Arn., Nux. vom.;) cardialgia when walking; *ascites* (after Acon.;) difficulty of breathing when walking fast, with continual disposition to draw a long breath; obstinate constipation (after Nux vom.;) *nose-bleed* in the place of the menses; *toothache,* aggravated by warm food, relieved by lying on the affected side, momentarily relieved by cold water, the teeth feel as if loose, worse in a warm room, in the evening and at night, or when walking; the pains are less in gloomy weather.

***Calcarea carbonica.** (Carbonate of lime.)

Acts chiefly upon the bones (with Silicea;) tearing and stitching in the limbs, the limbs incline to go to sleep, liability to feeling strained, the pains are worse during a change of weather, by working in the water, washing; *caries, curvature of bones; rickets;* scrofulous ailments; *epilepsy,* especially at night, with cries (with Caust.;) carcinomatous indurations in the mammæ (after Con ; humid and dry tetter; dry warts; polypus; fistulæ; ulcers; sarcoma; ganglia; *goïtre;* swelling and hardness of the cervical glands; adiposis; emaciation, with large bowels and good appetite; intermittent fever, after abuse of Cinchona, also of those who work in water; sensation of icy-coldness about the head; eruption on the head, on and behind the ears, in the face (mouth, nose, cheeks, after Sulph.;) slow closing of the fontanelles; hard hearing, with buzzing in the ears, cardialgia, vomiting of the ingesta, or sour eructations, nausea, yawning; obstinate constipation: sour-smelling diarrhœa of children; ascarides; menses too early and too copious (with Nux vom.;) milky *leucorrhœa,* previous to the menses; discharge of blood and mucus, when urinating; cough with copious expectoration, yellow, purulent; phthisis pulmonalis; *palpitation of the heart,* with feeling of coldness; delirium tremens (after Opium and Nux vom.;) sensitive to cold and damp air; toothache of pregnant females, with rush of blood to the head, from a cold, worse at night, even aggravated by cold and warm applications or food; fistula dentalis; difficulty of first dentition; morbid sensation as if the body were shrinking; softening of the internal organs.

Calcarea caustica.

Skin. Small vesicles filled with lymph and surrounded by a red areola, also smarting and itching, like scabies.

Sleep. Sleepless, tossing about, or restless sleep with dreams.

Fever. Violent chills, followed by great heat in the head.

Disposition. Peevish, slowness of thought, giddiness.

Head. *Stitches* from the forehead to the occiput; *dull headache* in the vertex; the headache is worse when stooping.

Eyes. Pressing weight in the eyelids; tearing and stitches in eyes; burning of the eyes when reading at candlelight; lachrymation in the open air; photophobia.

Ears. Stitching, tearing pains in the ears; ringing in the ears.

Nose. Dry nose; coryza, discharge of thick, tenacious mucous.

Face. Tearing in the malar bones; violent pains in the articulation of the jaws, with swelling of the cheeks.

Teeth. Dull, tearing, stitching pain in the decayed teeth, they feel elongated.

Mouth. Tongue thickly coated, greenish-yellow.

Throat. Stinging in the throat; difficult deglutition; phlegm in the throat, which it is difficult to hawk up; obstinate sore throat, with swelling of the tonsils; discharge of tenacious saliva; thickly-coated tongue; dull headache; small and hurried pulse.

Appetite, taste. Loss of appetite or else violent hunger; bitter taste in the mouth.

Gastric symptoms. Empty rising of air; regurgitation of food, with sourish-bitter taste; nausea, vomiting of sour fluid.

Stomach. Spasmodic contraction of the stomach.

Hypochondria. Stinging, tearing pain in both hypochondria.

Abdomen. Violent stitches in the small bowels, when stooping forward; pinching, contracting pains in the bowels.

Stool, Anus. Diarrhœic, slimy stools discharge of tænia; creeping or stinging tearing in the rectum and anus.

Trachea. Hoarseness, with pain in the throat; violent cough, with stitches in the chest, or expectoration of mucus and blood.

Chest. Stinging, tearing, pressing or pressing-tearing

pain in the chest or sides of the chest, worse when drawing breath; *influenza.*

Back. Tension in the back; stiffness of the nape of the neck; tearing in the posterior cervical muscles, in the back, small of the back, os coccygis.

Upper extremities. Stitching-tearing pains in the upper extremities.

Lower extremities. Stitching pains in the hip-joint when stepping; tearing and stitching in the knee.

Calcarea phosphorica. (Phosphate of lime.)

Arthritis, with swelling of the joints, curvature of joints, very painful.

Calendula officinalis. (Marsh Marygold.)

Applied externally and internally, this agent heals *large, deep, shaggy, profusely-bleeding wounds*, and favors the process of cicatrization, even if whole pieces of flesh should be wanting. This agent is also indicated if the wounds are painful, with raw feeling and stitches in the wounds, as if suppuration were to take place, with smarting around the wounds. Wound-fever in alternation with Acon. Inflammation of the eyes, after an operation, also in alternation with Acon.

*Camphora

Antidotes most homœopathic medicines, especially from the vegetable kingdom.

Sudden prostration of strength; excessive weakness, convulsions, tetanic spasms. *Cholera*, especially with violent cramps in the calves, coldness of the body, great anxiety, burning in the fauces and stomach, the pit of the stomach is very painful when touched; ascites, with complete suppression of urine, which may be caused by Cantharides; suppression of sexual desire, complete impotence, (after Nux V.,) sensitive to cold air; liability to taking cold, followed by chilliness, or colic with diarrhœa, discharge of brown and blackish stool.

Cancer fluviatilis. (Sweet-water Crab.)

Red, stitching eruption like measles, over the whole body; fever, with redness and heat in the face, internal chilliness, creeping chills when uncovering the body.

Cannabis sativa. (Hemp.)

Ailments arising from bodily fatigue; spots and obscuration of the cornea, cataract, epistaxis even unto fainting; long suppression of urine; painful emission of a few drops of bloody urine; inflammation of the bladder and kidneys; gravel, burning in the urethra when urinating; urethritis gonorrhœica; sterility; miscarriage in the third month of pregnancy (with Sabina); *stitches* in the lungs when drawing breath, talking, moving about; *pneumonia,* also with delirium, vomiting of green bile; shocks in the region of the heart; carditis.

***Cantharides.** (Spanish fly),

Acts chiefly upon the bladder; detention of urine, with spasmodic pains in the bladder; ineffectual urging to urinate, dribbling of the urine; *hæmaturia;* painful *gonorrhœa,* chordee; discharge of bloody mucus from the bladder; inflammation of the kidneys and bladder (after Acon.;) intermittent fever, with urninary difficulties, or with aversion to drink (with Bell.)

Capsicum annuum. (Spanish pepper.)

Laming stiffness of the knees and tarsal joints, especially when first getting up (after Rhus;) dread of motion. The pains are made worse by contact or in the open air; quotidian and tertian-fever, with chilliness prevailing; chill with violent thirst, followed by heat with or without thirst, sweat. During the chill: anxiety, restlessness, inability to collect one's self, intolerance of noise, headache, flow of saliva, vomiting of mucus, painful swelling of the spleen, back ache, tearing in the limbs, contraction of the limbs. During the heat: stitches in the head, bad taste in the mouth, colic with ineffectual urging to stool, pains in the chest and back, tearing in the limbs; fever after abuse of Cinchona; *home-sickness* with redness of the cheeks; hemicrania; angry tetter on the forehead; chapped lips; burning pimples on the inner cheek; spasmodic contraction of the fauces; sudden, sometimes bloody diarrhœa; discharge of fluid, tenacious mucus mixed with black blood; dysenteric diarrhœa; gonorrhœic discharge from the urethra; frequent urging to urinate; difficult urination, dribbling; burning in the urethra when urinating, also, before and after; *cough,* especially at night, with headache, as if the skull would split; violent stitches in the region of the heart, extorting cries.

Carbo animalis. (Animal charcoal.)

Arthritic stiffness of the joints; hard painful glandular swellings; burning chilblains; feeling as if abandoned by every body; vertigo with nausea, when rising from a stooping position; scald-head; otorrhœa; discharge of bright-red blood from the nose; burning swelling of the lips; bleeding of the gums; toothache, the teeth feel loose and elongated; weak digestion, nothing agrees with one; cardialgia, burning in the stomach; stool either hard or soft, like albumen; burning hæmorrhoidal tumors; premature menses with dark blood; burning-smarting leucorrhœa, tinging the linen yellow; painful nodes in the mammæ; cough with greenish expectoration; stitches in the right side; *suppuration of the right lung;* tetter or hard glands in the axillæ.

*Carbo vegetabilis. (Vegetable charcoal.)

Burning pains in the limbs, bones, ulcers, also in internal organs; eruption and humid tetter in the face; hard hearing, with dryness of the inner ear, especially after measles; cough, with soreness in the larynx and chest; phthisis larynxea; cough, with expectoration of whitish or greenish mucus; mucous phthisis; cardialgia, with sensation of burning pressure, flatulence and sensitiveness in the pit of the stomach (sometimes after Nux.;) ailments caused by fat food, after the unsuccessful use of Puls.; chronic ailments after the use of Mercury, looseness of the teeth, bleeding of the gums, etc.; stomatitis; piles; burning, bleeding tumors after stool; chronic hoarseness or aphonia; spasmodic cough with retching and vomiting of mucus; cold breath and collapse of pulse during cholera; swinging makes the pains worse. This remedy sometimes favors the reaction when not sufficiently excited by other remedies, (also Opium.)

Causticum.

Arthritic and rheumatic tearing in the limbs, less in bed and warmth; contraction and paralysis of the limbs; paralysis after apoplexy, especially on the right side, also with stuttering; hysteric spasms, epilepsy, chorea; bleeding, inflamed warts, especially on the nose; fistula rect.; aversion to sexual intercourse, in the case of females (with Baryt.;) racking cough, with spirting out of the urine; raging toothache; fistula dentalis, with painfulness and bleeding of the gums; chronic hoarseness.

Cepa. (Common Onion.)

Colic after eating salad, especially cucumbers; ailments induced by getting the feet wet, or by exposure to dampness or impure air; contusions and burns; ailments of children, such as, running of the nose, sore eyes, cough, rattling in the bronchia, colic, flatulence, worms, urinary difficulties; ailments of old people, dyspnœa, accompanied by or alternating with affections of the bladder and kidneys; toothache, relieved by cold, worse in the warmth; coryza, lachrymation, sensitiveness of the eyes, alternate heat and chills; the pains in the upper part of the body first appear on the right, then on the left side; in the lower part the reverse, are worse in the evening, less in the open air, worse again when re-entering the warm room.

***Chamomilla vulgaris.** (Common chamomile.)

Excessive sensitiveness of the senses, especially when caused by coffee and other narcotics; ailments induced by fits of chagrin; watery, greenish diarrhœa, or like stirred eggs, having a foul smell, during dentition; restlessness and spasms during the diarrhœa, the child draws up its legs; *crying* of infants without any apparent cause, abating when they are carried; dry cough from taking cold, hacking cough of children in the winter, with titillation in the throat-pit, worse at night; headache, after sudden suppression of sweat; *toothache*, by exposure to a draught of air, with otalgia, and as if the teeth were loose and elongated; *hoarseness* from taking cold; sore throat with sensation as if something had lodged in the throat which had to be hawked up; heat in the throat, with thirst; asthma millari; *angina pectoris* with suffocative symptoms, after a fit of chagrin; cardialgia, with pressure in the stomach as from a stone, relieved by drinking coffee, caused by a fit of chagrin; labor-like pains previous to or during the menses; uterine hæmorrhage, with discharge of fetid coagula; fever, with redness of one, and paleness of the other cheek.

***China.** (Peruvian bark.)

General *debility*, especially when caused by loss of fluids, onanism, depletions, nursing, suppurations, etc.; impotence; debilitating emissions; emaciation, especially of the limbs, atrophy of children; exhausting sweats, night or morning; pains in the limbs, aggravated by the least contact, *with disposition to perspire; intermittent fever*, especially in marshy regions, with absence of thirst during the chill and heat. The thirst generally sets in between the chill and hot stage, and increases during the sweat; *chlorosis*, frequently with swelling of the feet; *anasarca;* hæmorrhages, metrorrhagia; deficient or suppressed labor-pains; flatulence, fetid; constipation from debility; *diarrhœa* with feeling of weakness, discharge of undigested food, also after eating fresh fruit; cardialgia from debility; toothache, headache of nursing females or pregnant women; nocturnal enuresis of feeble children; involuntary stool and urine from debility; cough with granular expectoration; some pains are eased by shaking the head, (chief remedies for the china-cachexia, are: Ars., Ipecac., Ferr., Verat.)

Chlorum. (Water impregnated with Chlorine.)

Herpes; evening-fever; hurried pulse; difficulty of remembering the names of persons; impeded deglutition; malignant sore-throat; foul ulcers in the throat; nausea, vomiting; weakness of the bowels; colic, diarrhœa; sudden impotence with aversion to sexual intercourse, in the case of persons who had a passion for it; violent cough, hæmoptysis; ulcerative phthisis; nightsweats of phthisicky persons.

Cicuta virosa. (Water-hemlock.)

Soreness as if bruised; tetanic spasms; convulsions; epilepsy of children; suppurating eruptions in the face; going to sleep while sitting, the head bent forward, during the period of digestion or while listening to a dull sermon; vertigo when sitting up in bed, with obscuration of sight; weak sight, with dilatation of the pupils; photophobia; diplogia; hæmorrhage from the ears; vomiting while making an effort to raise the head when lying; worms; colic, with convulsions, in the case of children; involuntary discharge of urine, as from paralysis of the bladder.

Cina. (Worm-seed.)

Ascarides, lumbrici; pinching colic and irritating pain in the umbilical region, from worms; *spasms of children, from worms,* during which they dose with their eyes half-closed, and rub at the nose. Epilepsy, especially at night; whooping-cough, with worms; intermittent fever, with vomiting and canine; hunger; bluish color around the mouth.

Cistus canadensis. (Rock-rose.)

Tearing and drawing in the joints, especially in the toes and fingers; *swelling and suppuration* of the glands; scrofulous ailments, fetid otorrhœa; vesicular erysipelas in the face. *Caries* of the lower jaw. Swelling and looseness of the gums, they have an unpleasant appearance; the pains are worse towards morning, and after an unpleasant emotion.

Clematis erecta. (Virgin's-bower.)

Mercurial ailments; articular rheumatism in conse quence of mismanaged gonorrhœa; pustules over the whole body; *chronic, red and humid herpes,* itching in the warmth of the bed and after washing; scrofulous sore eyes; swelling and induration of the inguinal glands; *stricture* of the urethra; purulent gonorrhœa; swelling and induration of the testes; induration in the mamma, under the nipple. Arthritic nodes in the finger-joints.

Cocculus indicus. (Seeds of cocculus.)

Nausea when riding in a carriage, sea-sickness; cardialgia during and shortly after a meal; vomiting, worse when raising the head. Paraplegia, with numbness of the limbs, also proceeding from the small of the back; intermittent fever, with cardialgia or lameness of the small of the back; epilepsy, with involuntary discharge of urine during the paroxysms; menstrual abdominal spasms, also with cessation of the menses (after Puls.); angina pectoris of hysteric individuals. The pains are made worse by eating, drinking, sleeping, talking, driving, smoking.

Coccus cacti. (Cochineal.)

Dull, stinging, spasmodic pressing pain in the kidneys, increased by pressure and motion. Cutting pains in the region of the bladder; paroxysms of titillating, barking cough, especially night and morning. After a few turns of cough, the patient raises a large quantity of albuminous, tenacious, ropy mucus, white or yellowish-white, having a saltish taste, sometimes with gagging, or vomiting of the ingesta; *whooping cough.*

*Coffea cruda. (Raw coffee.)

The senses and nerves are very much *excited*, in the

case of lying-in females, especially when this state is caused by abuse of Chamomile-tea. Consequences of a paroxysm of sudden joy; anxious and weeping mood of hysteric females, crowding of ideas, acute thinking, arranging plans for the future, etc. Excessive labor-pains; protracted after-pains. Excessive excitability of the sexual parts. *Spasms* and diarrhœa during dentition, or from the abuse of Chamomile-tea.

Colchicum autumnale. (Meadow-saffron.)

Arthritic and rheumatic complaints, with tearing pains in warm weather, and stitching pains when the weather is cold; œdema and anasarca; nocturnal heat of the body, thirst; pulse 100; *vomiting* of bitter mucus or of food, excited or aggravated by motion; the abdomen is very much distended; fall-dysentery, with discharges of white mucus, tenesmus; bloody stools with discharges of patches of mucus. Scanty dark red urine, with burning and tenesmus in the urethra; cough at night, during which the urine spirts out involuntarily; hydrothorax; the pains are worse at night, when they are infense and last until day-time.

*Colocynthis. (Wild bitter cucumber.)

Hemicrania, with crampy pain, nausea and vomiting, every afternoon; colic, with violent pain in the umbilical region, causing the patient to cry out and bend double, the pain comes every few minutes and leaves the abdominal walls so sensitive that the pain is felt at every step; cardialgia with sensation of hunger which cannot be relieved by eating; yellow diarrhœa, excited by eating or drinking ever so little; vomiting and diarrhœa after a fit of chagrin; spontaneous limping.

***Conium maculatum.** (Spotted hemlock.)

Indurated mammæ, with violent pain; swelling and induration of glandular organs; caries of the sternum; cataract caused by injuries; impotence; chronic obstruction of the nose; tetter and spreading ulcers in the face; *cancer of the lip,* caused by a blow, contusion; swelling of the testicles, caused by a contusion; *cough,* only at night, especially shortly after lying down at night.

***Crocus.** (Saffron.)

Good for *metrorrhagia,* with tenacious, coagulated, fetid blood; the movements of the fetus are too violent.

***Crotalus horridus.** (Rattle-snake poison.)

Paralysis after apoplexy, especially of the right side; spasms and convulsions, also with violent cries and delirium; œdema of the whole body; oozing of blood from all the pores; black spots on the skin; blisters surrounded by a red areola. Ulcers arising from blisters; inflammatory fever, with pulse up to 130, first full and strong, afterwards feeble and scarcely perceptible; frequent attacks of erysipelas of the face; trismus.

***Cuprum.** (Copper.)

Dry cough, taking away the breath, like whooping-cough; *whooping-cough,* the children turn blue in the face, as if suffocating. Spasms preceded by weeping.

Asiatic cholera, especially if vomiting and diarrhœa are accompanied by convulsions of the extremities and pressure in the pit of the stomach, or preceded by spasmodic constriction of the chest, the liquids roll down in the œsophagus as if by their own weight (in alternation with Veratrum); *opisthotonos,* with discharges of urine; cramps in the calves; the convulsions begin at the toes and fingers; asthma, with difficulty of breathing even unto suffocation, and spasmodic vomiting at the end of the attack.

Daphne indica.

Rheumatic and arthritic pains in the muscles and bones; *bone-pains,* especially at night (in connection with Merc. and Aur.); palpitation, with inability to lie on the left side.

Digitalis purpurea. (Fox-glove.)

Blueness of the lids, lips, tongue, nails (cyanosis); slow pulse, down to 35; *dilatation* and diminished sensibility of the pupils; amaurosis; vomiting of bile or mucus; ash-colored stools: hydrocele; cough with expectoration resembling boiled starch; hæmoptysis; palpitation with slow pulse; hydrothorax and ascites, from organic disease of the heart.

Drosera. (Sun-dew.)

Whooping-cough with vomiting, the child feeling better during motion than during rest. The sweat is not cool, but rather warm (the opposite of Verat.);

whooping-cough with hæmorrhage from nose and mouth, pains in the hypochondria; nose-bleed, especially morning and evening, or when stooping; laryngeal phthisis, with rapid emaciation. The cough is made worse by singing, laughing, crying, smoking, drinking.

*Dulcamara. (Bitter-sweet.)

Diarrhœa, with colic, after taking cold; swelling and induration of the glands; catarrhal ailments (after Acon.); small, hard, dry warts (with Calc.); urticaria; humid and suppurating herpes, or dry, scaly tetter; ascites, hydrothorax; cough, with expectoration of tenacious mucus, and stitches in the sides of the chest.

Euphorbium officinale. (Spurge.)

Burning pains, especially in internal organs; rheumatic pains in the limbs, worse during rest; laming weakness in the joints; chronic eruptions; gangrene; erysipelatous inflammation of the head; chronic sore eyes, with suppuration; dimness of sight, objects seem too large, inducing one to raise the leg much more than the size of the object requires, in order to step over it; vesicular erysipelas of the face; œsophagitis; spasmodic cardialgia, burning in the stomach; papescent stools; urging to urinate, the urine passes off in drops; rigidity and burning pain in the extremities.

Euphrasia officinalis. (Eye-bright.)

Inflammation of the eyes, especially when caused by injuries (with Conium.) Inflammation and ulceration of the margins of the eyelids, with headache. Spots, ulcers and obscuration of the cornea; *lachrymation;* coryza with smarting lachrymation and photopbolia; heaviness of the tongue, causing difficulty of speech; colic alternating with sore eyes; figwarts; cough only in the day-time, with phlegm on the chest which it is difficult to raise; numbness of the fingers; *cramp in the calves* while standing.

*Ferrum. (Iron.)

Ailments arising from abuse of China and tea; milky leucorrhœa; smarting of the vagina during an embrace, deficient sexual feeling; metrorrhagia with labor-like pains; debility from loss of fluids (with China). Anasarca and ascites, caused by abuse of Cinchona or accompanied by liver-complaint.

Nitro-glycerine. (Glonoine.)

Headache, pressing in the vertex, or as if the brain were pressed asunder. Violent *rush of blood* to the head. Throbbing in the forehead as far as the nape of the neck. Stitches in the forehead or temples. During the headache the pulse is accelerated, the face red, the forehead moist. The eyes look red, stitches and heat in the eyes. Stitches and fullness in the ears. Pains and rigidity in the lower jaw. Throbbing toothache, with headache. Sensation as if the lower lip were swollen. Stinging and smarting in the swollen tongue. Gnawing in the pit of the stomach, colic, rumbling in the bowels. Oppression on the chest, throbbing of the carotids. *Pain, heat and chills down the back.* Numbness and weakness in the left arm and legs. Vertigo when walking.

*Graphites. (Black-lead.)

Humid tetter; scanty or delaying menses, with cutaneous eruptions. Chronic costiveness. Falling out of the hair (with Baryta and Lycop.)

Helleborus niger. (Christmas-rose.)

Anasarca, especially after suppression of an exanthem (scarlatina, measles, purple-rash); apathy to emotions; acute and chronic hydrocephalus. Aphthæ in the mouth. Swelling of the posterior cervical glands.

*Hepar sulphuris calcareum. (Sulphuret of lime.)

Arthritic and rheumatic pains, also with inflammation and swelling of the affected parts. Mercurial cachexia. Ulcerations and suppurations (in alternation with Merc.); panaritia (in alternation with Merc. or Sil.); Ulceration of the mamma; open chilblains; vesicular erysipelatous inflammations with swelling (with Rhus tox.); rhagades. Humid tinea; scrofulous ophthalmia with pimples on the lids; phlyctænæ of the cornea; fetid otorrhœa. Soreness in the groin. Croup (after Aconite, in alternation with Spongia); chronic hoarseness; chronic laryngitis; *laryngeal phthisis;* sore throat as if a pointed body were sticking in it; dyspepsia, with pressure in the stomach; sour, green diarrhœa of children; opalescent urine; leucorrhœa with smarting; sensation as if hot water were coursing through the swelling around the chest; ankles.

Hydrocyani acidum. (Prussic acid.)

In the last stage of cholera: 1. If the patient continues to spit continually without expectorating much saliva. 2. Heat in the head, with coldness of the limbs, vomiting of a black fluid, involuntary stools. 3. For cholera sicca (dry cholera) without diarrhœa or vomiting, with general cramps, at times in the calves, at other times in the arms and hands or in the masseter muscles, preventing the mouth being opened, with occasional involuntary shrieks, followed by prostration or fainting, 4. After the apparent cessation of all vital functions, with entire collapse of pulse (with Carbo. veg.) in the last stage (paralytic stage;) tetanus.

*Hyoscyamus niger. (Black henbane.)

Toothache, with flashes of heat towards the head; epileptic paroxysms, terminating in deep sleep; chorea; encephalitis (Bellad. being ineffectual;) grasping at flocks in typhus; consequences of unhapyy love, with jealousy; rage, with shameless manners, the patient goes about naked; spasmodic closing of the eyelids, squinting, diplopia, hemeralopia (in alternation with Bell.)

Hypericum perforatum. (St. John's-wort.)

Used externally and internally, this agent cures punctured wounds, cuts, bruises, lacerations of the fibre, if the pains are very violent, like toothache, proceeding from the injury along the limb. It is also useful, if children are affected with spasms after every slight injury.

*Iatropha curcas. (Barbadoes-nut.)

General prostration; coldness of the extremities, with blueness of the nails; vomiting of albuminous substances, with diarrhœa; *Asiatic cholera,* with frightful vomiting, constrictive or burning pains in the stomach, watery stools, violent cramps in the calves, coldness of the body (in connection with Cupr. and Verat.)

Ignatia amara. (St. Ignatius' bean.)

Spasmodic laughter and weeping, consequences of *grief, suppressed mortification, unhappy love;* convulsions after grief, fright, insults. Hysteric spasms, epilepsy (from similar causes;) menses premature and profuse, black and coagulated blood, (after Nux vom.;) cardialgia relieved by eating; uterine spasms, with contractive pressing pains; disposition to prolapsus of the rectum; hemicrania (clavus.)

Iodine.

Scrofulous ailments; swelling and induration of glands; œdema, anasarca; fever, alternate chills and flashes of heat, with delirium and subsultus tendinum, grasping at flocks; *hectic fever;* aphthæ, with ptyalism; continual vomiting; induration of the spleen; swelling of the inguinal glands; ovarian dropsy; metrorrhagia at stool; chronic, corrosive leucorrhœa; *inflammation of the larynx and trachea; croup* (in alternation with Acon.;) chronic hoarseness; cough, with white or bloody expectoration; *laryngeal* and *tracheal phthisis; goitre;* white-swelling of the knee, also inflammatory swelling, with violent pains and suppuration.

*Ipecacuanha.

Prostration, with loathing of food or drink; vomiting; *intermittent fever*, (especially after alloeopathic remedies had been used;) *cinchona-cachexia*, slight chills, a good deal of heat, gastric symptoms, oppression on the chest; gastric derangement after eating fat food (also Puls.;) *cholerine*, vomiting of mucus and bile (with Puls.;) rattling and vomiting of mucus, in the case of children; *hæmorrhage* from every orifice of the body; asthma millari, the pains are less in the open air.

Kali bichromicum. (Bichromate of Potash.)

Chronic rheumatism; pains shifting from one part to another; violent itching of the skin, followed by the breaking out of small pustules on the arms and thighs forming crusts; *secondary syphilitic eruptions.*

Apathy; irritable mood; vertigo on rising from a seat; stinging pains in the temples; throbbing headache.

Inflammation and swelling of the lids; chronic conjunctivitis; ulcers and spots of the cornea; optical illusions; stinging and ringing in the ears; *ozæna;* sponginess, polypi of the nose; *fetor* from the nose; loss of smell; plugs of indurated mucus in the nose.

Chapping of the lips; ulcers on the inner lips; painful ulcer on the tongue; yellow coating on the tongue; sensation as of a hair on the velum; sensation as if the food remained lodged in the œsophagus; small and excavated ulcer at the root of the uvula, with reddish areola, and secreting a yellowish matter; secondary syphilitic ulceration of the throat.

Sour or bitter taste in the mouth; heartburn; vomiting of blood or mucus; pains in the stomach aggravated by motion, relieved by eating, which leaves a feeling of oppression; boring pains in the bowels, relieved by pressure; habitual constipation, or occurring every three months; dysentery, with boring pain at the anus; scanty urine, with whitish pellicle and whitish sediment; rawness, soreness, itching and pustules of the pudendum; yellowish leucorrhœa, with weakness in the small of the back.

Dryness in the bronchia; painfulness of the larynx, with intolerable titillation, and dry cough day and night; or cough with expectoration of tenacious phlegm, or yellowish-gray phlegm; dyspnœa; tearing-lancinating pains in the whole left side of the chest; stitching-boring pains in the kidneys, with suppression of urine.

Tearing pains in the arms and hands; rheumatic pains in the hips, knees, also with trembling of the legs.

Kali carbonicum. (Carbonate of Potash.)

Bitter, sour, foul or sweetish taste; hoarseness, with sensation as of a plug in the throat; cough, with suffocative anguish, or with vomiting, especially in the morning; whooping cough with œdema of the upper lids; cough with purulent expectoration; dyspnœa, especially when walking fast; goitre.

Kreasotum.

Marasmus of children, with diarrhœa; swelling or induration of the neck of the uterus; incipient carcinoma.

Lachesis.

Paralysis, especially on the left side; epilepsy; twitching of the arms and legs, froth at the mouth; ulcers on the legs, secreting a fetid pus; inveterate fever and ague, especially after abuse of cinchona; sore throat; gangrenous ulceration.

Laurocerasus. (Cherry-laurel.

Tetanic and epileptic spasms; apoplexy, with loss of speech; hepatitis and induration of the liver; constipation, retention of urine, complete paralysis of the bladder; profuse menorrhagia during the critical period, with dark coagula; cough with copious gelatinous expectoration, also streaked with blood; slow, panting breathing; paralysis of the lungs; pains are less in the open air and at night.

Ledum palustre. (Marsh-tea.)

Nodous gout. Dry, itching herpes; swelling of the knee, with tension and stinging; inflammatory or œdematous swelling of the feet and legs.

Lycopodium clavatum. (Club-moss.)

Nodous gout; scrofulous and rickety complaints; curvature and softening of bones; mercurial bone-pains; paralysis; humid tetter; humid scald head; fistulous ulcers; chronic conjunctivitis; photophobia; ulceration of the Schneiderian membrane; freckles in the face; chronic hepatitis; *impotence;* cough with saltish expectoration; inveterate ulcers on the legs, with nocturnal tearing.

Magnesia carbonica. (Carbonate of Magnesia.)

Obscuration of the cornea; toothache of pregnant females; contracting or oppressive pains in the stomach, with sour eructations.

Magnesia muriatica. (Muriate of Magnesia.)

Schirrous indurations of the uterus; spasms of the broad ligaments.

Manganum. (Manganese.)

Nocturnal bone pains; chronic hoarseness and roughness of the throat; cough, with expectoration of green or yellowish mucus in little lumps; laryngeal phthisis.

Menyanthes trifoliata. (Buck-bean.)

Intermittent fever with feeling of coldness in the abdomen; otorrhœa after measles or scarlatina.

Mephitis putorius. (Skunk.)

Spasmodic cough, whooping cough.

Mercurius vivus and solubilis. (Quicksilver.)

Chancrous ulcers, especially when accompanied by drawing in the limbs; rickets, scrofulous and dropsical complaints; *swelling* and *caries* of bones, or inflammatory bone-pains, especially at night, also curvature and excessive brittleness of the bones; rheumatic or arthritic pains in the joints and limbs, becoming intolerable in the warmth of the bed, *especially at night, with perspiration which does not afford any relief;* scabies, or miliary itch, readily-bleeding small-pox (in alternation with variolin;) sequelæ of small-pox; tetter, especially *syphilitic;* spreading ulcers, spongy, blueish, *readily-bleeding;* inflammatory swelling of glands, parotitis; suppurations of various kinds; inflammatory fevers, with greatly hurried pulse and excessive sweat having a sour or foul smell; swelling of the head, eruption on the head; falling off of the hair; inflammation of the eyes and lids; tearing and stitching pains in the ears; purulent or bloody discharge from the ears; hardness of hearing, with roaring in the ears; inflammation and swelling of the nose, especially of the point; nose-bleed, the blood coagulates very speedily; tearing, stitching, jerking toothache, especially at night, in the roots of the teeth, shooting to the inner ear, aggravated by cold or warm drinks, or by inspiring cold air; also, with ptyalism and swelling of the cheeks; fetor from the mouth; aphthæ, ulcers in the mouth; *inflammation of the tongue,* swelling of the tongue, with thick coating of the same; excessive loathing of meat; desire for cold drinks, especially water; sore throat, with swelling of the tonsils and ptyalism; violent vomiting of bitter mucus; hepatitis, swelling and hardness of the liver; inflammation of the bowels and peritoneum; green diarrhœa, mucous, bloody, purulent, with cutting colic and tenesmus, continuing even after a discharge; sour or excoriating stool; protrusion of the rectum, it looks black and blood is spirted out; urine with white flocks, as if filled with pus and mucus; *hæmorrhage from the urethra; greenish gonorrhœa,* especally at night, with painful erections; balannorrhœa; hard swelling of the testes; prolapsus of the vagina; purulent, corrosive leucorrhœa; hard swelling or suppuration of the mamma; *catarrhal conditions* of various kinds, especially when attended with chilliness and aversion to the open air; *influenza;* dry, racking cough, as if the head and chest should fly to pieces; hæmoptysis when lying down; painful stiffness of the neck; exfoliation of the finger-nails; children refuse the breast; remedies against the excessive action of Mercury, are: Bell., Carb. veg., Hep. sulph., Nitri ac., Sulph., Lach., Lyc.

Mezereum.

Abuse of Mercury, chronic effects thereof, especially *caries* of bones; swelling of the parotid glands; humid scaldhead; excessive vomiting of green and bitter mucus, or bloody, chocolate-colored vomiting every day; burning pains in the stomach; *hæmaturia;* discharge of a few drops of blood after urinating; discharge of mucus from the urethra; balannorrhœa; albuminous leucorrhœa.

Millefolium. (Yarrow.)

This remedy is chiefly recommended for hæmorrhage from the various orifices of the body.

Moschus. (Musk.)

Hysteria and *hypochondria;* convulsions of males or females; tonic spasms; excessive vascular erethism; headache, as from a heavy weight on the head, with a sensation as if cold compresses were applied to the head; tearing in the right half of the head as if the head should be cut through; report in the ears, followed by discharge of a few drops of blood; vomiting every forenoon; pressure in the stomach, increased by drinking; throbbing in the region of the stomach; constipation relieved by coffee; violent sexual desire, with titillation in the sexual organs; spasmodic jerking of the hands and feet, followed by severe pains in these parts. Some of the pains abate in the open air.

Muriatic acid.

Foul ulcers on the legs; typhus, the patient settles down in the bed, fetid breath, aphthæ in the mouth, compressible and intermittent pulse.

Natrum carbonicum. (Carbonate of soda.)

Glandular swellings on the neck and in the groin; swelling of the feet, or coldness of the same.

Natrum muriaticum. (Salt.)

Intermittent fever, especially after abuse of Cinchona, quotidian or tertian, with bone-pains, great prostration, bitter taste in the mouth, backache, sallow complexion, ulceration of the corners of the mouth, loss of appetite, pressure in the pit of the stomach, with painful sensitiveness when touched, the paroxysms generally set in in the forenoon with thirst, even during the chill; falling off of the hair; lachrymation, especially in the open air, twitching of the lids, dimness of sight, blurred appearance of the letters, muscæ volantes, fiery points or streaks; hardness of hearing, with buzzing in the ears, ringing, otorrhœa. Swelling of the lips and cervical glands, scurvy, gumboil; sensation as of a hair on the tongue; vomiting of the ingesta, especially in the case of pregnant females; spasmodic cardialgia, afternoon to evening; chronic constipation or diarrhœa; prolapsus of the rectum, with burning in the anus and discharge of bloody ichor; tetter at the anus; painful hæmorhoidal tumors; gleet; scanty and retarded menstruation; acrid leucorrhœa, with sallow complexion; cough, caused by tickling in the throat or pit of the stomach; cough with vomiting of the ingesta; stitch in the chest when drawing a long breath or coughing; palpitation of the heart after the least exercise; irregular, intermittent beats of the heart; trembling of the hands when writing; dry and brittle skin on the hands; burning or coldness of the feet; the sweat of the feet which had been suppressed reappears.

*Nitric acid.

Chancre, gonorrhœa, figwarts, especially when complicated with mercurial symptoms; mercurial ulceration of the mouth; loose teeth and bleeding gums; inflammation and swelling of the testicles, the pain extending upwards along the spermatic cords; swelling and suppuration of the inguinal glands; affection of the kidneys, urinary complaints; flowing piles; chilblains; hardness of hearing (followed by Petrol.;) ulcerative phthisis (after Kali carb.); the pains are relieved by riding in a carriage.

Nitrum. (Nitre.)

Itching blotches on the body, *except on the hands and*

feet; headache after eating veal; nocturnal throbbing toothache, made worse by cold things; stitches in the chest when drawing a long breath; pneumonia; cough with purulent expectoration, after neglected pneumonia, or with expectoration of bloody mucus. The pains mostly appear in the afternoon and evening; those which make their appearance in the day-time, disappear in the evening.

Nux muschata. (Nutmeg.)

Consequences of exposure to dampness and cold; affections accompanied by drowsiness or disposition to fainting; intermittent fever with drowsiness, white-coated tongue, rattling breathing, bloody expectoration and but little thirst, even during the hot stage; *diarrhœa after the use of boiled milk.*

*Nux vomica. (Vomic nut.)

Cardialgia, pressure at the stomach with *sour eructations* and sour vomiting, flow of water in the mouth, *bloated bowels, backache;* sensation as if a band round the abdomen, as if it would fall off; bilious vomiting (with Puls.;) vomiting of dark, coagulated blood; ailments caused by the excessive use of coffee, wine, brandy, mental labor, talking, watching at night; dullness of the head as after intoxication; heaviness in the occiput; *delirium tremens* (with Opium;) nausea, foul taste in the mouth, especially in the morning; the pains are worse in the morning, after eating and during rest; hernia, prolapsus of the vagina and uterus, weakness of the uterine ligaments, pains in the bowels after confinement; pressing towards the womb; obstinate constipation and loss of appetite; hæmorrhoidal complaints, painful tumors, inflammation and induration of the liver; premature and excessive menstruation; yellowish leucorrhœa; desire to urinate; gravel, renal calculi; weakness of the small of the back, lameness of the lower extremities, bruising pain, formication, jerking of the lower extremities, dorsal consumption; excited sexual desire; tetanus after injuries, especially of the spinal marrow; impotence; consequences of onanism (with China.)

Cough, with soreness in the epigastrium, pain in the head as if it would split, aggravated by reading, thinking, etc.; restless sleep; intermittent fever, with pains in the stomach, blueness of the skin, excessive chilliness, backache, headache, nausea, constipation, desire for beer.

Headache in front and in the back part of the head; rush of blood to the chest; dryness and roughness of the throat, with sensation as of a plug in the throat.

Irritable mood, consequences of continued chagrin; disposed to find fault, to entertain thoughts of suicide; *hypochondria;* restless dreams; chiblains. If taken immediately after a cold, Nux may sometimes arrest the symptoms which otherwise require Aconite or Belladonna. This agent is especially suitable to individuals of a vehement temper.

Oleander.

Painless paralysis, especially of the lower extremities; deficient vital heat; sadness and diffidence in one's self; squamous or humid scaldhead; obscuration of sight when looking sideways; throbbing in the pit of the stomach.

*Opium.

Sopor, also in typhus. Stupefying sleep, unrefreshing, with the eyes half open, stertorous breathing. Dreamy, stupid sleeplessness (in opposition to sleeplessness from excessive wakefulness, which yields to Coffea); consequences of fright, trembling, jerking, convulsions beginning with rigidity of the whole body, loud cries; epilepsy; tetanus; painter's paralysis; expectoration of frothy blood when coughing. Dangerous pulmonary hæmorrhage; constipation from torpor of the bowels. Vomiting of fæces in ileus (with Plumbum). *Delirium tremens*. This agent is frequently suitable to drunkards and old people, and to persons upon whom other medicines are slow to act (compare with Carbo. veg.); colic of infants, with constipation; lead-colic.

Petroleum. (Rock-oil.)

Scrofulous ailments. Glandular swellings and indurations. Scaldhead, soft tumors on the head, painful when touched. Fistula lachrymalis (in alternation with Silic.); hardness of hearing, caused by paralysis of the auditory nerve (especially after using Nitri. ac.); itching and dampness of the scrotum, tetter between the scrotum and thigh (with Graph.); chapped hands; obstinate ulcers on the toes.

*Phosphoric acid.

Glandular ulcers (especially when burning); pain in the periosteum as if scraped with a knife; affections of

8

bones; ulcers. Diarrhœa, not weakening; mucus diarrhœa; diabetes; milky urine; *typhus* with taciturn mood, optical illusions, confused fancies, even when awake; consequences of silent grief (compare Ignatia), also of loss of animal fluids, onanism (after China); debility, emaciation. Impotence.

*Phosphorus.

Last stage of croup (in alternation with Bromine); nervous debility, emaciation (with impotence); mucous phthisis. Pneumonia, with stitches in the sides of the chest, rusty sputa, stage of hepatization (after Acon. and Bry.) Loss of blood during pregnancy. Smarting leucorrhœa. Chronic hoarseness, aphonia. Constant disposition to diarrhœa during cholera; glandular abscess and fistula, especially in the mammæ; dry, scaly tetter; affections of bones, with nocturnal pains; caries of the lower jaw; glandular swellings; zoomagnetic conditions; amaurosis, cataract, glaucoma; violet-odor of the urine (with turpentine); irresistible desire for sexual intercourse (in the male; aversion to it (in the female).

Platina.

Painfulness of the pudendum. Nymphomania, unnatural sexual excitement. Profuse and premature menstruation (with Nux and Calc.); induration and prolapsus of the womb. Hysteria.

Plumbum. (Lead.)

Paralysis of the extremities. Constipation. Hard, lumpy stools. Violent pains in the umbilical region.

Spasmodic retraction of the abdomen. Colic, relieved by pressure and bending double. Vomiting of fæces, in ileus (with Opium). Sweaty feet, smelling like decayed cheese.

Pulsatilla. (Wind-flower.)

Scanty and delayed menstruation. Amenorrhœa, especially when caused by a cold. Chlorosis. Irregular menstruation. Pains and cramps in the bowels, before or during the menses. Leucorrhœa; feeble labor-pains (also in alternation with Secale); after-pains; hastens the detachment of the placenta. Stoppage of the lochial discharge. Consequences of weaning, such as distention of the mammæ; stinging in the breast of young girls, with discharge of thin, acrid milk; fainting fits with deathlike pallor; epileptic spasms (especially when caused by menstrual suppression, or returning at every appearance of the catamenia.

Consequences of measles, such as hardness of hearing, otorrhœa, weak eyes, etc. A preventive against measles. (The principal remedy during the measles is Acon.) *Fistula lachrymalis*, or fistula generally. (Sulph., Hep. or Sil. may have to be given for the psoric taint or the affections of the bones); *ophthalmia*, also when of a scrofulous character, with pressure, stinging, lachrymation especially in the open air; dryness of the eyes. Stye on the eyelid; cataract; dimness of sight, diplopia, fiery circles; otalgia, jerking, stinging, tearing, humming, ringing in the ears; deafness caused by obstruction of the ears. Otorrhœa, especially after measles; nosebleed. Headache above the root of the nose. Catarrh with loss of taste and smell. *Dry coryza*, with ulcerated nostrils, discharge of foul, yellowish or green mucus.

Cough, with dryness of the throat, or cough with expectoration of yellow, bitter, salt or sweetish, blood-streaked mucus. Cough with desire to vomit. Cough with pain in the chest and stitches in the side; excessive accumulation of mucus.

Vomiting of mucus and bile. Pressure in the pit of the stomach; papescent, slimy, bilious, blood-streaked diarrhœa. Burning in the rectum. Fluent piles. Urging to urinate, with involuntary dribbling of the urine, discharge of mucus from the urethra; diabetes; wetting the bed, especially in the case of little girls; derangement of the stomach or other gastric derangements caused by eating fat, pastry (with Ipec. and Carb. veg.); cardialgia made worse by rapid walking. Flatulent colic and painfulness of the integuments when touched. Inflammation of the bowels (in alternation with Arsenic.); angina pectoris; suffocative paroxysms; constriction across the chest, with pain in the chest, especially when caused by the vapors of Sulphur; bitter taste; varices (in alternation with Arnica, which may likewise be applied externally). Erysipelas, shifting from one part to the other. Wandering gout (with Kali bichrom.); tearing in the limbs, relieved by uncovering the affected part). Chilblains. A characteristic symptom is the absence of thirst in all Pulsatilla-pains. This agent is especially suitable to females with gentle and timid dispositions, pale complexion, blue eyes, blond hair; in the evening the pains are worse, also during rest and in warmth, especially in the warm room; they abate in the open air, or when the patient is lying on the back or during moderate exercise.

Ranunculus bulbosus. (Crow-foot.)

Vesicular eruptions, as if scalded; flat, spreading ulcers with sharp edges and stinging-burning itching; ophthalmic affections, with immobility of the pupils; the pains are excited by contact or a change of position.

Ranunculus sceleratus. (Malignant crowfoot.)

Periodically-recurring pains, especially arthritic and rheumatic, *without sweat;* obstinate ulcers.

Rhododendron chrysanthum. (Siberian rose.)

Arthritic and rheumatic pains in the limbs, excited by rough weather, worse during rest and at night in bed, sometimes with swelling and redness of the affected parts (with Rhus tox.); hydrocele. Swelling of the knee.

***Rhus toxicodendron.** (Poison Sumach.)

Tearing and drawing, or stitching pains in the limbs *during rest, and at night,* worse when entering a room from the open air; rigidity of the limbs; numbness and tingling in the extremities; paralysis; ailments from getting wet; pain in the joints *as if sprained;* consequences of a strain or sprain (after Arnica;) sensation as if the flesh were detached from the bones; *vesicular erysipelas;* vesicular eruptions.

Nocturnal diarrhœa preceded by colic; dysenteric diarrhœa; diarrhœa alternating with constipation; panaritia with swelling of the whole arm; (compare Hep. and Sil.;) inguinal hernia; hydrocele (in alternation with Arnica;) removes the disposition to cramps in the calves.

Ruta graveolens. (Rue.)

Contusions and injuries of bones and of the periosteum; pains in the limbs, worse during rest, especially when sitting, relieved by motion; weakness of sight induced by much reading or sewing, (with Bell.;) prolapsus of the rectum; spraining the ankle-joint (apply also externally.)

Sabadilla. (Mexican barley.)

Intermittent fever, always recurring at the same hour; vomiting of lumbrici; tænia; pedicular disease (with Ars. and Merc.).

Sabina. (Savin.)

Prevents miscarriage, especially in the third month of pregnancy; metrorrhagia, the blood being bright-red.

Sambucus nigra. (Elder.)

For profuse sweat, especially after midnight; intermittent fevers with exhausting sweats; asthma millari.

Sanguinaria canadensis. (Blood-root.)

Violent headache, mostly on the right side, with nausea and vomiting of food or of bitter substances, recurring periodically, excited by a variety of causes, generally commencing in the morning, increasing during the day, relieved by sleep, aggravated by noise, walking, etc.; inveterate ichorous ulcers; spongy excrescences.

Secale cornutum. (Ergot, spurred rye.)

Deficient labor-pains (in alternation with Puls.;) detachment of the placenta; fetid metrorrhagia; protracted bloody lochial discharge; miscarriage; exhausting diarrhœic stools in rapid succession; colorless diarrhœa (during the cholera;) paralysis of the lower extremities, depending upon weakness of the spinal marrow; ergotism; sphacelus of the toes, in the case of old people.

Senega. (Rattlesnake-root.)

Spots on the cornea, or dimness and sponginess of the cornea; dry cough, or cough with difficult expectoration, wheezing breathing, racking pain through the whole chest.

***Sepia.** (Cuttle-fish.)

Is especially suitable to females (like Puls.;) scanty menstruation. Ailments incidental to the critical age; smarting leucorrhœa, also after the critical cessation of the menses; hysteria, flashes of heat, etc; ailments incidental to pregnancy, nausea and vomiting; humid herpes, with itching and burning; hemicrania with vomiting; boring pains somewhat relieved by rest and external pressure; cough with saltish expectoration (with Lycop).

Silicea.

Caries of bones; swelling and curvature of bones,

(rickets;) suppurating sores of various kinds, panaritia (in alternation with Hep.;) proud flesh; spongy excrescence in ulcers; gangrenous sores; ganglia; suppuration of the mammæ in the case of nursing females (in alternation with Hep. and Merc.;) inflammation of the nipples; carcinoma of the mamma; phthisis pulmonalis, especially of sculptors and stone-cutters, (with Calc.;) hectic cough with purulent expectoration; pulmonary fistula; fistula of various kinds, especially when bones are involved; glandular swellings, hard, painful, suppurating; tetter and eruptions with abscesses; yellow, brittle, distorted finger-nails (after Sulph.)

Ulceration of the big toes; suppression of sweat on the feet; swelling of the knee; deafness; otorrhœa; cataract; inflammation and swelling of the eyes; vomiting after drinking; intermittent fever, with predominance of the hot stage, (after Acon.)

Spigelia anthelmia. (Pink-root.)

Periodically-recurring headaches and face-ache of the left side, aggravated by motion and noise; carditis, enlargement of the heart; hydrothorax caused by organic disease of the heart; worms.

*Spongia marina tosta. (Burnt-sponge.)

Croup (in alternation with Hep.); goitre, with pressure and tingling in the swelling (with Iodine, also when a sensation of constriction is felt); hoarseness after singing; laryngeal phthisis.

Squilla maritima. (Squills.)

Fever with internal chilliness and external heat;

cough, with stitches in the side at every turn of cough, also with bloody expectoration; pleurisy and pneumonia.

Stannum. (Tin.)

Spasms during dentition; epilepsy in the evening; mucous phthisis.

Staphysagria. (Stave's acre.)

Chronic mercurial ailments; lupus; glandular swellings; cuts which refuse to heal; toothache in decayed stumps, with swelling of the cheeks; excrescences on the gums; small boils in the lids or along the edges.

***Stramonium.** (Thorn-apple.)

Dementia, (especially of drunkards;) illusions of the fancy; delirium; lascivious mania; proud mania; alternate ludicrous gesticulations and sad expression of the countenance; rage, with great violence; kicking and howling, crowing voice; catalepsy.

***Sulphur.**

Chief remedy for psora; herpes and eruption of various kinds; *itch;* rough and chapped skin; *warts;* sarcoma; acne; hepatic spots; ulcers; pancritia; spongy excrescences in sores; boils, (especially on the nates, with nitric acid;) intolerable itching; continually recurring erysipelas; anasarca; bone-pains, as if the flesh were detached; inflammation and swelling of bones; caries; rickets; arthritic tearing in the limbs, worse at night; paralysis; glandular affections; goïtre; affections of the eyes, ears, head, chest; vascular erethism, sweat, sour night-sweats; sweaty feet; intermittent fever of psoric patients; dry catarrh, or with discharge of burning water; hernia, prolapsus uteri (with Nux.;) prolapsus of the rectum; swelling of the scrotum; hydrocele; swelling and painfulness of the labia pudendi and of the vagina when sitting; labor-like pains above the os pubis; frequent urination; wetting the bed; irregular menstruation; acrid leucorrhœa; *piles* (with Nux, Carbo veg., Puls., Sep., Nitri ac.;) hæmorrhoidal colic; rumbling in the bowels; incarceration of flatulence with pressure in the sides of the abdomen; itching, stinging or burning in the anus; hard, lumpy stool; dysenteric stools with violent tenesmus; chronic *diarrhœa;* ascarides; inflammation and induration of the liver; pneumonia, stage of hepatization.

Cardialgia, burning in the stomach, digging in the pit of the stomach; loud or sour eructation; nausea, vomiting, heartburn; sweetish-foul or sour taste in the mouth; ravenous appetite; thirst all the time; vertigo, especially when sitting; epileptic convulsion, with creeping sensation proceeding from the anus or back.

This agent is especially indicated, if the patient had been at some former period troubled with the itch, or with ulcers, eruptions or suppurating sores. The pains are worse at night, in changes of weather, especially in damp and cold weather. The pains are relieved by warmth.

Sulphuric acid.

Consequences of bruises, contusions, etc., with echymosis of the injured part; aphthæ of infants; weakness and trembling after smelling coffee; incarcerated hernia; profuse menstruation; metrorrhagia; hæmoptysis; painful chilblains on the fingers.

Symphytum officinale. (Common comfrey.)

We apply the tincture diluted with water externally, (giving the potencies internally;) this agent is very efficacious in fracture of bones, contusions or injuries of bones and of the periosteum.

Tartar emetic. (Stibium.)

Pock-shaped eruption; intermittent fever with absence of thirst and sopor; vomiting of sour and bitter substances, also with diarrhœa and great debility.

Terebinthina. (Spirits of turpentine.)

Eruption resembling scarlatina; anasarca after scarlet fever, with discharge of dark urine, having the odor of violets; nephritis; hæmaturia.

Teucrium marum verum. (Wall germander.)

Nasal polypi; ascarides and ailments caused by their presence.

Thuya occidentalis. (Arbor vitæ.)

Figwarts, figwart-gonorrhœa; rough, shaggy and crusty warts, bleeding readily and having an offensive look; mercurial or mercurial-syphilitic ulcers; syphilis; slow recollection of ideas; indurations in the abdomen (with Lyc. and Lach.;) excrescences on the gums (with Staphys. and Lach.)

Urtica urens. (Nettle.)

Itching blotches; urticaria with headache and fever; anarsarca after suppression of cutaneous eruptions; swelling of the head; useful in burns, externally applied before blisters are raised.

Valeriana officinalis. (Valerian)

Pains which set in suddenly, with a racking fury, in a state of apparent health; morbid nervousness, with a feeling of lassitude pervading the whole body; intermittent fever with slight chill, followed by constant heat and dullness of the head, especially in the afternoon, and attacking children who have worms; hysteria; headache and faceache, breaking out suddenly, in paroxysms.

Variolin.

It is proposed to employ this agent as a remedy for small-pox and as a substitute for vaccination.

Veratrum album. (White hellebore.)

Cramps in the calves; whooping-cough, the children are weak, have some fever with cold sweat on the forehead, small, feeble and hurried pulse, great thirst; urine spirts out during the paroxsyms; pains in the chest, abdomen and groin; the children do not recover their natural brightness between the paroxysms, they are unable to hold their heads erect, they feel chilly, and are averse to talking. (All this is different when Drosera is indicated); aversion to warm feed; great desire for fruit and for sour things; unquenchable thirst; sudden prostration of strength. Debility and trembling. Debility after abuse of China (also removed by Ferrum). Coldness, numbness and formication of the extremities.

Tearing in the extremities, aggravated by damp and cold weather and by the warmth of the bed. Pains in the lower limbs, ascending to the abdomen, or else in the opposite direction; *tetanic spams*, the palms of the hands and the soles of the feet becoming bent inwards. *Cholera* (in alternation with Cuprum). Catalepsy, with flexibility of the limbs; epilepsy; intermittent fever, the coldness being only external, with internal heat, and violent desire for cold water.

Delirium. The memory is almost entirely gone. Confusion of mind, dementia, especially religious or amorous mania, with absurd acts; fancies himself a hunter, prince, minister, is proud of it; she boasts of being pregnant, etc. Paroxysms of pain causing delirium and mania for a short period. Bad consequences of fright.

Vinca minor. (Wintergreen.)

Tangling of the hair, with gnawing itching; plica polonica.

Viola tricolor. (Pansy.)

Crusta lactea with burning itching at night, and discharge of tenacious, yellow pus. The urine smells like cat's urine.

Zincum metallicum. (Zinc.)

Chronic eruptions of various kinds, especially tetter, and ulcerated tetter; ganglia; discharge of blood from the urethra, after urinating; pain in the chest when riding in a carriage. Chorea.

REMEDIES ACTING MORE ESPECIALLY ON THE RIGHT OR LEFT SIDE.

Left.	*Right.*
Aconite,	Agaricus,
Apis,	Alumina,
Arnica,	Belladonna,
Asarum,	Cantharis,
Calcarea carb.	Causticum,
China,	Crotalus,
Colchicum,	Drosera,
Colocynthis,	Hepar sulph.,
Crocus,	Ignatia,
Iodine,	Moschus,
Lachesis,	Plumbum
Mercurius,	Rhus tox.,
Nitric acid,	Ruta,
Nux vom.,	Sabadilla,
Rhododendron,	Sabina,
Spigelia,	Sanguinaria,
Sulphur,	Staphysagria.
Sulphuric acid.	

SPECIAL DIRECTIONS

FOR THE

TREATMENT OF ALL LEADING DISEASES.

Cholera. (Asiatic cholera.)

INTRODUCTORY REMARKS.

THE homœopathic treatment of cholera having produced such brilliant results, it seems very strange indeed, that it should not have been universally adopted. This is not owing to ill will, or to the jealousy of Old-School physicians, we cannot believe such meanness on the part of our professional opponents possible, when the object of our endeavors is to save human life,—no, it is simply owing to the old want of faith and to the old pride. Physicians cannot comprehend, and therefore refuse to believe, that such small agencies should produce such great effects. They imagine that their own wisdom is superior to nature's laws, and the result of their profound cogitations is the lamentable fact, as corroborated by the published mortality-bills of our city-authorities that fifty and even more of every hundred patients attacked with cholera, die.

Under homœopathic treatment one thousand four hundred and sixty-four patients out of one thousand five hundred and fifty-seven recovered in nineteen different cities, ninety-three only died, or six per cent. (See Dr. Buchner's "Results of allœopathic and homœopathic treatment according to official statements.") Where the spirits of Camphor and the higher potencies of homœopathic preparations were employed, only one in a hundred died as a general rule.

The official lists of cholera-patients in the district of Tischnowitz from November 7th, 1831, to February 5th, 1832, show that, under allœopathic treatment three hundred and thirty-one patients two hundred and twenty-nine were cured and one hundred and two died; under homœopathic treatment of two hundred and seventy-eight patients, two hundred and fifty-one were cured, twenty-seven died.

Dr. Baër of Prague lost under allœopathic treatment of one hundred and nineteen patients forty-seven—and cured seventy-two; under homœopathic treatment of eighty patients, he did not lose any.

Of seventy-one patients who were treated with Camphor without any other medicine, sixty were cured, eleven died.

Count Nadasdy of Daka in Hungary, in the absence of professional aid, treated his subjects with the spirits of Camphor. Of one hundred and sixty-one who were attacked, he only lost fifteen.

Dr. Schulz who had been my assistant in Cœthen, treated sixty-eight patients during the epidemic cholera of 1848, in Potsdam, and only lost nine, among whom were several scrofulous children and old men who had been diseased for some time; whereas the allœopathic physicians lost seventy in one hundred, and many died of other diseases following in the wake of cholera, especially typhus which was probably induced by the quantities of heroic and badly chosen medicines.

Why should physicians hesitate to try the truly curative method established by Hahnemann!

If physicians should continue to decline such experiments, laymen will institute them, and by their brilliant successes will cover the professional quacks with shame. I will show them in simple language how such brilliant results can be accomplished by Hahnemann's teachings. Any one who follows this advice, may cure his friends without first waiting for a physician, and will save their lives even if his hopes should have been very feeble.

PREVENTIVES AGAINST CHOLERA.

The best preventives against cholera are *Cuprum* and *Veratrum*, not Camphor. If they should cause rumbling in the bowels and even diarrhœa, these symptoms soon pass off again. It is, therefore, not advisable that persons in perfect health should take these medicines. They may be used during epidemic cholera as soon as the first unpleasant sensation is experienced in the bowels, such as rumbling, pinching or diarrhœa. In such a case six globules of *Cuprum* may be dissolved in six tablespoonfuls of water, of which a small swallow should be taken every few hours until the uneasiness ceases. If diarrhœa is present, the medicine may be taken after every attack. On a journey a globule may be taken dry on the tongue, instead of the watery solution.

During this period all acids should be carefully

avoided; otherwise it is well to continue one's regular mode of life, to eat and drink moderately, to avoid violent emotions, to overcome disturbing passions, to observe cleanliness and especially frequent washings with cold water, which strengthen and fortify the body.

An attack may be provoked by any violent and sudden change of diet, by the use of spirits of patent cholera-cordials, teas, etc. Travelers should endeavor to be perfectly regular in their meals and to use nourishing and simple food in moderate quantities.

Every body should keep the spirits of Camphor on hand (one part of Camphor to be dissolved in twelve parts of alcohol); this will afford the best help at the commencement of an attack, especially if tetanic spasms should be present, as will be more fully shown hereafter; the vial should be kept carefully closed lest the smell should injure the other homœopathic preparations.

During cholera, children are sometimes attacked quite suddenly with vomiting and diarrhœa, but without spasms; such an attack is speedily arrested by *Ipecacuanha*, five globules in six tablespoonfuls of water, of which a dessertspoonful may be given every fifteen minutes; the attack will cease in a few hours. The medicine should be given less frequently as soon as an improvement sets in, and should finally be discontinued. If Ipec. should be without effect, *Asarum* may be given; this cures vomiting of water with anxiety and diarrhœa without cramps. But if these symptoms should be complicated with cramps in the calves or bowels, *Cuprum* should be given as stated above; this will prevent the full development of cholera.

If cholera should actually break out, *Cuprum* and *Veratrum* may be given in alternation every fifteen minutes, and the danger may be averted.

If persons should be subject to continual attacks of diarrhœa or to a disposition to such attacks, without being much weakened thereby, the trouble may be arrested by *Phosphoric acid.*

The attack is sometimes ushered in by vertigo which may be removed by the following remedies; vertigo during a walk, especially when turning about: *Ipecac.;* vertigo obliging one to lie down, with heaviness in the head: *Secale;* vertigo when looking up, aggravated by motion, relieved by lying down: *Cuprum;* vertigo, everything seeming to turn around: *Veratrum;* vertigo, with disposition to fall, only when walking or when closing the eyes: *Arsenic.*

DIRECTIONS FOR THE MANAGEMENT OF CHOLERA.

The attacks of cholera are not always alike, but generally commence with tetanic spasm, without vomiting or diarrhœa; this may be termed the first stage. This stage has been less frequently noticed since 1849, when the attacks set in with the second stage and the use of Camphor became therefore unnecessary. The patient suddenly loses his strength he is unable to stand, his features become altered, the eyes look sunken, the face and hands look bluish, they are cold as ice, the rest of the body is likewise cold; his countenance has an expression of despondency and anguish as if he should suffocate; half stupefied and insensible, the patient moans and utters cries with a hoarse and hollow tone of voice, without making any distinct complaints unless asked; burning in the stomach and œsophagus, and cramp-pain in the calves and other muscles; he shrieks when the pit of the stomach is touched; he has no thirst, no nausea, vomiting or diarrhœa.

At this stage *Camphor* may still prove available provided it is employed at once by those present. The patient is placed into a warm bed, and takes a drop of the spirits of Camphor every five minutes, on a lump of sugar or in a small spoonful of water. The arms and legs of the patient are at the same time rubbed with the spirits of Camphor from above downwards, likewise the pit of the stomach and the abdomen. An injection of Camphor may likewise be administered, mixing two dessertspoonfuls of the spirits of Camphor in two tablespoonfuls of tepid water. The spirits of Camphor may likewise be evaporated from time to time upon a heated brasier, especially if the mouth is spasmodically closed, in which case the inhaled vapors may take the place of medicine taken by the mouth.

The more attentively these precautions are attended to, the more quickly and certainly the patients will recover. His warmth, strength, consciousness, quiet and sleep return: he is saved.

If this first favorable period should have been overlooked or neglected, the

Second Stage

Sets in, where Camphor generally proves unavailing. This stage is characterised by frequent watery discharges mixed with whitish, yellowish or reddish flocks; violent vomiting of quantities of similarly-looking watery substances, unquenchable thirst, loud rumbling in the bowels. increasing anguish, moaning and yawning, icy-coldness of the whole body, even of the tongue, mottled blueness of the arms, decreased action of all the senses, slow pulse, excessively-painful cramps in the calves and arms, and in the bowels.

If these symptoms are present, Camphor is of no avail, and it is best to remove the smell of Camphor, in case it should have been used previously, as much as possible by letting in fresh air, and thus preventing the Camphor from interfering with the medicines which will have to be prescribed at this stage.

Cuprum and *Veratrum*, six pellets of each, are now to be dissolved in separate tumblers of water, each containing about eight tablespoonfuls, and a small spoonful is to be given alternately every five minutes, or, in bad cases, even more frequently. If the watery solution should be inconvenient, a pellet may be given dry on the tongue, at a dose. As soon as the patient begins to feel better, the dose should be repeated less frequently, and if sweat and sleep should set in, all medicine is to be discontinued.

In some cases, after the disappearance of the dangerous symptoms, the skin becomes hot and the pulse full and bounding; in such a case *Aconite* should be given, six pellets in eight tablespoonfuls of water, a small spoonful every ten minutes; very soon the skin will be drenched with perspiration, sleep and recovery take place.

In cases where the attack seemed more obstinate, and the passages remain perfectly colorless, recovery has been effected by means of *Secale* alone, or in alternation with *Cuprum* or *Veratrum*.

If burning pains in the epigastric region or in the region of the spleen (on the left side below the ribs,) or in the bowels or anus were present, the above-mentioned remedies were unavailing; *Arsenic* had to be given, six pellets in water, a small spoonful every five minutes; if the patient complained of cramps in the calves, in alternation with *Veratrum*.

Some physicians have proposed *Iatropha curcas* for the following symptoms: projectile vomiting of quantities of a watery or albuminous substance, with spasmodic constriction of the region of the stomach, or burning in the stomach; watery diarrhœa, cramps in the calves, coldness of the skin. Dissolve six pellets in water, giving a spoonful every five minutes.

Hydrocyanic acid has been found adapted to the following symptoms in the last stage: 1. If the patient spits continually without expectorating much, (without this agent death soon sets in.) 2. Heat in the head, with coldness of the limbs, vomiting of a black fluid, involuntary stools. 3. Dry cholera, without vomiting or diarrhœa, cramps at times in the arms and calves, at others in the masseter muscles, so that the mouth is firmly closed; accompanied with frequent involuntary shrieking and subsequent prostration or fainting. 4. Apparent cessation of all vital functions, collapse of pulse, in the paralytic stage; tetanus.

Of course no other means, such as coffee, tea, fumigations, bleeding, or other medicines should be resorted to.

During the attack the patient should be kept warm, and the pit of the stomach, bowels and extremities should be rubbed with warm flannel or woolen cloth.

In many cases the patient feels relieved after a few doses of the right remedy, vomiting and diarrhœa cease. The desires of the patient should then be gratified with moderation. The best drink during and after the attack is a de.oction of oatmeal or fresh water, which should only be given in spoonful doses.

Another characteristic sign of Asiatic cholera is the loss of all tonicity of the skin which, if pinched up, remains without returning to its former condition.

Cases occur where, after the second stage has run its course, and the patient is about to die, tetanic spasms set in and the patient seems quite dead. Here *Hydrocyanic acid* or the spirits of Camphor may be given; the latter should be rubbed upon the skin with the palm of the hand, from above downward, and upon the pit of the stomach.

Patients apparently dead have likewise been restored to consciousness by means of an injection of tepid water and Camphor in the rectum, or by bathing the inner mouth with a mixture of oil and Camphor.

Sometimes cholera is transformed into a sort of typhus with delirium, especially under the use of violent and improper medicines. In such a case *Bryonia* and *Rhus tox.* should be dissolved in separate tumblers, six pellets of each in eight tablespoonfuls of water, a small spoonful to be given every thirty minutes alternately, and less frequently if symptoms of improvement should become apparent.

If typhoid symptoms should set in under homœopathic treatment, with stupid insensibility, optical illusions, confusion of the senses, *Acidum phosphor.*, six pellets in water, a spoonful every fifteen or thirty minutes, may be given. For dry heat, full and bounding pulse, anxiety, give *Aconite* alone, or in alternation with the former remedies.

Nobody should abandon himself to slavish fear, for fear alone brings on sickness and destroys all mental energy, No man should suffer the divine spark in him to be quenched by fear; every body should rely in full confidence upon the ruling Providence who governs the destiny of each of us. The mind, until it is absolutely prostrated by the disease, should sustain the body with vigor and by a strong and living faith. Let the physician, animated by this hope and intense faith, step to the bedside of the patient, and he will be able to effect wonderful changes for the better.

Croup. (Angina membranacea.)

INTRODUCTORY REMARKS.

In an attack of croup, it is of the utmost importance to afford help before the dangerous stage has set in. The mother who has the best opportunity of watching her child, may avert the danger by pursuing the treatment indicated in the following pages.

If a homœopathic physician should be at hand, he may be sent for, but the mother should at once administer the appropriate remedy, for by so doing she may pave the way for the physician's management without ever interfering with it. If no physician should be near, she may undertake the treatment in perfect confidence, being assured that thousands of children have been saved by the means which we here propose. It may be a satisfaction to every mother to know that the treatment which I recommend, has enabled me to save the life of every patient I have had charge of, and that, if, in accordance with the inscrutable designs of Providence, a little patient should die, he will not have been sacrificed by violent and destructive agencies. Many of our most experienced physicians have sanctioned my treatment, and I urge every mother never to lose a moment's time in adopting the means of cure which I here propose.

TREATMENT.

True membranous croup is not near as frequent as some persons imagine; most cases of croup would remain without any danger, if the proper treatment were at once pursued.

An attack of croup which sets in after midnight, may terminate fatally in a few hours, unless the proper remedies are at once resorted to.

If children are attacked with a hollow, barking cough, mothers are very apt to imagine that an attack of croup is impending. This is very frequently the case, and *Aconite*, six pellets in water, a small spoonful every hour or two hours, should at once be given.

Less dangerous is a scraping cough with roughness of the air-passages, which attacks children in cold or wet weather, especially in winter, when children get their feet wet by running in the snow. Sometimes a watery, greenish, fetid diarrhœa sets in. These symptoms yield to *Chamomilla*, a few pellets in eight tablespoonfuls of water, a small swallow morning and night.

But if the child should feel feverish, hot, or first chilly and then hot, restless and anxious, with heat about the head and forehead, heat of the palms of the hands, etc., *Aconite* may be substituted for Chamomilla, to be given night and morning, or even every hour, if the fever should be very violent. If the cough has a hollow or wheezing sound, *Hepar sulph.* may be given alone, or, if fever-symptoms should be present, in alternation with Aconite. Dose, six pellets of each in eight spoonfuls of water, a small spoonful every two or four hours in alternation. The child should be kept uniformly covered so as to prevent exposure and stoppage of the perspiration.

At such times children should never be left alone, nor should they be permitted during the winter to sleep in a very cold room, lest they should kick off the bed-cover and be attacked with a croupy cough, in which case the remedies which I have recommended, should at once be given.

Persons who have once heard the croup-cough will never forget it; those who have not heard it may know it by the following signs: It is very much like the hoarse barking of a common cur, sometimes shrill, crowing, sometimes deep and hollow, but rough. It is an anxious sound, and the cough occurs in paroxysms. The inspirations are long and labored, the expirations are interrupted and jerking. The little patients frequently toss about the bed in great agony, stretch their necks and bend their heads backwards. This should not be prevented, especially during the last stage, when the patients might suffocate in consequence of their heads being raised too high. The pulse is feverish, the urine deep-red.

These symptoms require *Aconite,* six pellets in a cupful of water, a small spoonful every ten or fifteen minutes, until the patient feels easier, after which the medicine may be repeated after every new paroxysm of cough. Warm and gentle perspiration is a good symptom. If the child falls asleep, let it sleep until morning, when a spoonful of a solution of six pellets of *Hepar sulph.* in a cupful of water may be given, to be repeated at night.

If Aconite produces no favorable change, the

Second Stage

Sets in, when the child complains of burning in the throat or grasps at the larynx which is sensitive, and sometimes swollen and hot. Suffocative paroxysms frequently set in, accompanied by fever and thirst. Sometimes the children fall asleep, but wake suddenly with aggravated symptoms. During the sleep the breathing is anxious and panting, and the head is bent backward. Do not wrap any woolen cloth around the neck, for this might cause renewed irritation, and aggravate the symptoms. The head should be kept free, the feet may be kept warm.

If Aconite produces no favorable change in one or two hours, *Hep. sulph.* and *Spongia* should then be given in alternation, six pellets of each in a separate cupful of water, an alternate dose every ten or fifteen minutes, and less frequently or only after a paroxysm, in case the general condition of the patient seems more satisfactory.

In the case of scrofulous children, with hard glandular swellings on their necks, *Iodine* should be given in alternation with *Aconite,* six pellets of each in separate cupfuls of water, a spoonful every ten or fifteen minutes.

In order to prevent the contact of cold, the spoonful of water may be poured into a larger spoon containing *tepid milk,* after which this medicated milk may be swallowed by the patient.

If children desire it, they may drink warm milk sweetened with sugar, or rice and oat-meal gruel as much as they please.

If the symptoms should get worse in spite of the

foregoing remedies, *Bromine*, six pellets in water, a spoonful every ten or fifteen minutes, should at once be administered. This is our chief remedy in the

Third Stage.

The pulse is small and accelerated. The breathing is exceedingly anxious, frequently wheezing or rattling; at every inspiration the abdominal walls are violently raised and depressed. During a paroxysm of cough, which is almost without any resonnance, the gagging frequently terminates in vomiting. The children look pale, the face is bloated and has a blueish look, the eyes protrude and are expressive of anxiety, the little patients seek to grasp at every thing near them.

If the patient had been treated homœopathically from the start, *Bromine* may then still save the child's life.

If the child should be very weak, or if violent allœopathic treatment should have prostrated the patient, *Phosphorus* and *Bromine* may be given in alternation, six pellets of each in separate cupfuls of water, a spoonful every ten or fifteen minutes, until an improvement sets in, after which the medicines should be given less frequently, until they can be discontinued.

SUBSEQUENT TREATMENT AND DIET.

After the cure, and more particularly, if the child had been under allœopathic treatment, a feeling of weakness is very apt to remain behind. This will yield to *China,* six pellets in water, a spoonful morning and evening.

If hoarseness remains, *Hep. sulph.* or *Bromine* should be given in a similar manner.

As a matter of course, all kinds of food or drink which are opposed to homœopathic medicines, should be avoided during and even for a week after the treatment of croup, more especially coffee, tea, wine, acids, spices, roots, etc.

These things should always be kept away from children with strict uniformity; children will never grow up to healthy and happy men, until the use of all unnatural compounds and spices is strictly and absolutely forbidden.

Every intelligent mother knows or should know that it is exceedingly improper to feed children on coffee or chamomile-tea; these beverages predispose the nervous system to all sorts of ailments, such as spasms during dentition, colic, etc. An excellent antidote to convulsions produced by chamomile-tea is black coffee, of which a few drops may be administered every few minutes until the spasms cease.

The best nourishment for children who are brought up by hand, during the first six months is a beverage composed of half milk and water, sweetened with a little sugar. Very weak children should have even less than half the quantity of milk, for the emaciation of children is very often owing to over-feeding or the use of too rich food. Very robust children may have a gradually-increased quantity of milk, and, if this should not satiate them, they may eat a little stale bread soaked in hot water, and slightly sweetened with sugar, and at times some very weak meat-broth without any fat. More solid food should not be given until the incisors are through.

Washing with warm water, which is still adhered to by so many mothers, is very weakening to children and should be abandoned. Children should be washed every day with fresh and cool water; this is truly invigorating. A fortnight or three weeks after the birth of the child, the use of warm water should be discontinued little by little, so that cold water is exclusively used at the age of five or six weeks. In the morning the back should be washed first by pressing water out of the sponge and causing it to flow down the spine; this may be repeated a dozen times, and the sponge may be passed over the back at the same time. After this proceeding the back is carefully dried, and if a mother wishes to strengthen her feeble infant, she may breathe upon its back from the head all the way down the spine; this will prove a pleasant stimulation to the tender nerves. The rest of the body should be washed in the same way by passing the sponge over it from above downward, and afterwards drying it carefully; after washing the back, the face, arms, chest and abdomen, and lastly the lower extremities should be washed in the same way. This mode of washing takes a little more time than bathing, but it is much more invigorating; and should not a mother be willing to make every effort to secure the health and vigor of her children? This natural system of education not only serves as a preventive against diseases, but, if the children should be attacked by illness, it will be found to be more manageable, because the nervous power had been adequately prepared to resist the inroad of disease.

Mothers should likewise be watchful in preventing their children from touching the private parts, or from putting their hands under the cover at night; for this might easily lead them to the dreadful practice of onanism which destroys both body and soul, and frequently entails incurable maladies, spasms, paralysis, epilepsy, consumption, upon its unhappy victims.

Let every mother keep the remedies which I have recommended for cholera and croup, in her house. How quietly may a mother retire to rest, if she knows that help is near in case her little darling should be attacked by these dangerous diseases! How many children are sacrificed by the use of violent emetics and by venesections! How many chronic ailments are entailed upon children by the use of large doses of Calomel! If croup is apparently cured by such remedies, the disposition to this disease is not removed, as may be inferred from the frequent recurrence of attacks of croup under alloeopathic treatment.

A mother should undertake the treatment with perfect confidence, otherwise she might neglect something. The result is undoubtedly in God's hand; if he has decreed the end of human existence, all human art and science must prove futile, and every true Christian will cheerfully and trustingly submit to the inscrutable, but wise counsels of Providence. It will be a consolation to a mother's heart to know that, if it should have been impossible to avert a fatal result, such remedial agents had been employed in her child's case as would have saved the patient's life, if this had been possible.

Toothache.

INTRODUCTORY REMARKS.

Those who are never afflicted with toothache, may deem it a very small matter, that much should be said on the subject; but persons liable to attacks of toothache will thank me for the trouble I have taken to show them the means of obtaining speedy relief from their sufferings.

In my clinic at least twenty patients are treated every day for toothache, and scarcely one in a hundred is not immediately relieved by smelling of the specific remedy. This successful mode of treating toothache requires a careful knowledge of the Materia Medica, for an apparently trifling circumstance sometimes points to the right remedy.

If a decayed tooth, for instance, is affected, and the pain is a throbbing and digging pain, involving even the eye, I hold the little vial containing *Pulsatilla* under the nostril of the affected side, and cause the patient to snuff up the emanations from the open vial with considerable force. In almost every case the pain yields at at once. If the toothache should be inveterate, and a second attack should set in, two or three pellets may then be dissolved in eight tablespoonfuls of water, of which a dessertspoonful may be taken every two or four hours, and after a while every morning and evening for some days only, lest the curative reaction should be interfered with.

If the pain should affect the whole left side as far as the ear, the tooth feeling loose and elongated, and exposure to a draught of air having caused the trouble, *Chamomilla* will relieve it.

If the patient is unable to point out the affected tooth; if the pain seems to affect the whole row of teeth, if they feel sensitive and elongated, and the head is hot, *Belladonna* will afford relief, either by smelling or in water.

The rule is, that if smelling should not be sufficient, a few pellets are to be dissolved in half a tumblerful of water, of which solution a small spoonful should be taken every two to four hours, and, after a few doses, every morning and evening for a few days only, avoiding all other remedies lest the proper reaction should be disturbed. If more than one remedy seems indicated, the two may be given in alternation. The tumbler should be covered, and placed in a dark spot; the spoon should be dried after being used. If the water becomes turbid, the solution should be renewed. All kinds of food or drink which interfere with the operation of homœopathic agents, should be avoided; meat, except fat pork, all ordinary vegetables, milk, simple farinaceous dishes, eggs, sweet fruit, etc., are permitted.

Coffee, tea, strong ale, spirits, acids and spices are forbidden. Perfumes should be avoided. I know by experience that the first spoonful of coffee may bring back the toothache after it had been appeased by treatment.

Persons afflicted with frequent attacks of headache or toothache, should never use coffee which is apt to excite these sufferings. Milk, cocoa, simple soups are far preferable.

Perfumed toothpowders or chemical tinctures for cleaning teeth should never be used; they remove the tartar, but they destroy at the same time the enamel.

The best substance to clean the teeth with, is sugar of milk or pulverised charcoal which removes all the impurities without affecting the teeth.

Morning and evening and after every meal the mouth should be carefully rinsed with fresh water; this will prevent the decay of animal matter between the teeth, and the formation of tartar.

The abuse of Kreasote and Opium during an attack of toothache should be guarded against; they may blunt the pain, but they at the same time attack and destroy the teeth.

It is very foolish to have a tooth pulled out for no better reason than because it aches or begins to decay. Proper homœopathic treatment may render this operation unnecessary.

I once treated a lady who had had all her teeth pulled out and was afterwards affected with the most intolerable pain in her jaws which yielded to treatment.

If the patient should not succeed in removing the pain, a good homœopathic physician should be consulted. In opening a vial, it should be closed again as soon as the patient has performed the operation of smelling. The first four of the following remedies are most frequently used:

Staphysagria.

a. If the pains proceed from decayed teeth or from stumps, even the head and ears are involved, the cheek is swollen but not hot, the pain is caused by inspiring cold air or by cold drinks; worse during or after eating, by touching the affected tooth, or only at night or after midnight.

b. Sudden blackness or decay, exfoliation of the teeth.

c. Tubercles or painful excrescences on the gums, liability of the gums to bleed (Compare sulphur.)

Belladonna.

a. If several teeth on one side are affected, so that it is impossible to point out the exact tooth; if the pain shifts about (rheumatic pain,) the teeth feel elongated, as if they would start out of their sockets.

b. The pain is aggravated by contact, or by cold or warm things.

c. There is determination of blood to the head.

d. Inflammatory or erysipelatous swelling of the cheek, when the medicine should be taken in water, as indicated in the introductory remark.

e. Simultaneous presence of neuralgic pain in one side of the face, especially the right side.

f. Glandular swellings, which disappear under the use of Belladonna.

g. Teething, the gums being swollen and red, the children are sometimes delirious. Spasms and convulsions may likewise be present.

Chamomilla.

a. The pain is caused by a draught of air, by sudden suppression of sweat; it affects the ear, causing earache.

b. The teeth feel loose and elongated.

c. The cheek and gums are swollen, the skin is not very red, (give the medicine in water.)

d. The pain is aggravated by warm drinks.

e. Teething, with watery, greenish, fetid diarrhœa, spasmodic symptoms.

Aconite.

a. Throbbing pain, with vascular erethism and nervousness, feverish symptoms.

b. If there are frequent attacks of vascular irritation, with heat and restlessness, the medicine should be taken in water as stated in the introductory remarks.

c. This should likewise be done when children are teething, and great heat and restlessness are present.

Arnica.

a. Arthritic-rheumanic toothache when caused by

sudden suppression of perspiration, a cold, wet, (see Rhus tox.)

b. The toothache is caused by a flow or contusion.

c. Toothache with pale and hard swelling of the cheek.

d. Pains subsequent to the extraction or filing off of teeth. In such cases great relief will be derived from rinsing the mouth with a solution of Arnica, the same as that recommended for internal use in the introductory remarks.

In using this and other remedies, the patient should carefully abstain from all exposure to draughts of air, wind, etc., which might check the perspiration.

Pulsatilla.

a. Throbbing or digging-pain, extending from the decayed tooth to the eye.

b. The toothache occurs while the menses are too feeble or suppressed; (in cases of menstrual suppression a few doses of *Puls.* may be taken in water.)

c. The pains are worse in the evening, in a warm room and at night in bed, especially before midnight; cold air relieves the pain.

Nux Vomica.

a. The pain is caused by the excessive use of coffee, wine or spirits.

b. Obstinate constipation.

s. Drawing and boring pain in a decayed tooth, as if wrenched out, with violent stitches now and then, which rack the whole body, especially when drawing in air, or if the pains commence or return in the morning.

d. It is an important remedy for all persons who lead a sedentary life and perform much mental labor.

China.

a. The toothache sets in in consequence of great weakness, after loss of blood, before or after parturition, or while nursing.

This remedy will often strengthen the nerves, if delicate females take it under the foregoing circumstances; it is also useful for the consequences of venesections and losses of animal fluids.

b. Tearing and drawing in the upper teeth, or stitching in the front-teeth, aggravated by the simple contact of the tongue.

Hepar sulphuris.

a. The pain is caused by an incipient gumboil.

b. Fully developed gumboils are removed by taking Hepar in water, a small spoonful morning and evening.

c. Fistula dentalis (with *Puls.*)

d. Looseness of the teeth, especially after abuse of Mercury.

Sulphur.

a. Chronic toothache, tearing, drawing, jerking, boring, stitching, with or without swelling of the cheeks. The teeth feel dull, loose, elongated. Aggravation at night.

b. The gums become detached and diseased (in alternation with Mercury, in water.)

c. Frequent bleeding of the gums.

d. Suppression of cutaneous eruptions by ointments or washes.

Mercurius.

a. Toothache with profuse ptyalism (not induced by Mercury).

b. Violent scraping pain in the cheek-bones; frequently the remains of some morbid matter which had been treated allœopathically (syphilis.)

c. Foul ulcers in the mouth, when the medicine may be given in water.

d. The pains are worse after midnight, frequently with profuse sweat which does not afford any relief.

Causticum.

a. Tearing, drawing and stitching in the teeth, especially when cold air is inhaled, with spasmodic closing of the jaws, like lockjaw.

b. The whole side of the face is affected, teeth, gums and cheeks, is especially adapted to the right side; less at night in bed.

These twelve remedies will be found sufficient to cure almost every case of toothache, provided the medicine has been well chosen. I will add three other remedies:

Bryonia, for stinging and throbbing toothache, yield ing for a while to the application of cold water; relief is obtained by lying on the affected side, aggravated in the warmth.

Sepia for the toothache of pregnant females (with China and Bell.), sudden decay and exfoliation of the teeth (with Staphysagria).

Kreasotum for drawing pains, especially in decayed teeth, extending to the temples and inner ear; also flashing downwards or towards the eyes (as in the case of *Puls.*), especially in the left side of the face; early on waking.

Phthisis. (Consumption.)

This general name is applied to a disease which may affect various organs. It is most frequently observed in the larynx and trachea, in the lungs, stomach, liver, bowels, mesenteric glands, kidneys, bladder and uterus. Whatever organ may be affected, there is always a waste of the tissues and a sinking of the bodily strength. Emaciation may likewise take place in other maladies; hence the necessity of ascertaining the true nature and seat of the malady. This is rather difficult for the lay-practitioner who is not acquainted with the structure of the human body. The following hints will enable him to see the danger to which the neglect of certain derangements may expose the sick.

1. Phthisis of the larynx and trachea. (Phthisis laryngea et trachealis.)

Consumption of the larynx and trachea generally occurs together, scarcely ever separately, and then only at the commencement of the disease, sometimes even after a simple, but neglected catarrh, especially in consequence of neglected influenza, or of badly-managed syphilis. The patient complains of a prickling, stinging or burning feeling at one spot in the larynx, as from the contact of a burning coal; sometimes the sensation is a feeling of pressure and constriction. If an ulcer has actually formed, deglutition becomes difficult, and the patient experiences a feeling as if an obstacle were in the way of the food. A continual irritation and inclination to cough sets in which is still increased by talking. The voice loses its resonance, becomes husky, and finally the patient loses his voice altogether and is only able to barely utter a sound. As the hoarseness increases, the cough increases likewise, the patient raises pus mixed with much mucus and saliva, which has a saltish or sweetish, bitter or foul taste. The inspirations become anxious and wheezing, with a peculiar rattling sound; the expirations are comparatively easier. Little by little the deglutition becomes still more painful, suffocative fits frequently set in, until finally the food taken into the stomach is ejected again with violent fits of cough. The patient is generally pale, and his looks are expressive of great agony. With the increasing emaciation hectic fever sets in, with a slight chill in the afternoon, violent heat towards evening, night-sweats and great thirst. The pulse is generally accelerated and the sleep restless. Towards the end the hair falls out, the feet swell, exhausting diarrhœa sets in.

If the disease is properly treated at the onset, a single dose of the appropriate remedy may frequently arrest it.

Phosphorus will be found adapted to the following symptoms: Great painfulness and sensitiveness of the larynx, hoarseness which is made worse by talking, complete aphonia; cough excited by titillation and scraping in the throat and chest, most frequently excited by drinking or laughing. Cough with expectoration of a quantity of mucus, of a white or greenish color, purulent in the more advanced stage of the disease, when it has a saltish or sweetish taste.

Hepar sulphuris calc. The larynx is very much affected, the voice is hoarse and faint, feverish chilliness down the back, flushed cheeks, sleeplessness, anguish, nervousness and emaciation. Cough caused by titillation in the throat, or by pain in the larynx, aggravated by talking or stooping, increasing towards evening and then ceasing all at once. There is a pricking sensation in the throat as from a bone.

In a case of syphilitic phthisis of the larynx, when the original syphilis had first been treated with Mercury, this medicine may be given first, and allowed to have its full effect, after which *Nitric acid* may be given.

Carbo vegetabilis. Hoarseness morning or evening, with inability to talk loud, the voice giving out when making the attempt; scraping and tingling in the throat; dry cough with pain in the upper part of the chest, or racking cough, with oppression and burning in the chest; cough with expectoration of purulent mucus having a whitish-yellow or greenish color. It may be given after the abusive treatment with Mercury.

Iodine. Pressure in the region of the larynx as from some swelling; the larynx is painful to external pressure. Hoarseness, especially in the morning after rising. Constant inclination to hawk up tenacious mucus, with creeping and tickling in the larynx. Cough caused by violent tickling in the throat and chest, with anxiety previous to the attack and great emaciation. Mucous rattling in the chest.

This remedy will probably be chosen first, if the disease springs from a scrofulous origin, especially if glandular swellings and indurations are present.

Causticum. Chronic hoarseness, also with complete loss of voice; cough caused by tickling in the throat or stooping, with soreness, rattling of mucus in the chest, and inability to raise the apparently loose mucus. This remedy may prove useful, if the disease owes it origin to neglected influenza.

Calcarea carbonica. Roughness of the throat or hoarseness, especially in the morning; accumulation of mucus in the chest or larynx, dry cough at night, or titillating cough as from fine feather-dust; cough with expectoration of yellow mucus, having a salt or sweetish taste, worse in the morning. Stitches in the head when coughing, soreness in the chest or sensation in the throat as if something were torn loose.

Arsenicum album. Rough and hoarse voice; feeling of dryness and of burning in the larynx; continual irritation and tickling in the larynx; short and dry cough as if caused by the vapors of Sulphur, with smarting in the chest as if excoriated, or soreness from the pit of the stomach upwards, with labored breathing, or with suffocative sensation and constriction in the larynx; all these symptoms are aggravated by drinking, especially by drinking without feeling thirsty.

The medicine adapted to each group of symptoms, should be given in water, six pellets in eight table-spoonfuls, of which a small spoonful may be given morning and night for four or five days, until the patient feels better; but if no improvement should take place after using the same remedy for several weeks, another medicine may be given. If fever should set in, with hot skin, thirst and a full and bounding pulse, *Aconite* should be given.

2. Pulmonary phthisis. (Phthisis pulmonalis.)

This disease which is frequently accompanied by laryngeal phthisis, involves a destruction of the pulmonary tissue. It has three stages which are not always clearly marked. In the first stage, the symptoms are frequently so obscure that it is not an easy matter to recognize the existence of pulmonary phthisis. In persons who are predisposed to this disease, breathing is not always easy, and becomes panting and hurried when such persons go up stairs or walk rapidly. They find talking and singing difficult, and a dry cough is frequently present which sometimes increases to violent attacks racking the head and chest and causing great prostration. After such paroxysms a feeling of fullness and oppression on the chest remains; many patients complain of drawing and stinging pains in the chest which suddenly come and go. After eating a flush is seen on the cheeks and ears, and the palms of the hands become hot and red. These symptoms are evanescent, but return frequently and become more and more obstinate. The oppression gradually becomes more perceptible and finally remains permanently, so that the patient complains of it all the time. The mouth and throat are frequently very dry, especially in the afternoon, after which tenacious mucus is hawked up in the morning. The cough is generally worse at night; in the day-time the condition of the patient is more tolerable. The appetite generally continues good and the digestion is undisturbed. Towards the end of this stage the voice becomes husky, and even hoarse. The muscular debility increases. The pulse becomes more frequent. The second stage is ushered in with fever which makes its appearance at noon or towards evening. The skin is dry and hot, the pulse hurried, a cooling perspiration breaks out in the morning. Gradually the cough becomes more violent, worse in a horizontal position of the body, and is frequently accompanied by pain in the chest and vomiting. The expectoration accompanying the cough is tenacious, opaque, and gradually assumes a greenish or yellowish tinge. The fever becomes more continuous, and during the paroxysm the cheeks of the patient exhibit a circumscribed bright-red flush. The breathing becomes more and more hurried. The voice is not so much hoarse as husky and hollow. The expectoration becomes ash-colored, has a foul smell, an acrid taste, and is frequently streaked with blood. In twenty-four hours the patient frequently raises a quart. Hæmorrhage from the lungs is not infrequent in this stage, and often terminates fatally. The body wastes away, the eyes become hollow, nose and chin become more prominent. The patients secrete a small quantity of dark urine which is sometimes frothy, and at other times is covered with an oily pellicle, and deposits a bran-like sediment after standing. The menses are either suppressed or scanty and irregular. The appetite generally continues good, although the digestion becomes irregular. The thirst torments the patients mostly only during the fever. The younger the patient, or the more rapid the course of the first and second stages, the sooner the third stage makes its appearance. The fever and perspiration now generally abate, in the place of which an exhausting diarrhœa sets in, which becomes watery and has a fetid smell. The strength decreases visibly, the pulse becomes soft, empty, exceedingly quick, the voice is thin, husky or hollow. The patient seems nothing but skin and bones. The breathing becomes shorter and shorter, and the cough more and more racking. At the same time the expectoration becomes less, and in its place the patient is tormented by excessive anguish. The tongue becomes cracked and covered with aphthæ, which impede deglutition. At times a sort of rash is seen on the chest. The diarrhœa becomes more and more frequent, alternating with night sweats. In spite of these discouraging symptoms the patients still continue to form plans for the future. Finally the feet become dropsical, and gradually the whole body is invaded by this change. Bedsores render the condition of the patients still more intolerable. Little by little the extremities become cold, the pulse becomes feebler and the patient passes away quietly in the full possession of his consciousness.

Like most other diseases, pulmonary phthisis is often curable if attended to in season, more especially by means of the following remedies:

Pulsatilla. If the fever is not yet fully developed, and the patient is not yet troubled with thirst. This remedy is likewise indicated, if the disease was caused by menstrual suppression; the patient is of a quiet, anxious, weeping mood, with pale complexion, oppression of the chest, shortness of breath, palpitation of the heart, cough with expectoration of bitter, sweetish, saltish or foul mucus, worse in the evening, at night or in the morning, less in day-time, sometimes accompanied with an inclination to vomit or actual vomiting. During the cough the patient complains of stitches in the shoulder, side or back. Hoarseness or very faint voice.

China, if the disease arose after venesections, or in consequence of excessive nursing or the loss of other animal fluids. Cough with expectoration of blood-streaked mucus, or of whitish mucus with blackish points; hæmoptysis; pulmonary hæmorrhage. This remedy may arrest the diarrhœa in the last stage of the disease when a cure is no longer possible, especially if the food passes off undigested; it is likewise useful, if the bedsores become gangrened.

Phosphorus. This agent is useful in the beginning of

phthisis as well as when the disease is fully developed, and patients still show a desire for sexual intercourse. Cough with expectoration of saltish and greenish mucus; watery, exhausting diarrhœa; general emaciation.

Calcarea carbonica. Especially indicated if the left lung is attacked, less adapted to the right lung, with stitches in the left side during a deep inspiration or when bending toward the right side; cough with expectoration of sweetish or saltish pus of a yellowish color, foul, worse in the morning; frequent attacks of hæmoptysis. Phthisis of stone-cutters, (see *Silicea.*)

Carbo animalis. Adapted to the right lung. Cough with expectoration of greenish or any other kind of pus; worse when lying on the right side.

Kali carbonicum. Suitable to women who have had many miscarriages, or who have nursed many children. (See China.) Racking cough, inducing vomiting, (especially after midnight.) Cough with purulent expectoration. This remedy is well adapted after Nitric acid or Silic. has been given, or in cases where the disease can be traced to neglected pneumonia.

Lycopodium. Likewise suitable if the disease can be traced to neglected pneumonia. Cough with expectoration of saltish mucus or pus, having a gray or greenish color, (suitable after Calc., Phosph., Silic.)

Millefolium. The disease commences with, or is accompanied by occasional hæmorrhage from the lungs. *Chlore* may likewise prove adapted to this condition.

Silicea. The disease is caused by the inhalation of stone-dust, stone-cutter phthisis, (with Calc.)

Stannum. Mucous phthisis, with expectoration of quantities of colorless mucus.

Sambucus nigra. In cases characterised by profuse and exhausting sweats.

Sulphur. The disease is traceable to the suppression of some cutaneous eruption or sore. If the patient is very weak, give *China* first, or in alternation with Sulphur.

Aconite should always be given, if acute fever-symptoms develop themselves.

In no case should the medicines be given in too rapid succession; I generally allow a month and even two months to pass by before resorting to a new remedy.

3. Consumption of the Stomach.

This disease may be caused by the use of cold drinks while the body is heated, and likewise by the abuse of acrid medicines. The following symptoms have come under my own observation: Oppression of the stomach, generally continuous, but worse after eating; vomiting of the ingesta, afterwards vomiting of bitter, tenacious, whitish mucus; the region of the stomach is swollen and sensitive; cough sets in, which soon becomes permanent, with expectoration of a little yellowish mucus, which gradually changes to quantities of purulent mucus, and lastly to vomiting of liquid pus.

The principal remedy in this disease is *Pulsatilla*, although *Coccus cacti* may be useful at the commencement when no pus is yet raised.

4. Consumption of the Liver.

This not very frequent disease is generally traceable to neglected inflammation of the liver. The liver is swollen, but not hard. If the abscess is seated on the surface of the liver, a soft tumor may be felt which fluctuates on pressure. The abscess may discharge in various directions, and thus endanger the patient's life, If the pus is discharged into the lungs, it is expelled by cough. The pus is qualitatively distinguished from that of other organs. It is friable like wine-dregs, and contains an admixture of bile. General symptoms are: Jaundiced color of the skin, rapidly-increasing emaciation of the whole body, and a fever peculiar to hepatic phthisis, setting in every other day and sometimes twice on the same day. If the disease is curable, *Sulphur* is the main remedy; this is to be followed by *Silicea,* next by *Mercurius* and lastly by *Lachesis.*

Each medicine is dissolved in water, six pellets in half a tumblerful, of which a small spoonful is taken morning and night for six days in succession, after which no medicine is taken for several months, unless an acute attack should render some intermediate remedy necessary.

5. Intestinal phthisis. (Consumption of the bowels.)

This disease is recognized by the following symptoms. The patients complain of periodical paroxysms of colicky pains in the bowels. The pain is generally burning and is mostly felt during the night. The pain is aggravated by pressure upon the abdomen. A characteristic symptom is nocturnal diarrhœa with copious discharges. Afterwards the diarrhœa likewise takes place in the day-time, but the nocturnal attacks are always more violent. The nature of the discharges is characteristic. If received in a tumbler, they deposit flocks of blood-streaked or dark-red or brown-red pus, and have a very fetid smell. The other symptoms peculiar to phthisis develop themselves with great rapidity, but especially the emaciation becomes so great that the patient is often reduced to a skeleton in one fortnight. The disease is likewise characterised by a filiform and rapid pulse, and by night-sweats.

The main remedy in this disease is *Arsenicum*. If this remedy has exhausted its action, *China* or a few doses of *Phosphorus* may be given. *Mercurius, Pulsatilla, Antimonium crudum* may likewise be given.

6. Mesenteric consumption. (Phthisis meseraica.)

Scrofulous children are especially liable to this disease. It is characterised by distention and hardness of the abdomen, increasing emaciation of the whole body, more particularly of the extremities. The skin of such patients is strikingly pale, wrinkled, and scales off in the shape of fine, shining scales. Upon examining the abdomen, moveable tumors are distinctly felt, which are somewhat painful to pressure. At first the patients complain of costiveness, but afterwards diarrhœa sets in, and is particularly troublesome at night. The dis charges are frequently mixed with whitish flocks. The fever is considerable, and the pulse frequently rises to one hundred and twenty beats.

The main remedy in this disease is *Arsenicum*, which removes the danger in most cases. The disease being rooted in a scrofulous disposition, it will be found impossible to effect a cure without the alternate use of *Sulphur* and *Calcarea*, provided that each of these remedies is allowed to act for several months.

7. Renal consumption. (Phthisis renalis.)

This disease is characterised by the following symptoms: The patients complain of aching pain either in one or both kidneys; very rarely however in both kidneys; in which case the pain in one kidney is, nevertheless, more acute. The pain is worse during motion, especially on bending forwards. An examination frequently reveals an elastic swelling of the region of the kidney. The pain which is dull and drawing, extends through the ureters down to the bladder. The emission of urine is attended with a burning and pressing pain. The urine is mixed with pus which is distinctly visible through a microscope. The sediment is frequently mixed with blood. The symptoms characteristic of consumption generally, are also present, such as, frequent pulse, violent heat towards evening, exhausting diarrhœa, rapid emaciation and prostration.

The most appropriate remedy for this disease, which has indeed been cured by means of it, is *Cantharides.* Next we recommend *Terebinthina,* and the treatment may be closed with *Lycopodium.*

In treating consumption, it is of importance to allow a dose of the right remedy to act its full length of time. By dose I understand three to five pellets dissolved in a small tumblerful of water, of which a dessertspoonful should be taken morning and evening for five days. If acute symptoms should show themselves, they will have to be met by specific intercurrent remedies

Inflammation of the brain. (Meningitis, phrenitis.)

This disease is exceedingly dangerous, not only because its issue is dubious, but because it is so easily confounded with other diseases. A mistake in the treatment may be productive of fatal consequences. By carefully observing the existing symptoms and selecting a remedy accordingly, it will not be difficult to save the patient's life.

Like other inflammations, the disease sets in with chilliness followed by heat, or with violent boring pains and heat in the head, beating of the carotids and temporal arteries, deep redness of the face, anxiety, restlessness, sadness, sometimes, however, striking mirthfulness, disposition to laugh and sing, a remarkable degree of listlessness, shyness or boldness. Other symptoms are: A wild or staring look, or else obscuration of sight, vertigo or restless, unrefreshing sleep, general emaciation, trembling of the limbs, loss of appetite, nausea and vomiting, occasionally nosebleed. The fever has the character of a violent inflammatory fever, attended with continual, burning, tensive, tearing or lancinating, constrictive, throbbing pains, either on the surface or in the interior of the brain, but chiefly in the occiput or at the vertex. These pains frequently extend to the nape of the neck and even down the spine. The patient bores with the head into the pillow, is extremely sensitive to light and noise. The pupils are contracted, the eyes look fiery and red, the look is wandering, the eyes are rolled wildly in their sockets; the patient complains of humming and buzzing in the ears, there is wild delirium, or constant talking, screaming, howling, laughing, sometimes there are spasms or convulsions, more particularly spasms in the œsophagus and other hydrophobic symptoms.

Some cases of meningitis resemble typhus. The patient complains of a dull pain or excessive weight in the head, moans, grasps at the head, tosses his limbs, or seems unconscious, in a state of torpor or bland delirium. The symptoms of local paralysis are sometimes present, as if the patient had been struck with apoplexy. These symptoms often set in at the onset, or else follow the first mentioned symptoms, or alternate with the latter. Meningitis is frequently accompanied by severe gastric symptoms, such as frequent and violent vomiting of acrid mucus, or of green fluid bile, constipation and retention of urine.

The last-mentioned symptoms may lead an inexperienced observer to overlook the inflammation of the brain, and to mistake the disease for a severe gastric disorder.

This disease may be induced by a variety of causes which should be carefully considered in the treatment.

The determination of blood to the brain which is so frequently present during dentition, is one of the causes of meningitis. The symptoms are those above mentioned; the children moreover thrust their fingers into their mouths, or move the jaws as if they were masticating. *Aconite,* six pellets in a cupful of water, a dessertspoonful every hour, is frequently sufficient to remove the danger in twelve hours. If no change for the better takes place in six to eight hours, *Aconite* and *Belladonna* should be given in alternation every hour, Bellad., to be prepared like Aconite.

Children who have worms, frequently manifest symptoms resembling meningitis, with dryness and heat of the skin, hurried and soft pulse, sopor with the eyes half open, spasmodic twitching of the arms and hands, boring with the finger in the nose until it bleeds. *China,* a few pellets in water, may be prescribed, to be preceded by a few doses of Aconite until the skin has become moist. But if the above symptoms are accompanied by perspiration at the onset, *Mercurius* should be given.

In hot weather, persons whose bare heads are exposed to the rays of the sun, are frequently attacked with inflammation of the brain. This is termed sunstroke. The disease often terminates fatally in less time than it required to develop it. In such a case the *spirits of Camphor* should be given, a few drops every five or ten minutes until the danger is over. Each dose is to be given in a spoonful of water or on sugar. After this, *Belladonna* is often indicated by the modified symptoms.

An inflammation of the brain may likewise be caused by the influence of intense cold. In this case *Aconite* and *Bryonia* may be given in alternation every fifteen minutes, in water, according to the above described rule.

If meningitis is caused by the sudden retrocession of erysipelas, *Belladonna* has to be given in a case of the common, smooth erysipelas, and *Cantharides*, if the erysipelas was of the vesicular variety.*

Meningitis induced by the sudden retrocession of scarlatina, yields to *Belladonna*; by the retrocession of measles, to *Pulsatilla*; the last-mentioned remedy is likewise required, if the disease arises from the suppression of otorrhœa. The medicine should be repeated every hour.

Meningitis induced by a blow or fall on the head,

* In such a case *Rhus tox.* is recommended by most practitioners. Cantharides are far more homœopathic to such a form of meningitis, as may be seen by any one who chooses to consult his Materia Medica. I have not only cured vesicular erysipelas with *Cantharides*, but likewise with *Euphorbium*, especially if the patient felt rheumatic pains which abated during motion.

requires *Arnica,* which may be alternated with *Aconite* every hour.

In order to facilitate the selection of a remedy, I subjoin the symptomatic indications of each particular drug:

Aconite, at the commencement of the disease; chill followed by continual dry heat, burning skin; full, hard pulse, congestion of blood to the head, heat and redness of the face, fullness and oppressive weight in the forehead, with sensation as if the forehead should split; lancinations and throbbing in the head; burning pains in the head as if the brain were agitated by boiling water; delirium; vomiting of green bile.

Belladonna. Boring with the head into the pillow; *excessive sensitiveness to noise and light;* stinging, boring, burning, lancinating, throbbing pains in the head; red, sparkling eyes, with furious look; red, bloated face; visible throbbing of the carotids; sopor, with half open eyes and distorted eyeballs; loss of consciousness and speech, or inarticulate muttering, violent delirium with howling and screaming; small, quick, intermittent pulse; spasmodic movements of the limbs, spasm in the œsophagus with impeded deglutition; vomiting, involuntary emission of urine and discharge of fæces.

Bryonia. Chill, followed by violent heat, unquenchable thirst; redness and puffiness of the face; tossing about, sopor with delirium and frequent starting; sudden and frequent starting from sleep, with a shriek; vertigo and extreme weakness when rising in bed; excessive weight and violent pain in the head, burning and aching, or compressive from temple to temple, also with dull pains in the occiput; dark redness of the eyes bilious vomiting, constipation or diarrhœa, unconscious discharge of urine, quick and feeble pulse. A characteristic indication for Bryonia is a movement of the jaws simulating mastication, a dangerous symptom when occuring after the period of dentition.

Cantharides. Meningitis after the sudden retrocession of vesicular erysipelas; violent aching, tearing, pulling, lancinating pains in the head, with sensation as if the head were pressed from behind forward, and if the brain would press out at the forehead; rush of blood to the head, with redness and puffiness of the face; protruded and sparkling eyes, with fixed and staring look; sleeplessness with tossing about, or starting up from sleep; delirium; spasm in the œsophagus with impeded deglutition, especially when attempting to swallow liquids; *aversion to liquids;* vomiting with violent straining; constipation and retention of urine; full and hard pulse.

Glonoine. Sunstroke, violent determination of blood to the head, throbbing in the forehead, temples and vertex; soreness of the brain, especially when shaking the head; redness of the face, sweat on the forehead, hurried pulse, eyes protruded, fierce look.

Hyoscyamus. Constrictive or stupefying pain in the forehead, or undulating-throbbing sensation in the brain; red eyes, dilated pupils, diplopia; delirium, at times bland, at others violent, the patient talks about his affairs; sopor, starting of the limbs, grasping at flocks; spasmodic constriction of the throat, with inability to swallow; aversion to drinks; vomiting of bile, retention of urine, with constipation; hurried, intermittent pulse.

Opium. Weight in the head, especially in the occiput, causing the head to fall backward; tension in the head, or pain as if the brain were torn; pressure in the forehead from within outward; rush of blood to the head, throbbing of the arteries; red, staring and glistening eyes; dark redness and bloating of the face; *sopor with the eyes half open;* frequent vomiting, retention of stool and urine, quick and hard pulse.

Stramonium. Violent throbbing headache, with rush of blood to the head and sparkling eyes; restless sleep, the patient wakes crying and moaning; *delirium with frightful spectra;* redness and puffiness of the face; spasm of the œsophagus, impeding and even preventing deglutition; aversion to liquids; vomiting of bile, with starting of the limbs; constipation, retention of urine, intense heat of the skin, small and quick pulse.

Sulphur may be given as an intercurrent remedy every three or four hours, in the case of scrofulous subjects, provided the symptoms justify its use.

Asthma, Dyspnœa.

This disease manifests itself in various forms, because it may be induced by a variety of causes. It may be caused by a defective structure of the thorax, by curvature of the spine, or it may be symptomatic of some other disease, such as hydrothorax. In such a case the asthma cannot be cured unless the cause is removed. Sometimes the disease exists independently of any other disorder, and its dangerous character is proportionate to the peculiar form or intensity of the paroxysms. Without complicating my remarks by the names and pathological distinctions of Old School physicians, I will content myself with indicating the various symptomatic forms of this disease, and their appropriate treatment.

1. Asthma from determination of blood to the chest is chiefly observed among plethoric young people, among girls whose catamenia have become arrested, or among females in consequence of the suppression of the lochia. The patients complain of difficulty of breathing during exercise, of pressure, fullness and constriction of the chest, of anxiety and palpitation of the heart, and noctural aggravation of all the symptoms. Very frequently cough with dark-brown or bloody expectoration is present; the patients feel easier after raising mucus. The pulse is generally full, the face red and puffed. Headache is almost always present.

Aconite is here the chief remedy, if the attack is induced by the least emotion, characterised by the presence of heat and restlessness, inability to take a long breath; the attack befals children who are suddenly roused from sleep by a paroxysm of suffocative cough, with a barking, hoarse sound of the voice, spasmodic constriction of the throat and chest, and labored breathing.

Belladonna, suitable for the same symptoms as Aconite, or in case Aconite should not be sufficient, with vertigo when rising from a recumbent position.

Bryonia; the patient is disposed to draw a long breath, but is unable to do so, with stitches in the chest when making the attempt. The symptoms are worse when the patient is lying down, talks or moves about; momentary relief when rising from a recumbent posture.

Pulsatilla. Suitable to females, when the asthma is complicated with, or can be traced to, menstrual suppression or scanty and delaying menses. This remedy is generally useful, if the symptoms are better in the open air.

Nux vomica, suitable to persons who lead a sedentary life, undergo much mental labor, use much wine, coffee, spirits, or in whom the attack sets in after suppression of the piles. The menses are profuse and too frequent.

2. The *spasmodic asthma* of adults is a paroxysmal disease without fever. The paroxysms generally set in at night, but they announce themselves even in the afternoon by a feeling of fullness in the stomach, restlessness, anxiety, headache, and heaviness in the extremities. Towards evening the pulse becomes more frequent, the breathing more labored, and a violent and dry cough frequently supervenes. The anxiety increases until midnight, when it reaches the highest degree. The patient experiences a constrictive sensation across the chest, pants, gasps for air, and is unable to remain in bed. The breathing becomes wheezing, rattling. The pulse becomes small, intermittent, the hearts beats violently and irregularly.

The limbs become cold and perspire. Fainting fits, vomiting, cough with frothy and bloody expectoration frequently supervene. At the commencement of the disease, the paroxysms only last a few minutes, but recur for several nights in succession, after which they cease for three or six months; but if the disease continues, the paroxysms become more violent and continuous, until they finally take place every night. They terminate with cough and mucous expectoration, the pulse again becomes regular, the skin warm and moist, and the watery again assumes its normal color. Unless proper remedies are employed very speedily, other disorders may supervene, until hectic fever, apoplexy, suffocative catarrh terminate the patient's sufferings.

The following remedies are suitable for this affection:

Arsenicum; cough as from the vapor of Sulphur, with a feeling of suffocation in the bronchial tubes, obliging the patient to sit up. Moreover labored breathing, panting and wheezing, with great anxiety, restlessness, violent palpitation of the heart and cold perspiration, small and intermittent pulse, aggravation in a warm room, or by exercise, such as getting into bed; the attacks are excited by rough weather.

Belladonna; dry and spasmodic cough at night, labored breathing, with stitches under the sternum, constant gasping for air; constriction and painfulness of the larynx when turning the neck, with suffocative sensation, expression of anxiety in the face, and convulsive movements of the limbs.

Bryonia; labored breathing, especially at night and towards morning, with stitches in the chest and urging to stool, frequent coughing and pain in the hypochondria.

Cocculus; the paroxysms intermit for some days, and then recur with renewed violence after midnight, with constrictive sensation in the region of the larynx; anxiety, racking cough, moaning, disposition to start, tremulous weakness (especially suitable to hysteric females.)

Cuprum; the paroxysms set in during the menstrual period, with spasmodic constriction of the chest, mucous rattling in the air-tubes; labored, hurried, wheezing breathing, with suffocative paroxysms and short and spasmodic cough; chiefly suitable to hysteric females.

Nux vomica; the paroxysms set in every fortnight, or at every change of moon, with anxiety, heat, palpitation of the heart, racking and dry cough which be comes somewhat loose towards morning; spasmodic constriction of the lower portion of the chest, relief from the distress in a recumbent possure.

Pulsatilla; spasmodic constriction of the throat and chest as from the vapor of Sulphur, worse when lying on the back, less when sitting up; the attacks may have been caused by the vapors of Sulphur.

If the existing paroxysms have been shortened by the specific homœopathic agent, the treatment had better be continued for some time longer in order to perfect the cure. The patient may take *Sulphur,* five pellets in a cupful of water, of which a dessertspoonful may be taken morning and night for six days. This remedy is especially indicated, if the patient had been treated for the itch or some other eruption with ointments or washes. This remedy should be allowed to act for several months.

3. *Asthma Millari,* which attacks children between the years of two and eight (seldom infants at the breast and full-grown persons), is very similar to cramp. The attack almost always sets in in winter, in consequence of a cold, first at night, suddenly, without any distinct premonitory symptoms, and sets in at once with the most violent symptoms of suffocation, without any rattling or wheezing. The pulse is hurried and small. If cough sets in, it is short, rough, without gagging or expectoration; the voice is hoarse, deglutition difficult. However the child does not complain of a local obstacle in swallowing or breathing, or of pain in the larynx or trachea, but of a dull pain or spasmodic drawing throughout the whole chest, as if caused by suffocating vapors. Slight spasms and changes of color are noticed, a general erethism of the circulation and nervous system, scanty and pale urine having a sweetish odor.

The patient is suddenly roused with a fearful cry and an expression of anxiety in the altered features. The voice is deep, barking, hollow-sounding, husky, very rarely wheezing or crowing. During the convulsive movements of the chest, the labored inspirations are suddenly followed by a noisy expulsion of the air. The face becomes dark-colored, the eye becomes staring and protruded, the veins of the neck and temples swell. If the attack does not destroy life, it ends in a few hours with sneezing, eructations and vomiting. The breathing becomes easier, the peculiar sound disappears, and amid a general subsidence of the symptoms the children fall into a quiet slumber, from which they wake exhausted and desponding. Generally a second attack sets in in the following night, more violent than the former, with increasing fever. The danger of suffocation is greater, the face and lips become blue, mottled, the shoulders are raised, and all the muscles of the thorax are violently worked. The face becomes more and more distorted, the nostrils dilate, the pulse is very rapid and intermits. The patient tosses about, is covered with cold or lukewarm perspiration, fæces and urine are passed involuntarily, but the consciousness is undisturbed; finally the patient dies of suffocation amid convulsions. Only a few children survive more than one attack; death almost always sets in during the third or fourth attack. The attacks never terminate with expectoration.

Asthma Millari cannot well be confounded with croup, if we remember that in croup the larynx is always sensitive to pressure, and that the patients bore their heads into the pillow, whereas in this disease the children sit erect, and do not complain of pain in the larynx, but of spasmodic constriction of the chest. In croup the breathing is fine and crowing, in asthma Millari it is deep and hollow. If the disease is speedily recognized, subsequent attacks may be averted, and existing attacks may be alleviated by one of the following remedies:

Ipecacuanha; sudden paroxysms of suffocation at night, with a sensation of violent constriction in the chest; short and anxious inspirations, and sudden and jerking expirations; pale, bloated face with blue margins around the eyes; peevish mood.

Sambucus nigra; sudden starting up from sleep with a shriek, anxiety and trembling; sudden wheezing inspirations which sometimes intermit; deep, hollow, rough or else crowing voice; blueish puffiness of the face and hands; protruded eyeballs with the mouth half open; anxious tossing about, heat without thirst, hurried and tremulous pulse; torpor towards the end of the attack, and copious, mostly cold sweat.

On comparing these indications with the symptoms of the disease, it is readily seen that *Ipecac.* can only be given at the commencement of an attack, and that, if the disease attains to its full development, *Sambucus* has to be given. If the attack should set in again in the night following, nothing can be expected of this agent, and it will be advisable to give *Arsenicum.* All these remedies have to be given in the form of a watery solution, every five to ten minutes.

Other varieties of asthma can be most frequently controlled by Arsenicum.

For asthma caused by the inhalation of the vapors of Sulphur, we give Pulsatilla.

Asthma caused by a fit of anger or by a cold, yields

to *Chamom.* or *Nux vom.*, the latter being more particularly indicated by a vehement disposition.

For asthma caused by the inhalation of stone-dust, in the case of stone-cutters, sculptors, etc., we give *Calc. carb.*, *Silic.* or *Sulph.*

Calc. carb. is a main remedy for chronic asthmatic complaints, with disposition to draw a long breath, and sensation as if the breath were arrested between the shoulder-blades. The distress is relieved by raising the shoulders. Mere stooping causes the breath to give out; frequent paroxysms of dry cough, especially at night.

In attacks of acute asthma, *mesmerism* sometimes proves exceedingly useful. A robust and healthy man makes a pass with the extended hand over the chest from above downwards, and likewise over the back of the patient some ten or twelve times, after which the effect should be watched. See *mesmerism* at the close of the work.

The medicines should be administered in water, six pellets in a cupful, of which a dessertspoonful is to be taken morning and night for six days.

Scarlet-fever. (Scarlatina.)

This disease is more especially a disease of childhood. Full-grown persons are only attacked by this disease if they had remained free from it in their childhood. The disease is somewhat similar to the smooth form of erysipelas, and may appear under various modifications which expose the inexperienced practitioner to the danger of confounding scarlatina with some other disease. In whatever form, the scarlet-exanthem may show itself, it always sets in with certain precursory symptoms. The patients complain of heaviness and dullness of the head, nausea, vomiting and chills. These chills frequently alternate with flashes of burning heat which finally become permanent. This heat is burning and dry, and often accompanied with a troublesome prickling in the palms of the hands. The pulse varies, but in most cases it is full, moderately hard and extremely hurried, (one hundred and twenty beats, sometimes double-beating.) In this stage the patient complains of vertigo, headache, pains in the limbs, thirst. The patients feel exhausted, are irritable and very restless. The fever increases towards evening. The heat reaches its acme and is accompanied with occasional delirium. Mouth, tongue and fauces are dry, tense and hot. Deglutition and speech are very muck impeded. The submaxillary or parotid glands begin to swell and become painful. By giving *Aconite* and *Belladonna* in water, an alternate dose every hour, the course of the disease will be very much modified. Nose-bleed sometimes sets in at this period, to the great relief of the patient. The alvine discharges are generally retarded. The urine deposits whitish clouds, some of which adhere to the bottom of the vessel; or the urine may be dark-colored and has a strong smell. Some patients are troubled with a constant urging to urinate, without discharging much urine. The cutaneous exhalations have a peculiar odor, which it is difficult to describe, and which some physicians compare to the odor of herring-brine or musty bread. An experienced practitioner may recognize the existence of scarlet-fever by its smell, which is exceedingly characteristic.

Amid a progressive increase of the pains, an exanthem makes its appearance on the third day (seldom sooner, and still less frequently later,) consisting of bright-red, diffusive spots. These spots are somewhat angular, rounding, not raised, they disappear under pressure, but the redness reappears as soon as the pressure ceases, from the margin to the centre. These spots first break out on the uncovered or slightly covered parts of the body, the face, neck, chest, and thus down to the feet; the skin is dry and hot, and this dryness is characteristic. The peculiar smell is most fully perceived during this period; it lasts from three to six days, during which the redness gradually disappears in the order in which it broke out, from above downwards. The fever abates in the same proportion, and finally ceases with the other symptoms.

As soon as the redness appears, we give *Belladonna*, six pellets in a cupful of water, a teaspoonful every hour or two hours, and if the fever is intense, we alternate this drug with *Aconite*.

The skin now begins to peel off, and this constitutes the third period of the disease. Soon after the disappearance of the redness, and in some cases even a considerable length of time after this takes place, the skin peels off in large flakes, sometimes several times in succession. The patients seldom complain of any pain during this period, except of a troublesome itching of the skin.

The disease does not always run such a regular course as we have described; its development is sometimes arrested by external influences, or the disease is complicated with inflammation or dropsy of the brain, croup, typhoid-fever, etc. These diseases set in at the onset or in the second stage of the disease, and prevent the regular appearance of the exanthem which sometimes remains entirely suppressed. Even after the regular termination of the disease the patient is still in danger, until the desquamation is accomplished. Until then, the patient should not be taken into the open air, or be permitted to sit on the floor.

I will now mention the more prominent forms of scarlatina, and their appropriate treatment.

1. Smooth scarlatina. (Scarlet-fever.)

The redness is smooth and shining, without any unevenness; arising from small, red spots, which keep increasing in size until they run together; the redness is at first of a rose-color, gradually changes to that of boiled lobster, and finally becomes of a dark scarlet. The chief remedy in this form is *Belladonna,* as stated above, to be alternated with *Aconite,* if the fever is very high.

2. Scarlet Rash.

The whole body, or the larger part of it, first becomes red, and soon after rough and uneven. A careful examination shows a very fine vesicular rash, the vesicles being sometimes closely grouped together. The vesicles may likewise spring up on parts of the skin which are not red. In this form, *Belladonna* is not sufficient, and has to be alternated with *Aconite,* both in water, every hour or two hours. *Dulcamara* may likewise prove useful.

Pustulous Scarlatina.

Small vesicles spring up upon the spots, which gradually run together, assuming the appearance of vesicular erysipelas. They are filled with a yellowish fluid, break in about eight days, and then form crusts. This form requires the alternate use of *Aconite* and *Belladonna*, and, if the pustules are fully formed, *Rhus tox.*

4. Masked Scarlatina. (Scarlatina larvata.)

This form varies. Some patients pass through the first stage, but no eruption appears, only a violent itching, after which the skin peels off in patches. Other patients exhibit the following symptoms: Depression of spirits, dull, staring look, obscuration of sight, cold and pale face, lameness of the extremities, difficulty of swallowing, with stinging pains in the parotid glands, headache, etc. In other cases the exanthem is entirely wanting, but the disease takes the form of a violent angina, with swelling and bright-red inflammation of the tonsils, uvula and fauces. These symptoms require *Belladonna* in water, every hour or two hours, and for the violent angina *Belladonna* and *Merc.*, in alternation, sometimes *Arsenicum*, (see below.)

If the eruption comes out too slowly or retrocedes, *Bryonia* may be given in water every hour, and if it does not suffice, it may be alternated with *Apis*. If the fever is high, we give *Aconite;* scrofulous patients require *Sulphur*.

If the eruption remains pale and faint, and the children toss about in great anxiety, we give *Arsen.* If the exanthem looks blueish, *Veratrum* is required; if the breath is cold, *Carbo veg.*

Other modifications of the above-mentioned forms may take place; in order to facilitate the selection of a suitable remedy in such cases, I subjoin the following symptomatic indications:

Aconite; dry heat with thirst; full and hurried pulse; congestion of blood to the head, with red and puffed face; vertigo which is worse when raising the head after lying down; throbbing headache; delirium and sudden starting up from sleep; colic with bilious vomiting; painful and anxious urging to urinate, with difficult discharge of small quantities of dark urine; painful, dry cough; nose-bleed, hæmoptysis.

Belladonna; smooth scarlatina, the affected parts are hot and swollen. Vertigo with obscuration of sight, nausea, worse when rising from a recumbent posture; violent headache, lancinating or tearing, worse when looking at the light; inflamed eyes; *inflammation of the tonsils, uvula and fauces,* with stinging and constrictive pain; violent fever, with delirium, intense thirst, also aversion to liquids; inability to swallow liquids; sleeplessness, restlessness; *frightful spectra* when closing the eyes; sudden starting up from sleep; this remedy is a preventive against scarlatina, if children take a few pellets every evening for five days in succession, and then again after a pause of a fortnight. In scarlet-rash *Belladonna* and *Aconite* have to be taken on alternate evenings.

Ammonium carbonicum; in smooth scarlatina, if the upper half of the body is attacked, the lower half remaining free, with *heat in the head,* cold feet and moderate sore throat.

Arsenicum album; violent vomiting at the onset of the attack, sudden prostration, burning heat and thirst, or else absence of thirst and cold hands; anxiety, altered features; *gangrenous angina;* foul, burning ulcers; desquamation of the skin in large flakes, with burning itching; also in dropsy after scarlatina (also *Apis.*)

This powerful medicine has sometimes to be given in the first stage, but more frequently in the third, when it will carry the patient through all danger.

Bryonia; this remedy is indicated, if only a few spots make their appearance here and there, after which the eruption becomes arrested, and is superseded by pneumonia (see this article;) Bryon. may also be given after the retrocession of the eruption (with Apis).

Mercurius; violent angina, with swelling of the glands, ptyalism, ulcers in the mouth; also with swelling of the inguinal glands which sometimes takes place in scarlet-fever (in alternation with Arsen.)

Phosphorus; tongue and lips are dry and hard, covered with blackish crusts; loss of speech and hearing: difficult deglutition; inability to retain his urine; *falling off of the hair.*

Rhus tox.; small vesicles spring up upon the scarlet spots; they gradually increase in size, become filled with a yellowish fluid.

Sulphur; this remedy may be given whenever a correctly selected remedy is not followed by an improvement, especially in the case of scrofulous persons (it may be repeated every two, four or six hours, in alternation with *Acon.*, if the fever is high); it is also indicated by obstruction of the nose, by a dry, cracked, red tongue, or a tongue lined with brownish mucus.

After-diseases (sequelæ) of Scarlet-fever.

Chief remedies for these ailments are: *Bell.*, *Hep. sulph.*, *Merc.* and *Apis.*

One of the most common after-diseases of scarlet-fever is dropsy, the main remedy for which is *Arsen.* in water, a spoonful four times a day. Sometimes the disease seems to get worse under the use of this remedy for the first few days, but after this period an improvement begins to set in. This agent is particularly suitable in ascites depending upon enlargement of the liver or spleen. It will also be found serviceable in hydrothorax and anasarca. If Arsen. does not effect a cure, *Helleborus* will be found suitable. In dropsy of the brain after scarlatina, *Belladonna* remains the chief remedy; if it has no effect, *Helleb.* may be given; some recommend *Apis.*

Dropsical swellings of the scrotum and penis yield to *Rhus tox.*

For otorrhœa and otitis, *Bell.* is the main remedy if insufficient, *Merc.* and *Hepar sulph.* may be given.

Inflammation and swelling of the parotid glands require *Merc.* and *Bell.*, in bad cases *Sulph.* and *Baryta carb.*

For glandular abscess, *Calc. carb.* is suitable; for open abscesses, *Kali carb.* is recommended by Dr. Hering of Philadelphia.

Ulceration of the Schneiderian membrane and of the nasal cartilages requires *Aurum.*

Inflammation of the eyes yields to *Bellad.*, in alternation with *Acon.;* if the cure is not complete, *Apis* and *Sulphur* may be given.

In regard to diet and hygiene, I have to observe

that the temperature of the room should be regulated by the intensity of the fever; if this is high, the room should be kept cool, at a temperature of fifty degrees F.; if the fever is moderate, the room may be a little warmer, say sixty degrees. Care must be taken to prevent the patient from uncovering himself. During the period of desquamation, every exposure and washing with cold water should be carefully avoided. For the latter purpose bran-water should be used with great precaution. Fresh linen should not be put on the patient without having been previously aired by the fire.

Fresh water may be allowed at all times during the disease, but in moderate quantities at each imbibition; water and milk may likewise be used, or water and strawberry-juice, water and sugar, thin oatmeal-gruel, rice-water, cracker-soups, etc. Sweet apple-sauce or baked apples may be used, but nothing fat.

The sick-room should be kept comfortably dark from the commencement of the disease. The room should be ventilated several times a day. During this time the patient's bed may either be carried into an adjoining room having the same temperature, or else the patient may be covered with a cloth as long as the windows are open and even a few minutes after they are closed again, until the former temperature of the room is restored. It is well to favor the movement of atmospheric currents in the room, by agitating the air with a handkerchief.

All the natural wants of the patient should be gratified in the bed, by means of appropriate utensils.

Whooping-cough. (Tussis convulsiva, pertussis.)

This cough generally lasts eighteen weeks, and under

bad treatment with quantities of medicine, still longer; it may even pass into larygnitis, pneumonia, croup, etc., its course may be shortened or its intensity moderated by proper homœopathic treatment.

The first or catarrhal stage, which is characterised by peevishness, depression of spirits, irritable temper, catarrhal cough, redness and weeping of the eyes, slight fever, etc., is often arrested by one of the following remedies:

Aconite; dry, shrill or wheezing cough, most violent at night, sometimes attended with fever and dry heat, burning pains in the wind-pipe. Dose: three to five pellets in a cupful of water, a spoonful every few hours.

Pulsatilla; loose cough with scanty expectoration, hoarseness, vomiting of the ingesta or of a fluid white mucus; *worse towards evening;* mucous diarrhœa. Dose same as for *Acon.*, but only twice a day for five days, then stop.

Nux vom.; dry, racking cough, worse after midnight and in the morning, with vomiting, anxiety, suffocative symptoms, bleeding from the nose and mouth. (Same dose as Puls.)

Ipecacuanha; cough with great anxiety, suffocative symptoms, blueish face, vomiting of mucus, the symptoms are the same at all periods of the day. (Same dose).

Coccus cacti; cough excited by constant tickling in the windpipe, coming in paroxysms, *terminating in the expectoration of quantities of an albuminous, tenacious, ropy mucus,* sometimes attended with gagging, and vomiting of food after a meal. Urinary difficulties are often present.

Arnica; paroxysms of whooping-cough commencing

with weeping or crying; this continues often during the attack.

Carbo veget.; suitable when the cough passes into the second stage; frequent paroxysms of spasmodic cough in the day-time, especially in the evening until midnight, also with gagging and vomiting, painful stitches through the head, redness and irritation in the throat, pain on swallowing, soreness and burning in the chest. (Same dose.)

If this remedy does not arrest the passage into the second stage, and no other remedy is indicated, *Kali carb.* may afford relief.

Second or spasmodic stage. (Whooping-cough in a more particular sense.)

The cough breaks out in repeated paroxysms in longer or shorter intervals. The inspirations are long and anxious, of a panting and spasmodic character, followed by five or six shrill turns of cough, during which the inspiration of air becomes impossible. Finally, while the rima glottidis is spasmodically contracted, the patient succeeds in performing a long, anxious and wheezing inspiration, after which a second and even a third series of coughing fits may take place, until the whole paroxysms, which sometimes lasts two or three minutes, terminates in vomiting of mucus and food, and blood is sometimes discharged from the nose and mouth. At the onset of the paroxysms the children rise in great anxiety, run to the mother, or hold on to something as if in great distress, in order to support the upper part of the body.

The paroxysms are frequently excited by emotions

and after meals; hence it is necessary to treat such patients with great kindness, and to overlook many of their derelictions. They should eat light but nourishing food, such as boiled rice, stewed apples, gruel, sago, stewed fruit sweetened with sugar, milk fresh from the cow in any quantity, or milk diluted with tepid water.

If the weather is unfavorable, and the children have to be kept in the house, the room should be frequently ventilated, or else they have to be frequently taken from one room into another. When in the open air, they should take moderate exercise, not get heated by running and jumping, lest the paroxysms should return.

The following remedies seem to be best adapted to the spasmodic stage of whooping-cough:

Veratrum album; the children are very much exhausted, do not recover entirely after an attack, have to lean the head against something for support. Fever with cool or cold perspiration, especially on the forehead, intense thirst, small and quick pulse; emission of urine during the paroxysms; they return when rising from bed, cease on lying down; vertigo, with pain in the head, chest and abdomen, especially in the inguinal region. Give three to five pellets in water, a small spoonful morning and night for five days, then stop. By this means I have cured children who were near death, and had become reduced to skeletons.

Drosera; after the most violent paroxysm the children recover perfectly, jump about as if nothing were the matter; they feel better when moving about than during rest; no thirst during, but after the chilliness. The perspiration is warm or hot, and breaks out mostly at night. The cough has a shrill sound, the children become red and blue in the face during the paroxysm, they are threatened with suffocation; pain under the ribs as if violently constricted, the children obtain relief by pressing upon these parts, generally the paroxysms terminate in vomiting of blood or nose-bleed. One dose of this remedy, two pellets dry on the tongue, is sufficient.

Cuprum metallicum; the paroxysms are quite frequent, the children become blue in the face, quite rigid, lose their breath, until vomiting of mucus sets in, with trembling of the limbs, and continued mucous rattling in the air-passages. The paroxysms frequently occur at night quite suddenly, amid convulsions. Give the medicine in water, five pellets in a cupful, a spoonful morning and night for five days.

Cina; the children become stiff during the paroxysms, gasp for air, turn pale, a gurgling sensation is heard from the throat to the stomach. This remedy is especially indicated when worms are present, as may be inferred from the existence of great paleness, bloated abdomen, frequent colic, itching of the anus and nose, canine hunger, rising of water, vomiting of mucus, flatulence. To be taken like Cuprum. *Cina* and *Bellad.* are said to be efficient, when given in alternation.

In this stage the following remedies have sometimes proved useful:

Coccus cacti; when a ropy mucus is coughed up.

Arnica, if the attacks begin with crying.

Conium, in the case of scrofulous children, the attacks are very violent, with flushed face and bloody expectoration.

Compare also *Hyoscyam.*, *Bell.*, *Ignat.* and *Ipec.*

Of the third stage, that of expectoration, scarcely

any thing is known in homœopathy, If much mucus should be expectorated, and the cough should continue an undue length of time in consequence of careless management, we may have recourse to

Hepar sulph., if the larynx is very sensitive to cool air; the cough is dry, has a hollow and rough sound, with disposition to vomit after the attack; there is oppressed breathing, chills along the back, hot cheeks and hands, emaciation. Dose: Same as for Verat.

Sulphur, when the larynx is sensitive to damp and cold weather; racking cough, with gagging, vomiting, pain in the larynx. The voice is husky, with wheezing breathing and oppression on the chest. The children look pale and haggard; it is especially suitable to scrofulous and rickety children. (Same as Verat.)

Compare *Sepia, Puls., Carbo veg., Dulc.*

Physicians will do well to institute frequent examinations of the chest, especially in obstinate cases, when the cough will be frequently found complicated with pneumonia, pleuritis, pericarditis, tuberculosis, etc.

A change of air is particularly beneficial after the cough has ceased; mountain or sea-air, or at least pure country-air is of great use in removing the habitual irritation of the nervous system, and completing the restoration of health.

Affections of the Liver.

These affections manifest themselves either in an acute form, or else in a chronic form which takes the place of the former. We are most frequently called upon to treat

1. Inflammation of the Liver. (Hepatitis.)

This inflammation is recognized by a continuous, seated, stitching pain in the right side under the short ribs, sometimes ascending to the right shoulder, and causing both in the right arm and right lower extremity a sensation of numbness. The more the inflammation spreads, the more the lungs become involved, and the lancinating pain is not only aggravated by motion, but likewise by deep breathing, sneezing and coughing. The pain is not always a stitching, but sometimes a tensive, lancinating, burning or aching pain. Intense fever is generally present, consisting of dry heat, thirst, accelerated pulse, restlessness, anxiety. When placing the hand upon the region of the liver, a throbbing is perceived. The patient feels somewhat relieved when lying on the back.

As a general rule, acute hepatitis is speedily cured by *Acon.* in alternation with *Nux vom.*, or *Sulph.*, or *Merc.*, but other remedies are sometimes required, a list of which will be found subjoined; six pellets of each remedy may be dissolved in a cupful of water, a dessertspoonful to be given every hour, and, as soon as the symptoms begin to abate, every two or four hours.

Aconite; violent heat with thirst, restless tossing about, fear of death, stitches in the region of the liver.

Nux vomica; stinging and throbbing pains in the region of the liver, aggravated by motion and contact; bitter and sour taste, nausea or vomiting, pressure in the hypochondria and stomach, short breathing, thirst, red urine, headache, vertigo, paroxysms of anxiety.

Mercurius; pain in the region of the liver with sensitiveness to contact; stitches in the liver, impeded respiration and eructations; painful pressure from within outwards, the patient is unable to lie on the right side; continual chilliness, jaundiced color of the skin and sclerotica; bitter taste, loss of appetite.

China; aching and stinging pains, worse every other day; swelling and hardness of the region of the stomach and liver, headache, bitter taste and coated tongue.

Chamomilla; dull aching pains in the liver not modified by external influences, oppression of the stomach, jaundiced color of the skin, yellowish coating of the tongue, bitter taste. If the disease is caused by a fit of chagrin, *Cham.* may be given in alternation with *Acon.*

Belladonna; aching pains in the region of the liver, extending to the stomach, chest and right arm; headache with congestion of blood to the head, twinkling before the eyes, thirst; restless tossing about.

Bryonia; aching pains, tension in the hypochondria oppression of the chest with hurried, anxious breathing, yellow coating of the tongue, constipation, aggravation by motion.

Pulsatilla; stitches in the region of the liver as from an ulcer; frequent attacks of anxiety, especially at night, with diarrhœa, consisting of green mucus. Tendency to vomit, bitter taste, coated tongue, absence of thirst, oppression of the chest, tension in the hypochondria, pressure at the stomach.

Lachesis; stitches in the right side, with contractive sensation, as if a lump were forming; in obstinate cases this remedy may be given in alternation with *Merc.* or *Bellad.*

Sulphur; this remedy may be given in water, four doses a day, if the inflammation does not readily yield to the above-mentioned remedies, or if the patient is scrofulous or affected with eruptions; it is indicated by pressure in the liver immediately after eating, and at night (with yellowish color of the sclerotica), stitches in the liver and right groin, especially when walking; pinching and boring pain; throbbing and twitching from time to time, also on one of the lower ribs, relieved for a while by external pressure; burning and burning stitches on the lower ribs when bending forward while sitting.

Lycopodium; excoriation-pain in the region of the liver, when stooping sideways, or drawing a long breath; contractive pain; clutching pain, dislocation-pain; painless twitching in the region of the liver, when coughing; itching in the liver.

In chronic hepatitis the doses should of course be repeated much less frequently than in the acute form, more especially when such powerful agents as *Sulphur* and *Merc.* are administered.

2. Swelling and Induration of the Liver.

These disorders may arise from a variety of causes, such as mechanical injury by a blow, fall, or improper treatment of acute hepatitis with large doses of Calomel, or mismanaged fever and ague. If the liver is enlarged and indurated, the patient feels an uncomfortable fullness in the right side, and a dull pain is caused by pressure. If the liver is simply swollen, it yields to pressure with the hand, whereas an indurated liver resists pressure. Such an affection is generally complicated with other disorders, such as bitter taste, eructations, oppression of the stomach, constipation. The following medicines have proved most useful in this affection:

Arnica; if the affection is caused by a fall or blow, and the pains are hard and aching as if a stone were pressing on the liver, the pains are particularly felt when lying on the left side, both during an inspiration and expiration.

Arsenicum; induration of the liver after the abuse of cinchona; pressing in the liver when walking in the open air.

Calcarea carb.; swelling and induration of the liver after abuse of cinchona; pressure in the liver when making a step, or stitches in the liver when stooping.

China; swelling and induration of the liver after treating hepatitis with venesections; pressure and stitches, made worse by contact.

Nux vomica; swelling and induration, the patient complains of bitter taste and bitter eructations, oppression of the stomach, constipation, morning-aggravation of the symptoms; also after abuse of cinchona. This remedy is especially adapted to drunkards, and savants who lead a sedentary life.

Mercurius; swelling and induration, with jaundice; for these conditions *Merc.* affords speedy relief; but if it had been taken in large doses under allœopathic treatment, it must not be given, but *Sulphur* will have to be administered.

Sulphur; chronic hepatitis, swelling and induration of the liver. Jaundice; pressure, stitches and tension in the region of the liver; also useful after abuse of cinchona; this medicine may also be given after other remedies, to complete the cure.

In all chronic cases the medicine should be given in water, a dessertspoonful morning and evening for five days, then stop.

3. For abscess of the liver, the most important remedies are *Hepar sulph.*, *Merc.*, *Lach.* and *Sil.*, (Compare Ulcers.)

4. For biliary calculi give *Sulph.*, *Calc.*, *Hepar. sulph.*, *Sil.*, *Lach.*

Acute Dropsy of the Brain. (Hydrocephalus.)

This disease may befall persons of all ages and sexes, but children are especially liable to it, It consists in an effusion of serum and coagulable lymph into the ventricles of the brain, consequent upon a previous determination of blood to the meningeal membranes and blood-vessels, such as occurs in all acute inflammations.

Acute hydrocephalus may be induced by a variety of causes, such as: Violent treatment of the head during delivery; the abuse of Opium or Morphine in diseases; too tight bandaging of children; dentition or worms; concussion of the brain; suppression of cutaneous eruptions by external means; abuse of Opium, Hyoscyamus, Belladonna and other narcotic medicines, abuse of spirits.

In the course of this disease we observe four stages: 1. The congestive stage. 2. The inflammatory stage. 3. The stage of exudation; and 4. The stage of paralysis.

First stage.—Children who are habitually cheerful, become irritable, averse to company, even to objects and persons of whom they used to be fond. The healthy color of the face begins to fade, the eye becomes dim, the muscles lose their tone, the body becomes more angular and the motions become awkward and heavy;

and if the second stage sets in with much violence, the face exhibits even at this period an increased redness. The appetite is less, the alvine and urinary discharges are less frequent and copious. The patients wake from their restless slumber more exhausted than before. On rising from bed, or when sitting up in bed, older children complain of vertigo and a passing stupefaction, whereas younger children express this vertigo by balancing the head to and fro, or by a sudden silence in the midst of their cries. Older children likewise complain of rheumatic pains, especially in the nape of the neck, in the calves and soles of the feet; younger children indicate this distress by moving their hands to the occiput, and by crying. The pulse, which as yet does not vary much from its ordinary rhythm, sometimes slackens by a few beats, or intermits entirely. It is generally the seventh, ninth, sixteenth, seventeenth or thirty-first beat, which is felt by the exploring finger, or which beats more feebly than the rest. The skin even now is perfectly dry. The children now frequently look as if they were sunk in reverie, from which they are roused with a deep inspiration, when they look round with an expression of anxiety or concern and amazement. At times the color of the face undergoes frequent changes, and they complain alternately of flashes of heat and creeping chills. Their gait is vacillating, labored, like that of a drunken person; when making a step forward, they sometimes raise the leg as if they would step over a high object.

In the case of young children it is much more difficult to recognize this stage of the disease than in the case of older children, since very young children frequently vomit and start from sleep without being very sick. Sopor may supervene in consequence of a simple derangement of the stomach, and the pulse may be altered without any striking cause. The following symptoms may reveal the presence of the disorder even in very young children: sleeplessness, constant screaming until the breath gives out, head and trunk being bent backwards; the gentlest contact causes them to start; excessive sensitiveness to light and noise, the slightest noise rouses the little patients from their slumber; they refuse the breast; they cry when gently moved, and they become suddenly silent when the movement is sudden and violent; frequent grasping at the occiput; scanty urine, darker than usual; less copious passages which assume a dark-green tint soon after the evacuation; deficient emission of flatulence, increased warmth on the forehead and back of the head, or of the whole head.

These symptoms most frequently characterise hydrocephalus in little children; sometimes however the symptoms are much more violent. After a sudden feeling of lassitude, stupefaction, vertigo, violent headache, gastric disorders, white-coated tongue, disposition to vomit, the children are suddenly attacked with fever, with a full and hard pulse and generally attended with spasmodic symptoms.

Second stage.—The symptoms of the previous determination of blood now disappear, and the symptoms of an inflammatory affection are fully developed. Older patients complain of violent aching pains in the forehead, extending to the neighbourhood of the temples, are most violent above the eyes, and change about with colicky pains in the bowels. Other symptoms supervene, such as pains in the limbs, tension in the nape of the neck, and an internal anxiety which deprives the patient of all rest. The look becomes wandering, the eyeball retreats into its socket, squints upwards, the eye is half closed as if afraid of the impinging rays of light; it is entirely open only in the dark. The patient's head is hotter than heretofore, especially on the forehead and occiput; the carotids throb violently. The face now looks pale, sunken, in few cases puffed; in either case the features are characteristically altered. The nose and the chapped lips are dry, the latter look pale or pale-red. The tongue has a dirty-whitish or brown coating. The appetite is generally gone, but the thirst is unquenchable in all violent cases. In the course of twenty-four hours the patients vomit four or six times; the vomiting does not continue long, but may be increased by motion and by raising the head. The region of the liver and stomach exhibits signs of pain when strongly pressed upon. The abdomen which was large and distended before the attack, now caves in, which is likewise characteristic of acute hydrocephalus. The bowels are obstinately constipated, and the scanty passages are like glue, tenacious and brown. The urine is voided only in small quantities, is dark-colored, and deposits a whitish, slimy sediment. The breathing is frequently interrupted by moaning. The ear is exceedingly sensitive. During a restless slumber the patients grit their teeth, and cry out. The pulse is slow and intermittent, but sometimes quite regular in patients of only a year old. The dry skin becomes quite relaxed, and assumes a dingy-white color. As a rule the patients now like to lie on their side, with the hand of the side upon which they are resting, under the head, the other hand being at times extended, and at other times moved towards the forehead and vertex, at other times again hidden between the thighs as if to cover the private parts.

Third stage.—Many of the symptoms which we have described so far, now give way to opposite conditions, other symptoms become still more marked. The patients are no longer able to leave their beds, or to sit up. They continually lie on their backs, kicking off the cover with one foot or the other. They continue to grasp at the head, mouth or nose; while boring with the finger in the last-named organ, their legs vacillate to and fro. All the senses become blunted, except the hearing which still continues sensitive. The eyes which had been sensitive to the light and turned up, are now turned down, with the pupils dilated, and insensible to the light. The visual power is moreover feeble and illusory; the patients see double or fancy the objects more remote than they really are, in consequence of which they miss objects when attempting to seize them with trembling hands. Sometimes they suddenly open their eyes quite wide, but close them again as suddenly. Almost at every inspiration the patients moan and groan, and their features express a sombre earnest. The emaciation now increases at a fearful rate, so that the patients often resemble a mere skeleton. The skin continues dry, except in some parts which exhibit signs of moisture. The urine is voided involuntarily, but the alvine discharges cease. The pulse becomes more and more irregular and feeble, the breath is foul, and the general debility increases. The sopor from which they no longer wake as heretofore, with a cry, now increases to complete stupor and loss of consciousness.

Fourth stage.—At the close of the third stage the consciousness returns for a moment, after which the patient again relapses into the previous stupor, and the following symptoms likewise supervene: general convulsions which are soon followed by paralysis (most frequently of the right side), violent spasm which draws the head backwards and causes a horrible distortion of the face and limbs; violent fever with irregular, intermittent, but exceedingly hurried pulse. The burning head is drenched with sweat, while the rest of the body is cool. The visual power is extinct, the eyeball in spasmodic motion, the pupil is exceedingly dilated (but sometimes very much contracted), and cornea is generally covered with mucus; the eyeball is no longer as deeply sunken as before. Deglutition is more difficult; the urine is voided involuntarily, and has a deep-yellow color. The pulse becomes smaller and smaller, wiry, at last imperceptible; the inspirations likewise become shorter and more hurried, and the breath becomes cold. The feet now begin to swell, and death puts an end to all these sufferings.

Although all ages and sexes are liable to this disease, yet it most frequently attacks children, but often remains unrecognized. In many cases where children are said to have died of convulsions from teething, hydrocephalus was the cause of their destruction, the timely removal of which might perhaps have saved the child's life.

It is true, there are diseases with which hydrocephalus might be confounded; but this can never take place, if not single symptoms but the totality thereof are constantly held in view. It is very frequently confounded with worm-fever, the characteristic differences of which two diseases I will now proceed to describe.

Acute hydrocephalus never terminates before the thirteenth and very rarely after the twenty-first day, generally attacks florid, and healthy children, never shows a marked remission of the symptoms, is characterized by a striking alteration of the features, sets in with violent frontal headache, loss of appetite, constipation, scanty discharge of a milky, turbid urine, and is accompanied by sleeplessness or restless sleep. At first the pulse continues regular, then slackens and becomes intermittent, and lastly assumes a febrile type. The patients are very restless, toss about, grasp at their heads. At the commencement of the attack the eyes are sensitive to light, but afterwards lose this sensibility entirely. Almost during the whole course of the disease the hearing remains very acute, but becomes dull towards the end of the disorder. The nose remains dry, the head hot. The patients become visibly thinner, a peculiar eruption makes its appearance around the mouth and on other parts, and in every case the abdomen becomes depressed.

The worm-fever, on the contrary, runs an irregular course, sometimes continuing beyond thirty days; it mostly attacks sluggish, over-fed children with large bowels; the features remain unaltered; the pain is strikingly limited to the bowels; the patients eat a good deal, have copious stools; the sleep is sound; the pulse is from the start irregular, feverish, never slower than in healthy days; the children lie quiet; the eyes are not abnormally sensitive to the light, nor do they lose this sensibility; the hearing is not unnaturally acute, the nose is moist and itches; the patients do not become thin, and the abdomen increases in size.

TREATMENT

For many years I have found the following treatment of this disease the most successful: In the first and second stages I give *Aconite* and *Belladonna*, alternately every two hours, commencing with Aconite, a dessert-spoonful of a solution of six globules of each in a small tumblerful of water, until an improvement sets in. If the patient comes under my treatment at the close of the second, or at the commencement of the third stage, I have frequently succeeded in effecting a cure by the alternate exhibition of *Belladonna* and *Mercurius* every fifteen minutes. At the close of the third or in the fourth stage, a cure is rarely possible; the symptoms may however be moderated by the alternate use of *Belladonna* and *Opium*.

In order to facilitate the selection of a specifically-appropriate remedy, I here subjoin the symptomatic indications of each particular drug.

Aconite: Sleeplessness with restlessness and constant tossing about rushes of blood, or frequent chills with dry heat of the skin; heat in the head; peevish and irritable temper; dread of men, tendency to start, appearance as if sunk in reverie; vertigo, with or without nausea, worse when raising the head; frontal headache, photophobia; sensitiveness to noise; colicky pains in the abdomen; suppression of stool and urine; rheumatic pains in the nape of the neck when moving the neck; vacillating gait.

Belladonna: Sleeplessness with tossing about, starting up from sleep with a shriek, or sopor; chilly creeping when touched by the least current of air; heat in the head, with throbbing of the carotids and temporal arteries; pulse full and slow, or small and slow; tendency to start, apathetic mood; vertigo when rising from a couch, or when walking about, with tendency to stagger as if drunk; frontal headache, over the eyes; spasmodic bending of the head backwards; photophobia, the eyeballs are distorted or spasmodically rolled about; diplopia; intolerance of noise; excessive dryness of the nose; paleness of the face, with distortion of the features; dry and chapped lips, they look dark-red; vomiting of mucus or bile; colicky pains; constipation, suppressed or retarded secretion of urine; rheumatic pains in the limbs and nape of the neck.

Bryonia: Sleeplessness or restless sleep, starting when on the point of falling asleep; heat in the head; frontal headache; vertigo when sitting up in bed, with nausea as if the patient should faint; photophobia, dry nose, pale and bloated face, dry and chapped lips, bilious or watery vomiting, especially directly after drinking; constipation; discharge of urine with colicky pain; moaning breathing.

I have found this remedy useful in hydrocephalus only if the face was pale and bloated, and the vomiting, which is peculiar to this disease, set in directly after drinking.

Helleborus: Sopor, with the eyes half open and turned upwards; heat of the whole body, especially the head; slow and small pulse; staring at one point; pale face, forehead drawn into wrinkles; scanty discharge of stool and urine.

Mercurius: Restless sleep, gritting of teeth; alternate

chills and flashes of heat, heat in the head, pressing pain in the occiput and forehead; pulse feeble, slow and tremulous; the eyes are sensitive to the light, pupils dilated; twitching of the lids; pale face, altered features, livid nose, perspiration on and around the nose and lips; the tongue is thickly coated with white mucus; vomiting of bitter mucus; sensitiveness of the region of the stomach and liver to pressure; constipation; white and cloudy urine, as if flour had been stirred in it; rheumatic pressure in the nape of the neck, increased by moving the neck; drawing pain in the thighs and legs; emaciation, prostration.

This remedy may not only be indicated in the second and third stage, but sometimes even in the first, especially during the period of dentition, when it may have to be given in alternation with *Aconite* and *Belladonna.*

Opium: Stupor, sopor, depression of the lower jaw, moaning, hurried breathing and feeble pulse; sunken and altered features, distortion of the muscles of the face; the eyes are partially closed, pupils dilated and insensible to light, (may palliate the symptoms in the fourth stage.)

Sulphur: Indicated if the disease is owing to sup pression of an eruption, whether spontaneous or by external applications; it should be given at once in alternation with *Aconite,* both in water, giving Sulphur every fourth dose, and a dose of Aconite every hour.

All these medicines have to be given internally; but if the disease is caused by external injuries, a fall, blow, etc., *Arnica* may be given internally and externally. Six drops of the strong tincture may be mixed in a cupful of water, and a cloth soaked with this solution may be applied to the head fresh every two hours;

internally the pellets should be given every two hours; in water, in small spoonful doses.

Stool may be promoted by daily injections of tepid water, and the urinary discharges may be facilitated by frictions on the lower abdomen with the palm of the hand.

If the patient has to be moved, it should be done gently, and the head should always be supported with the hand; all noise must be avoided, and the room is to be kept dark.

If these dietetic and therapeutic indications are properly and seasonably attended to, a cure may be expected in almost every case.

Dropsy. (Hydrops.)

By dropsy we understand an effusion of the water in the tissue or in the interior of organs. Such an effusion is most commonly the result of some other derangement, which has to be carefully ascertained, if a cure is to be expected. Diseases of the brain, lungs, liver, spleen, ovaries, uterus, may terminate in dropsy; acute eruptions may likewise change to this disease. We distinguish the following forms of dropsy:

1. Hydrocephalus. (Chronic Dropsy of the Brain.)

By hydrocephalus we understand any morbid accumulation of fluid under the scalp, or in the cavities of the brain; the former is designated as external, and the latter as internal hydrocephalus.

In the external form, the water is either in the cellular tissue of the scalp, or else between the pericranium and the bones.

In internal hydrocephalus the water is either in the cerebral tissue or else in the cavities of the brain.

This disease either runs an acute or chronic course.

The acute internal form has been described in the preceding chapter, which may therefore be consulted; acute external hydrocephalus is generally the result of external injuries, and appears in the shape of an external swelling, involving the whole head, and sometimes even the forehead and nape of the neck. This form requires *Arnica* internally and externally, as stated under acute hydrocephalus.

Chronic hydrocephalus affects only children, between the ages of one and seven years; it is a symptom of scrofulosis, and may be a congenital disease. The disease is known by the following symptoms: The children become peevish and dull; if they had commenced using their legs, they lose their power, and their speech likewise becomes inarticulate; if they had not yet acquired the faculty of walking and talking, they do not acquire it at all. Such children are unable to hold their heads erect, which fall forwards or sideways; if the head is raised suddenly, vomiting is frequently the result. Striking changes are perceived about the head. The fontanelles do not close, but present fluctuating tumors. Pressure on these tumors may provoke spasms. Proceeding from these localities the size of the head increases uniformly in every direction, until it protrudes beyond the line of the face, which assumes an oldish, sunken appearance. Symptoms of paralysis gradually supervene, and are first noticed in the sensual organs. The eye is turned downwards, the pupils become dilated and vision becomes extinct. Taste and smell likewise vanish, the sense of smelling remains longest. The extremities likewise lose their motor power. The patients are unable to stand or walk; the feet are turned inwards. At a later period the rectum and bladder become involved in the paralytic weakness. Towards the last the patients are seized with suffocative fits about dusk, during which the breathing becomes short, panting, rattling, the face looks bluish, until the patients are relieved by vomiting tenacious mucus.

If this disease, which may last several months, or even years, is not too far advanced, it is curable, provided the right dietetic and therapeutic means are strictly used against it. The first remedy to be given is *Sulphur,* six pellets in a cupful of water, of which a dessertspoonful is to be given morning and evening for five days, after which the medicine is discontinued until a change in the symptoms indicates some other remedy. This is generally *Calcarea carb.*, which is given in the same way as Sulphur. Children who are very much emaciated, with afternoon or evening-fever, may take *Silicea* after Calcarea. This treatment will most generally arrest the further accumulation of fluid, and pave the way for a cure. But other medicines may have to be given, in case the disease should assume a more dangerous and acute form. In such a case we may have to resort to

Arsenicum, for excessive swelling of the head, pale and old-looking face; general emaciation and prostration; *vomiting is provoked by the least attempt to sit up in bed;* retention of stools and urine, or else involuntary discharges. Suffocative fits in the evening or night. Wrinkled skin.

Th: vomiting on sitting up in bed, and the suffocative paroxysms are characteristic indications for this drug, A spoonful of a watery solution of six pellets may be given every six hours, until an improvement takes place.

Belladonna; the disease manifests itself suddenly, and the symptoms resemble those of acute hydrocephalus in the second or third stage. In such a case, this medicine will only afford temporary relief, and should be given in water, every two hours.

Helleborus; at a later period of the disease, if the following symptoms make their appearance: sopor, with the eyes half closed, pupils turned upwards; tossing about in bed; loss of consciousness; complete suppression of stool and urine; spasmodic movements of the limbs, paralysis; rash.

The medicine should be given in water, a dose every two, four, six or twelve hours, according as the symptoms are more or less violent.

Mercurius; the swelling of the head is considerable, and the patients are troubled with profuse sweats which afford them no relief. This remedy is given in the same way as the former, morning and evening, unless the acute character of the symptoms should require a more frequent exhibition of the drug.

2. Hydrothorax. (Dropsy of the chest.)

This is an accumulation of water in the chest, either in one part or in the whole chest; it is acute or chronic.

In the acute form, violent dyspnœa may set in quite suddenly, sometimes in a few hours. This soon increases to such a degree that the patients can only breathe in a sitting posture and by stretching their necks forward. The intercostal spaces very frequently swell, and bulge out. A violent cough supervenes which is generally dry, or at most results in the expectoration of a small quantity of albuminous mucus. The lips and cheeks look bluish, and the features are expressive of the great anguish which the patients experience in consequence of the want of air. At first the skin is burning-hot, the pulse full, hard and tense, thirst very great; afterwards the skin of the extremities becomes cold, the pulse small, feeble, compressible. The skin now becomes dry, except on the forehead where it is covered with cold, clammy sweat. The dark-red, fiery urine is secreted in small quantities.

Acute hydrothorax may prove fatal in twelve to twenty-four hours, but may last four to seven days. In conducting the treatment we have first to moderate the fever by means of *Aconite,* six pellets in a cupful of water, of which a dessertspoonful may be given every half hour, until the fever abates; if no such improvement should take place in a few hours, one of the following remedies should be selected at once, and should either be given alone, or in alternation with some other suitable remedy.

Arsenicum; excessive anguish, with dread of dying; dullness and heaviness of the head altered features, expressive of anguish; bluish lips; thirst, the patient drinking frequently, but little at a time; suppression of the urinary secretions, or scanty urine; suffocative dyspnœa, with superficial breathing which can only be accomplished by bending the chest forward; palpitation of the heart; small, feeble, intermittent pulse; clammy sweat.

This remedy is most useful, when the disease has

reached its acme, and then only, if it can be traced to the sudden and violent suppression of a cutaneous eruption; it is scarcely ever applicable at the onset of the attack. We give it in the same way as Aconite.

Bryonia; generally after Aconite, if the fever is not modified by the latter, or if the disease depends upon previous inflammation of the lungs, or is complicated with it. For the symptomatic indications we refer the reader to "pneumonia."

Cahinca; hydrothorax setting in after scarlatina or measles, with hot skin which feels dry and unyielding like parchment, accelerated pulse, unquenchable thirst; scanty urine; shortness of breath when lying down, relieved by sitting up; quick beating of the heart, with suffocative distress when lying down; drawing, pressing and tension in the left breast.

This remedy is frequently suitable after Aconite, and should be given in water.

Digitalis; the ordinary symptoms of hydrothorax are accompanied with increased action of the heart and slowness of the pulse. Dose: every hour, in water.

Helleborus; dyspnœa, the patient gasping for air; it may be repeated in water, every fifteen minutes, until the patient feels easier.

Spigelia; hydrothorax after inflammation of the heart; the least motion, raising the arm, brings on a suffocative fit. In water, every half hour.

Chronic hydrothorax comes on very gradually. At first the patients complain of dyspnœa, but only after fatiguing exertions, going upstairs, or talking continually. Other patients are periodically troubled by a severe dyspnœa which increases towards evening and disturbs their sleep. This may continue for weeks and months, it may pass off again with expectoration and profuse perspiration, but returns again worse than before, and finally remains permanently. The patients find it impossible to lie down, have to sit up in bed, and finally are compelled to sit on the edge of the bed with their legs hanging out. Cough supervenes, at first dry, but afterwards with expectoration of large quantities of tenacious, purulent mucus. The patient's face has a bluish cast, especially the cheeks and tongue, sometimes also the hands. These local symptoms finally become complicated with the symptoms of general anasarca. The feet swell, and the swelling speedily spreads to the private parts. The skin remains dry, and is cold, especially on the extremities. The urine is generally secreted in small quantities, is dark-red and deposits a thick sediment.

The treatment of hydrothorax is accompanied with many difficulties. The course of the disease cannot always be correctly ascertained, and the perceptible symptoms are so little characteristic that it is very difficult to select the right remedy In all such cases it is of great importance that the prescribing physician should gather all the information concerning the disease which the patient's relatives or friends are able to impart. It may even be necessary to trace the whole history of the patient as far back as his earliest childhood, to find out what diseases he had been attacked with, what impressions they had left upon his body and mind, and to determine the share they may have had in bringing about the present derangement. After these preliminary remarks I subjoin a list of the most appropriate remedies in hydrothorax; they may be given in water six pellets in a cupful, a dessertspoonful morning and evening for five days, after which we discontinue the medicine until a change in the symptoms calls for a new remedy or a repetition of the former.

Arsenicum; the same symptoms as those of acute hydrothorax, especially in cases where the disease arose after the excessive use of Cinchona; both the hands and legs are swollen, and a burning distress is experienced in them, the extremities at the same time feel cold to the touch, the skin looks shallow, the symptoms are periodically worse or better.

China; the disease develops itself after frequent depletions, and the patient has frequent attacks of suffocation; wheezing and rattling breathing; nocturnal paroxysms of suffocative cough, with aching pain in the chest and scapulæ, difficult expectoration of a partly, tenacious and sometimes blood-streaked mucus; violent palpitation of the heart; scanty, dark-colored urine with brick-dust sediment.

Dulcamara; the disease has a catarrhal origin, and the patient feels worse in damp weather.

Kali carbon.; oppression of the chest, labored breathing, *pressure and stitches in the back, especially in the rena region* (a chief-symptom); the dry cough is worse after midnight.

Senega; dry cough with expectoration of tenacious mucus; oppression as if the chest were too narrow; stitches in the chest, especially when coughing and drawing a long breath; burning soreness in the chest; drowsiness and chilliness in the day-time; the pains are worse in the day-time.

This remedy is especially indicated, if the disease sets in after mismanaged catarrh.

Sulphur; this remedy may be given whenever the

disease sets in after the spontaneous or artificial suppression of a cutaneous eruption, or in cases where remedies, although apparently homœopathic, have no effect.

3. Ascites. (Dropsy of the Abdomen.)

In a general sense we understand by ascites any accumulation of fluid in the abdominal cavity, no matter what organ may be the seat of it. This general definition, however, is too vague for curative purposes; for a cure cannot be achieved unless we know the starting-point of the disease. Hence we have to be acquainted with all the morbid phenomena immediately preceding the disease, and with the exact organ where the derangement was first experienced by the patient. If the disease had its beginning in the kidneys, the treatment has to be conducted with different remedies than if the disease originates in the liver or spleen. This inquiry into what is the primarily-affected organ, is of great importance, for the simple reason that the symptoms do not always reveal it at a more advanced period of the disease.

Ascites is characterised by the following striking symptoms; gradually the abdomen swells from below upwards, the swelling varying with the position of the body; in a standing posture the swelling presses downwards and forwards; if the patient lies on the back, the swelling shifts to the groin, directly above the crest of the ilium. If the patients make a rapid motion, they as well as those near them hear the murmur of the fluid. The constitutional symptoms which are generally present in dropsy, now begin to supervene, such as diminished quantity and altered quality of the secretions, swelling of the lower extremities, etc. At first, when the accumulation of fluid is not yet considerable, it is not very easy to diagnose it. In order to obtain some certainty regarding its presence in the abdomen, we cause the patient to stand with the trunk bent forward, so that the trunk is at a right angle with the pelvis, or else the patient may kneel down, supporting himself upon his hands. Placing one hand upon one side of the abdomen, and striking the other side gently with the other hand, the fluid in the cavity is felt like a wave striking against the abdominal integuments. This examination should never be omitted, lest a simple swelling of the abdomen should be mistaken for dropsy.

These symptoms may be accompanied by many others, according as the disease, is more or less obstinate or depending upon other organs. The disease in its acute form assumes symptoms differing a good deal from those in its chronic form.

In acute dropsy the patients complain of burning and stinging pains in the abdomen, which are not, however, very severe. The abdomen becomes distended, the swelling being rather moderate, but the tension of the integuments quite considerable. The abdomen is quite sensitive to the touch. Percussion yields an indistinct fluctuation of the fluid which is accumulating in the abdominal cavity. Constipation, disposition to vomit and actual vomiting supervene. The skin is dry, warmer than usual, the abdominal integuments are sometimes even quite hot. The pulse is hurried, rather hard, either large or small, spasmodically contracted. The lower extremities are swollen and hard. The urine is scanty, dark-red, fiery or brown. The tongue exhibits a whitish coating, the thirst is intense.

This form of dropsy is frequently met with in connection with other forms of dropsy, and most frequently occurs in consequence of the sudden suppression of some cutaneous eruption.

In most cases we commence the treatment with *Aconite*, or *Aconite* and *Bryonia* alternately. They may be given in water, an alternate dessertspoonful every two hours. If no improvement takes place after a few doses, we may have to resort to *Belladonna*, especially if an acute cerebral affection had preceded the disease, and if the extremities become cold, *Arsenicum* should be given in water, a dessertspoonful every two to four hours.

The following medicines may likewise have to be used in the treatment of acute ascites.

Arnica, if the disease is caused by a blow or fall upon the abdomen, or by suppression of the cutaneous exhalation. *Aconite* and *Arnica* may be given in alternation. I continue these medicines every two to four hours alternately for eight days, then wait eight days, and resume the same treatment unles another remedy should be indicated; but if the improvement should be very marked, I wait even longer.

Cahinca; hot, tense and dry skin, quick pulse, violent thirst; nausea or vomiting with aching pain deep in the right hypochondrium. Painful distention of the region of the liver; drawing and pressing in the kidneys from within outwards; painful distention of the abdomen, with pressure upwards, as if there were not room enough; scanty secretion of urine.

If the ascites sets in after suppression of an acute

eruption, or after neglected hepatitis, this medicine will be found very serviceable; (see Sulphur.)

China; dropsical swelling of the abdomen, with swelling and induration of the liver and spleen or dropsy brought on by copious depletions. The urine is dark-red, deposits a brick-dust sediment, there is cough and dyspnœa.

This medicine may be given in alternation with *Arsenicum.*

Helleborus; the ascites is accompanied by stinging pains in the limbs, diarrhœa, partial suppression of urine, sopor.

Dulcamara; ascites caused by the suppression of the cutaneous exhalations in consequence of exposure to wet and damp weather.

Mercurius; ascites after mismanaged inflammation of the liver, with swelling and hardness of this organ; heat all over, violent sweat, short and racking couch, scanty and dark urine. Ascites that had been treated with large doses of calomel, has to be treated with *China,* or with *China* and *Mercurius* in alternation.

Chronic Ascites.

The abdomen swells from below upwards very slowly; gradually a feeling of tension and coldness in the abdomen supervenes, especially if the patient stands up; the lower portion of the abdomen seems to be pressed forwards and sideways. Upon examining the patient in the manner indicated for the acute form of ascites, fluctuation is soon perceived. The digestive functions are disturbed at the very commencement of the disease; for besides a feeling of pressure and tension in the abdomen, the patient complains of eructations, flatulence and sluggish stool alternating with diarrhœa. The lower extremities swell in the day-time, the swelling goes down again over night. At a later period the swelling remains permanent; gradually the swelling spreads beyond the calves and reaches the private parts. In the case of females the lips of the vulva swell, and in the cases of males the scrotum. The skin of the extremities is cold and pale. At first the urine is secreted in the usual quantity, but its quality is very much altered. The urine looks pale and greenish, an analysis yields a quantity of albumen; the pulse is small, feeble, empty, wiry.

Besides the remedies which have been recommended for acute ascites, and which may likewise be used in the chronic form, if indicated by the symptoms, the following medicines may likewise be required in some cases:

Kali carbonicum; excessive dryness of the skin; pressure in the abdomen as from a load; chilliness and fluc tuating sensation in the abdomen as if full of water; hard or loose stool; pale, greenish urine, with burning during and after a discharge; pulse slower than usual.

Lycopodium; ascites preceded by swelling of the feet; flatulence with aggravation of the symptoms. I have cured several cases of ascites with *Lycopodium*, which commenced with swelling of the feet or had resulted from the drying up of old sores on the legs; the symptoms seemed worse in the afternoon, and the patients felt better in the open air.

Sepia; ascites from menstrual suppression, especially at the critical age.

Sulplur; ascites preceded by suppression of cutaneous eruptions.

Ovarian Dropsy.

On one side of the abdomen, generally on the right side, where the horizontal ramus of the pubic bone joins the crest of the ilium, a tumor with drawing-stinging pains, gradually shows itself, causing at first only a feeling of pressure and weight, and being scarcely felt through the abdominal integuments, until it increases in size when it becomes distinctly perceptible, and causes an irregular distention of the abdomen. The tumor is immovable, and the patients, if turning rapidly from one side to the other, experience a sensation as if a globular body were rolling from side to side, which is caused by the changes in the position of the ovary resulting from a corresponding change of position of the body. A vaginal examination shows that the uterus is pushed out of place to the opposite side, so that the fundus of the uterus is pressed towards the left side if the right ovary is the seat of the dropsy, and *vice versâ*. The uterus is always drawn up, so much so that it is sometimes impossible to reach it with the finger. With this change in the shape and situation of the abdominal viscera, other symptoms gradually become combined, such as a feeling of numbness in the extremity of the affected side, which sometimes alternates with a drawing and tearing pain; nausea, vomiting, frequent urging to urinate, difficulty of urinating, constipation, flatulence, etc. After the disease has lasted some time, the patient's face looks pale, the pulse is small and quick, the skin feels dry, and finally the legs and private parts begin to swell.

Until recently our efforts to cure this disease, have been crowned with but limited success, even in the sphere of homœopathy. *Apis* may perhaps prove valuable in this disease. A patient who had been treated by two alloeopathic physicians and was given up to die, was cured by me by taking *Apis*, five pellets in a small tumblerful of water, a dessertspoonful morning and night for eight days; the improvement which set in progressed uninterruptedly without any further treatment, and the patient has been perfectly well for more than a year. The symptoms were: distinctly perceptible swelling of the right ovary, with sensation of pain and swelling when pressing upon the part; when the patient lies on her back, the right half of the abdomen is perceptibly raised; nausea and frequent disposition to vomit; frequent urging to urinate, scanty discharge of slimy urine; hard stool only every six days; complete dryness of the skin; small, hurried pulse; prostration; menstrual suppression.

Dulcamara and *Sabina* have been recommended by same physicians.

Dropsy of the Uterus.

This affection manifests itself with the following symptoms: The menses cease, after which the abdomen begins to swell. This swelling does not increase progressively as during pregnancy, but much more rapidly, so that in a few weeks the abdomen is as large as in the seventh month of pregnancy. If the dropsy proceeds more gradually, the increase is nevertheless more irregular than in pregnancy. An exploration shows that the vagina is cold, the womb is pushed out of its place, higher up into the larger, or lower down into the smaller pelvic cavity. On making pressure upon the lower side of the uterus, the fluid contained in its cavity is distinctly felt. Gradually the lower extremities, and finally the lips of the vulva swell, the extremities become cold, the skin is brittle, the urinary secretion is diminished, the pulse small, feeble, filiform and empty.

The disease most frequently befals women who have had many children in quick succession, or who have been debilitated by great uterine losses. Hence *China* is a main remedy for this disease, especially if the disease is caused by severe uterine hæmorrhages, and assumes an acute form. *Sabina* may be given, if the patients complain of contractive pains in the uterus, with pressing downwards from the small of the back, resulting in discharge of blood, or if the disease sets in after a miscarriage. *Sepia* may prove useful, if the effusion sets in after menstrual suppression at the critical period, or in cases where other medicines had effected relief, but no perfect cure. In one case of five months' standing, where the disease set in after artifical delivery, *Sepia* effected a cure within six weeks.

4. Anasarca, or general Dropsy.

This is an accumulation of watery fluid in the subcutaneous cellular tissue. In proportion as this accumulation increases, the cells become distended and increase in size. The consequence is that the affected part becomes enlarged, having a soft and doughy feel. The skin loses its elasticity, so that it remains pitted on pressure. It becomes pale, transparent, and feels cold and dry. The water transuding into the interior of the sheaths and substance of muscles, diminishes their motor power, whence it is that the patients become indolent and are averse to motion. As in other forms of dropsy, so in this form, the excretions and secretions are very much diminished in quantity. As a general rule the dropsical effusion does not take place uniformly over the whole body, and one side alone is first affected, the swelling beginning at the ankles and gradually travelling upwards until it reaches the private parts. General dropsy of the whole body does indeed occur, but generally only in connection with some other disease. If anasarca sets in suddenly, it is accompanied by fever; the chronic form is without any marked fever.

It must be the first object of treatment in this disease to restore the cutaneous action, for no cure is possible without a free and unimpeded action of the skin. Hence, if the skin is dry and the pulse hurried, *Aconite* will have to be administered in water every two hours. If the disease is caused by the suppression of some cutaneous eruption, with coldness of the skin and especially of the extremities, *Arsenicum* should be administered in water, a dessertspoonful four times a day. *Bryonia* is to be given in this same manner, if the dropsy sets in suddenly, the skin looks red, and Aconite is found insufficient. *Dulcamara* may be administered in this manner if the affection is caused by exposure to damp and cold weather. If Arsenic only produces partial relief, *Helleborus* may be given, and if the disease becomes chronic, and develops itself after the suppression of a cutaneous eruption, *Sulphur* may be given in alternation with some other remedy, if necessary.

The diet to be pursued in this disease, should be conformable to the general rules laid down for patients under homœopathic treatment. Dropsical patients may drink as much cold water as they please ; it is cruel to deprive them of the beverage and liquids generally which they so much crave. Milk fresh from the cow is very beneficial; meat-broth and all kinds of light but nourishing food are perfectly proper and advisable.

Typhus.

By typhus we understand fevers of a continuous type where the nervous system is chiefly involved. It is sometimes impossible to point out the precise cause of such fevers. We distinguish various forms of these fevers, each of which is characterised by peculiar symptoms. A pathognomonic sign of all these fevers is the frequent change and antagonism of the symptoms, such as: dry mouth without thirst, full development of the disease without any distinct consciousness of the same. We distinguish

1. Acute typhus.

This form is characterised by symptoms which point to the brain as the chief seat of the disorder. It attacks most frequently plethoric young subjects. After having complained for some days of dullness of the head, vertigo, headache, restless sleep with uneasy dreams, the patient is attacked with creeping chills followed by heat over the whole body, which continues all the time and is accompanied by dryness of the skin. This heat is generally attended with delirium, a disposition to escape, dread of visionary figures, or with sopor. On waking the patient shows a certain hurriedness in all his motions, and complains of buzzing in the ears. The pulse is variable, at times full and not much accelerated, at other times small, feeble, soft and hurried.

These symptoms might lead us to confound the disease with meningitis, but a careful comparison of their respective symptoms will enable us to avoid such a mistake.

At the very onset of the attack *Aconite* is the best remedy, if the following symptoms are present: great heat, with burning dryness of the skin; it can only be exhibited until the fever abates. If this result is not speedily obtained, one of the following remedies will have to be prescribed in accordance with the existing symptoms: *Bell.*, *Bry.*, *Rhus*, *Phosphoric ac.*, *Hyosc.*, *Op.*, *Stram.*, *Verat.*, *Cham.*, *Lycop.*, *Mur. ac.*, *Nux vom.*, *Camph.*

Of the selected remedy we dissolve six pellets in a cupful of water, and give a dessertspoonful every two to four hours. If two remedies are to be given in alternation, the same remedy may be repeated every four hours, giving a dose of medicine every two hours alternately.

2. Lentescent typhus.

This form of typhus runs an indefinite course, which may however be distinguished into two stages.

The first stage is very easily overlooked on account of the imperfectly marked character of the symptoms: At first the patients feel tired and heavy, and do not exactly know how to account for it; the face looks pale and puffed; the breathing becomes short and anxious, the pulse is variable, generally hurried. Sleep is restless, so that the patient does not always know whether he slept at all.

The second stage commences with chills which alternate with hot flashes. Fainting fits set in, during which cold sweat breaks out; diarrhœa likewise supervenes. Towards evening the symptoms get worse; the fever becomes more intense, the pulse more hurried, the respiration impeded, the sleep more restless. Even at this period the prostration of strength is very great, the features are somewhat altered, and express anxiety and restlessness. In the further course of the disease the consciousness which had been undisturbed heretofore, becomes impaired. The eyes are dim and without lustre, the tongue is dry and tremulous. The last named organ and the lips become gradually covered with a brownish crust. Even where the disease assumes a favorable turn, a crisis is seldom witnessed. The patients recover slowly, sleep and appetite return, the tongue cleans off, and a moderate perspiration breaks out over the whole body.

This form of typhus requires principally *Mur. ac.*, *Lach.*, *Ars.*, *Op.*, *Rhus*, *Verat.*, *China*, *Cocc.*, *Nux vom.*, *Arn.*, *Sulph*, *Merc.*

I here subjoin a few general remarks on typhus.

Every catarrhal, inflammatory fever of the mucous membranes may pass into typhus, although it is fair to assume, in such a case, that the typhoid character existed from the very commencement of the attack. If the typhoid type threatens to set in, it generally announces its advent by the following group of symptoms: Weariness even after rising, with heaviness in the limbs, irresistible drowsiness and disposition to lie down; the patient is sad, seems apathetic or absorbed in reverie. Oppressive headache, especially in the forehead, aggravated by thinking. Several paroxysms of heat and chilliness every day. Blue margins around the eyes. Loss of appetite, aversion to food and drink. Eructations tasting of musty air. Nausea, distention of the abdomen. Drawing and tearing in the bowels, especially low down, from right to left. Frequent small passages having a foul smell. Pains in the limbs as if bruised.

As soon as these symptoms show themselves, *Cocculus* should at once be given, to be accompanied with an occasional dose of *Aconite,* if dry heat and a full and hard pulse are present.

If typhus is epidemic, *Cocculus* may be taken as a preventive; it should be taken only if the least indisposition is experienced. The presence of the above group of symptoms, under such circumstances, would be an additional indication for Cocculus.

The disease commences with a chill which is first felt in the spinal column, whence it spreads over the whole body, alternating with hot flashes for six or twelve hours, after which the heat becomes permanent. The organs of the senses lose their power, the eyes become dim, the pupils fixed and dilated, the voice husky and hollow. The hearing is dull. The features lose their expression, the skin is hot, covered with a clammy, fetid perspiration. The occiput feels heavy, the dizziness of which the patient complains, proceeds from this part of the brain. Sopor and delirium set in, stool and urine are passed involuntarily. Finally the patients begin to grasp at flocks, the senses and respiratory organs become paralysed.

Warm weather, humidity of the air and want of cleanliness seem to favor the development of typhus. This is the reason why typhus so frequently breaks out in crowded hospitals, in prisons, on ship-board and in narrow and damp, dirty dwellings. If typhus prevails, the usual mode of life should not be departed from; but no cathartics should be taken which only tend to weaken the body; artificial tonics and stimulants should likewise be avoided, and persons should take a good deal of exercise in the open air. If a violent and destructive epidemic prevails, the rooms should be fumigated every day with vinegar, and ventilated in order to secure an abundance of fresh air.

All fear of contagion should be banished, and perfect faith and confidence should be had in the ruling of an all-wise Providence.

As regards the treatment of the different forms of typhus, it is of importance to bear in mind that these forms are mere modifications of the general type, and that therefore the same remedies are applicable to all. I shall indicate the chief remedies in the order of their importance, and the others alphabetically.

If the cause of the disease is known, it should be carefully considered. If the disease is caused by the continued abuse of spirits, by long watching, by excessive emotions, the most important remedy is perhaps *Nux vomica.* If care, grief, disappointed love are the determining causes, we give *Acidum phosphor.* Among the medicines which may be required by the various modifications of this disease, the following may be found sufficient: *Acid. phosph., Cocc., Laches., Lycop., Nux vom., Op., Verat., Phosphor., Puls., Hyoscyam., China, Ignat., Canth., Carbo veg.*

Although it may be well to treat every case of typhus agreeably to its own particular symptoms, yet it will often be possible, in cases where the cause of the disease cannot be fully ascertained, and where the symptoms are as yet indistinctly developed, to arrest the disease by the alternate use of *Bryon.* and *Rhus,* which may be given in alternate doses every two to four hours, in water, and less frequently *if an improvement* takes place.*

Before proceeding to enumerate the remedies which are used in this disease, I will allude to the management of bedsores which so frequently occur in this disease, and affect more especially the parts which support the weight of the body, viz.: the back and sacral regions, sometimes also the heels. We gain a good deal by preventing the breaking out of this disorder as long as possible, for we do not always succeed in preventing it entirely. To this end we place a basin of fresh water under the patient's bed, which has to be renewed every day; if it can be had, a deerskin may be laid under him, with the tail downwards. Care should be had to spread the bed-sheets very evenly and to avoid all wrinkles. If bedsores should break out in spite of these precautions, linen compresses should be dipped in a solution of five drops of the tincture of Arnica in a

* In prevailing epidemics, one medicine will sometimes be found to contain among its effects the whole series of phenomena which characterise the various modifications of the disease; but it requires an experienced eye in order to ascertain this specific curative agent. In 1853, I succeeded in curing every case of fever and ague which came under my notice in the district of Coethen, by means of *Rhus tox.*, except two cases, one of which yielded to Bryonia, the other to Tartar emetic.

cupful of water, and should be applied to the sores, taking care to prevent the dripping and to renew them frequently in the course of the day. If this does not heal the sores, on the contrary, if they should become suppurating and offensive, the linen compresses should be moistened with a solution of five pellets of China in a cupful of water. If the sores become gangrenous, a weak decoction of Peruvian bark may be applied. If the patient has made himself unclean by the involuntary passage of fæces or urine, his sheets should at once be changed, but no fresh sheets should be used unless they are perfectly dry, well aired and soft. Let us now proceed to study the symptomatic indications of the medicines which may have to be used in this disease:

Aconite; at the commencement of the disease, if the symptoms present an inflammatory type, with great heat, burning dryness of the skin, violent thirst, red face, or else alternate redness and paleness of the cheeks, nervousness, restless tossing about, moaning, anxiety, rush of blood to the head, vertigo and fainting fits when sitting up in bed. Nocturnal delirium. Tendency to start, apprehension of dying; obscured vision, dilated pupils; photophobia; painful sensitiveness of the abdominal integuments to pressure. If no improvement takes place in twenty-four hours, or if new symptoms supervene, one of the following remedies will have to be chosen.

Belladonna; alternate chills and heat, or else general heat with flushed face. Furious delirium, dread of visionary figures which the patient fancies he sees near him, disposition to escape; sleeplessness, tossing about, or sopor with grasping at flocks; the pulse is either full and strong, or small and hurried; vertigo on raising the head; violent headache, especially in the forehead; sparkling eyes, with dilated pupils; photophobia; buzzing in the ears, hardness of hearing; impeded or painful deglutition; chapped lips, ulcerated corners of the mouth; tongue dry and red, or covered with yellow mucus; loss of appetite, loathing of food; constipation; scanty, bright-yellow urine, the urine is scarcely ever dark or brown-colored; hurried, anxious breathing; faint, indistinct speech; lassitude, pains in the limbs; petechial spots on the skin.

Bryonia; chills followed by dry heat all over, with flushed face and thirst; violent delirium, the patient talks about his business and seeks to escape; quick, irregular and even intermittent pulse; sleeplessness, sopor, grasping at flocks; vertigo on raising the head; frontal headache, aggravated by moving the eyes; dim, glassy eyes, or sparkling and weeping eyes; hard hearing as if the ears were stopped; dry tongue, having a brownish coating; chapped and ulcerated lips; loss of appetite, loathing of food; constipation, also involuntary stool; scanty, red or brown urine; hurried breathing; stitches in the chest or sides; paralytic weakness of the limbs as if bruised; rash and petechiæ.

Rhus tox.; restless sleep, or sopor with stertorous breathing, muttering delirium, grasping at flocks; dry heat, anxiety; small and quick pulse; delirium, desire to escape, occasional clearness of consciousness; vertigo when turning about; flushed or pale face, with sunken cheeks, blue margins around the eyes, painted nose; hard hearing; parched lips, with brown crusts on the lips; dry red or brown tongue; bloated bowels; violent colicky pains; diarrhœa; dark urine; prostration; pains in the limbs; petechiæ.

Phosphori acidum; slow typhus, caused by grief, care, disappointed love, loss of animal fluids, with the follow- symptoms: alternate chills and heat, or heat all over without much thirst; irregular pulse, moaning during sleep, picking at flocks, at times sad, and at others smiling expression of the countenance, with distortion of the partially opened eyes. Apathy, aversion to talk; optical illusions, spectra when closing the eyes, headache on waking made worse by noise; dim, staring look, the eyes have lost their lustre; ringing and humming in the ears; blue margins around the eyes; pale face, dry tongue, watery diarrhœa mixed with undigested food; dark urine which deposits a sediment; prostration; if the disease originated in loss of animal fluids, this medicine may be usefully alternated with *China.*

Muriatis acidum; the patient lies on his back, *and settles downwards in the bed; every third beat the pulse intermits;* tongue heavy and if too long, so that the patient is scarcely able to raise it; dryness of the mouth and fauces; prostration, fetid urine.

Lachesis; dry heat with small pulse; sopor, muttering delirium, collapse of features, parched and cracked tongue, impeded deglutition, white-coated tongue.

Nux vomica; the fever is caused by the continued abuse of spirits, watching, mental labor, with the following symptoms: starting during sleep, or sleeplessness; burning heat in the whole body; small and even intermittent pulse; muttering delirium; sensitiveness to noise and light; irritable temper; vertigo and frontal headache; pale, haggard countenance; parched and blackish tongue, dry lips, loss of appetite, aversion to food and drink; bitter or foul taste; pressure in the stomach; constipation; red urine with brick dust sediment; laming and bruising pain in the limbs.

Cocculus; slow typhus, when resulting from severe diseases such as cholera; anxious starting in sleep, with hurried breathing, spasmodic motions of the head, eyes and hands; dry heat and small, hurried pulse; frontal headache; frequent fainting fits; hiccough; nausea, oppression of the stomach, laming weakness of the limbs.

Arnica; the patient lies motionless, or in a state of sopor with delirium and picking at flocks; starting during sleep, involuntary passage of stool and urine.

Arsenicum; tossing during sleep, or sopor with delirium, picking at flocks; starting and loud moaning during sleep; dry, burning heat; pulse small and hurried, also intermittent; sunken features, pale face, depression of the lower jaw; dry, cracked, black lips; parched, trembling, black tongue; involuntary stool and urine; watery diarrhœa; prostration; parchment-like dryness and coldness of the skin; petechiæ.

Camphor; cadaverous face, with open and staring eyes, or violent delirium with dullness of the head, cold and clammy skin, prostration, clammy and exhausting sweats, disposition to diarrhœa; feeble pulse. This remedy is sometimes suitable after *Rhus tox.*, but has to be repeated every fifteen minutes on account of the shortness of its action.

Cantharides; dry heat, hurried, small pulse, pale and sunken face, dry mouth and lips, tremulous voice, aversion to liquids, bloated and sensitive abdomen, watery and bloody stool, or consisting of bloody mucus; retention of urine.

Chamomilla; after a fit of chagrin, when the ordinary symptoms of typhus are accompanied by spasmodic colic, diarrhœa.

China; the disease is caused by loss of animal fluids, diarrhœa, onanism, sexual excesses, etc., with the following symptoms: Alternate chilliness and heat, weakness of the lower limbs; feeble and rather slow pulse; apathy, intolerance of noise, vertigo; headache, humming in the ears, pale and sunken features; parched lips, blackish tongue; loss of appetite; watery or yellowish diarrhœa mixed with blood; may be given in alternation with *Acid. phosph.*

Carbo vegetabilis; in the last stage of typhus, when the bowels are bloated, and the patient passes foul wind and cadaverous stool; coldness of the tongue, with cold breath.

Lycopodium; constipation, peevish mood, or nervousness, with hot head, flushed cheeks, prostration, sweats which do not afford any relief.

Mercurius; sleeplessness, starting and moaning during sleep; alternate chilliness and heat; hurried pulse, little or no delirium; listlessness; frontal headache; dim eyes without any lustre; buzzing in the ears; livid complexion, altered features; dry lips, brown-coated tongue; foul taste; aversion to solid food; desire for cold drinks; great sensitiveness of the pit of the stomach, of the region of the liver and abdomen; pressure in the right side of the abdomen, inability to lie on this side, the bowels feel as if pressed upon; diarrhœa, consisting of bloody mucus, green, yellow, also watery, spirting out; dark, red or brown urine; burning dryness of the skin, or copious, clammy, exhausting sweats. Mercurius, if given at the right time, will sometimes prevent the ulcerative process in the intestines; unfortunately this medicine is seldom indicated at the onset of the disease.

Natrum mur.; prostration, loss of consciousness, unquenchable thirst, dry tongue.

Opium; muttering delirium; *sopor and stupor with stertorous breathing,* the mouth being open and the eyes distorted.

Phosphorus; restless sleep, from which the patient wakes with a shriek; constant heat, small and hurried pulse; vertigo, stupor, headache; hard hearing, dimness of vision, pale face and sunken eyes, dry and cracked lips and tongue, loss of appetite, copious urine with whitish clouds, dyspnœa, stinging and rattling in the chest, oppressive cough with discharge of blood.

Pulsatilla; loss of recollection, delirium, sopor, crying as if in great distress, small pulse.

Stramonium; the whole body feels hot; small, hurried, tremulous, intermittent pulse; violent delirium, *frightful spectre,* disposition to escape; illusions of sight and hearing; the patient sings and prays with a devout mien, or talks in a foreign language; throbbing headache, especially on the top of the head, dilatation and insensibility of the pupils; altered features, impeded deglutition, dry and rough tongue, it trembles when put out; inarticulate speech; suppression of stool and urine.

Sulphur; if previously administered and well chosen remedies have no effect, which may be the case if the disease originates in the suppression of some cutaneous eruption, or is complicated with some other chronic affection. It is indicated by the following symptoms: Dry heat with thirst and hurried pulse, worse in the evening. Sleeplessness; delirium, with the eyes wide open; picking at flocks; pale and haggard face, with blue margins around the eyes; dry and brownish tongue; hard stool; scanty, dark-red urine, soon becoming turbid.

Veratrum album.; last stage of lentescent typhus, with coldness of the skin, and cold sweats covering the skin of the whole body; pulse slow and almost extinct; cold, cadaverous countenance, with pointed nose and sunken cheeks; sopor; almost imperceptible breathing; delirium, the body being cold, the eyes open and the face having a cheerful look; mental alienation, amorous or religious mania, thinks himself a preacher, prince, hunter; feins blindness, a cancerous disease, pregnancy, etc. This remedy is often suitable after or in alternation with Arsenic.

The patient's wants have to be attended to with great care, especially during the time of convalescence, when an indiscretion in diet may bring on a relapse. The patient should be restricted to light, readily-digested food, and should avoid all stimulating drinks. If the weakness of the patient should continue obstinate, he may take for four days a dose of China, morning and night.

The following cases show that typhus may be cured with a few doses of the specific remedy.

Two persons in different parts of our city were taken sick at the same time. I was informed by their friends that they complained of a dry, glowing heat, flushed and bloated face, and that they had had violent delirium over night, and had to be kept in bed by force. They had humming in the ears, weariness, luminous vibratory appearances before the eyes; lips and mouth were dry, the tongue red and burning; they had violent thirst, and the deglutition was impeded; bowels bloated and the abdominal integuments sensitive to contact. Frequent diarrhœic stools. I gave *Aconite* and *Belladonna* in alternation every hour. Towards evening I visited the patients and found that the delirium had subsided and that a gentle perspiration had broken out. I ascertained that one of these patients, on closing his eyes, saw a confused collection of luminous circles and points, and the other a multitude of forms which came and went. Both took *Phosphoric acid* in water, a spoonful every two hours, and on the following morning both felt well, and were able to rise and eat something, but had to walk with canes; but after the lapse of three days they paid me a visit and were able to attend to their business.

Mrs. B., residing in an adjoining village, was taken ill quite suddenly. She had a violent cough, which became worse at night, with expectoration of yellow, blood-streaked mucus; watery diarrhœa preceded by violent urging and spirting out with violence, dry and glowing heat. I sent her *Pulsat.*, *Merc.* and *Acon.*, to be taken in alternation. Next morning the diarrhœa had ceased, the cough was much less, not blood-streaked, but violent delirium had set in; the patient was constantly talking about her business; the tongue cracked and blackish, likewise the lips and nostrils; there was restless tossing about; the eyes looked glassy; the skin was dry as parchment; the lower jaw depressed, the speech heavy and inarticulate, with picking at flocks; hard hearing; stitches in both sides of the chest; the body keeps settling downwards in bed, she lies on her back with her knees bent double and pointed upwards; frequent starting. I gave *Arsenicum, Bryonia* and *Muriatic acid* in alternation, every hour.

Two days after, the following change was reported: tongue moist and clean, the black color of the lips and nostrils had left; the lips were moist, the eyes bright, speech intelligible, the picking at flocks had ceased, the hearing was better, the lower jaw was no longer depressed, and the body did no longer settle down. She feels stronger, is still slightly delirious morning and evening, and when coughing she complains of stitches in the side. These few symptoms yielded to *Bryonia.*

Yellow Fever.

This disease is peculiar to tropical countries, and manifests itself with the following symptoms: Chills, nausea, headache, especially in the forehead, generally precede the breaking out of the disease, the tongue speedily becomes coated with a thick layer of mucus, although it remains comparatively clean in some cases. The bowels at first are constipated, after which the stomach becomes so irritable that any thing the patients eat is expelled again by the mouth or rectum. After these symptoms have lasted three or four days, blood begins to ooze from the gums, nose and other orifices of the body, the face assumes an expression of reverie, the sclerotica has a dingy-red look, the eyes look glassy as in the case of drunkards; the breath is foul, almost cadaverous, the blood becomes brownish and viscid, sometimes almost black, and often has a bad smell.

The unacclimated residents of tropical regions are more especially liable to being attacked by this scourge. Among the determining causes we notice more particularly the hot days followed by cool and damp nights;

abuse of spirits, overloading the stomach with food to which one is not accustomed, such as pine-apples, bananas, etc. The disease may also be engendered on ship-board, if the air becomes vitiated in consequence of deficient ventilation, overcrowding, the use of bad water, unwholesome food, etc.

In localities where the disease prevails, *Arsenicum* in water, a small spoonful every few hours, may serve as a preventive, against the invasion of the disease, if taken as soon as the premonitory symptoms are experienced. If the disease should break out nevertheless, and the patient should complain of heat, and be restless, anxious, toss about, *Aconite* should be given in water, five pellets in a cupful, a dessertspoonful every ten to fifteen minutes.

If delirium sets in, with heat in the head, frontal headache, wild and anxious expression of the countenance, *Belladonna* may be given in alternation with *Aconite* every fifteen minutes, and less frequently if an improvement takes place. Very often this treatment proves sufficient to arrest the further progress of the disease. If it should progress toward the subsequent stages, the medicines which have been recommended for typhus, may be consulted, with any of which *Aconite* may be given in alternation, whenever the skin becomes excessively dry and hot. The following medicines may prove more especially useful:

Nux vomica, for nausea, vomiting, constipation, and excessive irritability of the stomach.

Arsenicum album, for burning in the epigastric region, with great prostration; vomiting of a blackish or brown fluid, (a spoonful of five pellets in a cupful of water may be given every five minutes.)

Veratrum album, for coldness of the extremities and the rest of the body (may be alternated with any of the other medicines, if necessary, every five to ten minutes.)

Mercurius may be serviceable, when the gums, nose, etc., bleed.

Crotalus is recommended by some physicians.

A friend has sent me the following notice of an attack of yellow fever, which is very apt to be brought about by exposure to wet, by excessive labor, etc.

The commencement of the attack varies: In some it sets in with headache; in others with a feeling of weariness, soreness and lameness in the extremities, sometimes with creeping in the tips of the fingers, blueness of the nails. Excessive prostration. Constipation in many cases, with disposition to vomit. Sopor, delirium, congestion of blood to the brain; hurried pulse (one hundred to one hundred and twenty beats).

If vomiting sets in, it is always mixed with bile. After the fever is cured, foreign residents retain a sallow complexion and remain debilitated for a long time; this weakness very frequently terminates in fever and ague.

For the premonitory symptoms, such as: tingling in the tips of the fingers, blueness of the nails, etc., *Rhus tox.* is recommended by this writer, in water, a spoonful every two hours. If the fever breaks out, and the pulse is hurried, with delirium, determination of blood to the head, hard stool, *Bryonia* may be given every hour. For bilious vomiting *Ipecac.* or *Nux vomica* may prove serviceable, or *Pulsat.*, if there is an absence of thirst. If great weakness remains, *China* may be administered in water, a spoonful morning and evening, for five days.

Sea-sickness.

This disease is caused by the balancing motion of the ship, and is characterised by nausea, headache, heat in the head, or paleness of the face, vertigo, vomiting or diarrhœa; all these ailments disappear of themselves as soon as the passenger lands on firm ground.

This disease may not only be moderated, but sometimes prevented by homœopathic agents.

Similar symptoms are sometimes induced by riding in a carriage. These symptoms can be controlled by *Cocculus*, five pellets in a cupful of water, of which a few spoonfuls may be taken some hours previous to the moment of departure, and likewise on the journey as soon as the traveller begins to feel sick at the stomach. A few pellets may be kept dissolved in a well corked vial and a small swallow may be taken whenever the least nausea is experienced.

If this should not be sufficient, and a watery diarrhœa should set in, *Arsen.* may be given in alternation with *Cocculus.*

If nausea sets in without vomiting or diarrhœa, with stinging pains in the occiput, buzzing in the ears, aversion to meat and boiled food, with a feeling of weakness, *Petroleum* may be given in the place of Cocculus.

Sulphur has been recommended for similar symptoms, with trembling of the hands and feet; and for vomiting of water and mucus, if the patient complains of heat and pressing in the forehead, with cold hands and feet, *Kreasotum* may prove most efficient.

Persons should not leave port with empty stomachs; they should take their meals regularly, eat good and nourishing food, remain on deck as much as possible, and look upwards at the sky rather than at the sea, especially if the motion of the ship is more violent than usual.

Strength of will is a most essential requisite in combating or preventing the disorder. All fear must be banished, the mind should always preserve its sway.

Inflammation of the lungs. (Pneumonia.)

This disease occurs most frequently in dry and cold weather, especially in mountainous districts, it is a most dangerous disorder, which may be excited by a keen north or north-east wind, by taking a cold drink when over-heated, by violent emotions, excessive exertions of the lungs, such as loud talking, especially against the wind, singing, running, dancing, carrying of heavy burthens, injuries, etc.

Pneumonia sets in with a violent chill which is followed by a continuous dry heat. Pain in the chest soon supervenes, especially towards the left side. A peculiar oppression deep in the chest, which afterwards changes to a stinging or aching pain, renders the breathing short, hurried and anxious. The expired air is burning hot. The face is very much flushed, and the carotids are distended. If both lungs are inflamed, the thorax is either little or not at all raised during an inspiration; if only one lung is inflamed, the thorax on the sound side is alone raised. In such a case the stinging or lancinating pain is only felt in one side of the chest, whereas, if both lungs are inflamed, the pain is felt in the whole cavity of the thorax; the inflamed portion is hotter than the other. The patient is unable to draw a long breath, because this causes violent stitches in the lungs; he prefers performing the act of inspiration with the abdominal muscles which are indeed visibly raised during it. At first the cough is dry, after a while a transparent, tenacious, and frequently reddish mucus is expectorated. The bowels are constipated; the urine is burning, and has a reddish or brownish color.

This is the first stage, in which *Aconite* is given, six pellets in a cupful of water, a dessertspoonful every two hours, or more frequently according as the disease is more or less violent. The use of Aconite is continued, until the fever is moderated, and sweat breaks out.

In order to obtain a correct knowledge of the intensity and extent of the inflammation, it is indispensable to institute a physical exploration of the chest. Percussion is performed by placing a thin tablet of ivory, or two fingers of the left hand upon the patient's chest, and striking upon them with the right index-finger. The tissue of sound lungs being filled with air, it must necessarily yield a clear sound on percussion; if this is not the case, they are either filled with blood, as in the second stage of pneumonia, termed the stage of hepatization, or with pus as in tubercular phthisis. The duller the sound, the more the lungs are filled with blood. For purposes of auscultation, the ear is likewise a much better instrument than the stethoscope. All physical signs should be principally observed on the back part of the patient's chest; for, independently of some forms of pneumonia, such as the asthenic form, occurring principally in the posterior portion of the lungs, the hepatized lungs, (or lungs which have become infiltrated with blood), especially on the right side, likewise naturally incline by their own weight to press towards the posterior wall of the thorax.

The more the cells of a portion of lung become filled with blood instead of air, the more the ordinary respiratory murmur which resembles the crepitation of common gold-foil, will disappear, and will be replaced by the so-called bronchial murmur, a sound which may be aptly compared to the slow enunciation of the German guttural "ch" and which seems to proceed from a greater depth in proportion as the disease increases in intensity and extent.

If the presence of these physical signs is announced by an increasing dyspnœa and an increasing desire to draw a long breath, if the stitches become more and more violent and the expectoration accompanying the short and hacking cough, is more and more tinged with blood, the second stage of pneumonia has set in, and we now give *Bryonia* in alternation with *Aconite,* both in water, an alternate dose every hour or two hours, until the expectoration ceases to be bloody. *Bryon.,* may already be given before this time, as soon as the fever begins to abate under the use of Aconite.

If in the progress of the disease the expectoration assumes the color of rust, we give *Phosphorus* in water, a spoonful every half hour, and less frequently as the symptoms improve.

In case there should be an excessive accumulation of mucus on the chest, with much rattling, dyspnœa, danger of suffocation, *Tartar emetic* may be substituted for Phosphorus.

For pneumonia resulting from the suppression of a cutaneous eruption, we give *Aconite* and *Sulphur* in alternation, in such a manner that *Acon.,* is given every fifteen to thirty minutes, and *Sulphur* every four hours.

If the patient is able to resume his business, but still complains of a feeling of weight and weakness on the lungs, we may derive much benefits from the use of *Sulphur*, *Lycopodium* or *Phosphorus*, according to circumstances.

If the fever should not yield to *Acon.* and *Bryon.*, and violent delirium should set in, *Bell.* is very frequently of great use, and produces even an abatement of the fever. If typhoid symptoms should supervene, *Rhus tox.* must not be lost sight of.

If we should be called to a pneumonic patient who had been bled for this disease by an allœopathic physician, we may give him *China*, one globule upon the tongue, and afterwards give *China* and Aconite in alternation, in teaspoonful doses of a watery solution every two hours.

Old-school physicians describe two forms of pneumonia which deserve a mention in this place, pneumonia notha and malignant pneumonia. Pneumonia notha or spurious pneumonia is characterised by the following symptoms: soft but hurried and small pulse, slight stinging pain in the side which is only felt when drawing a long breath; great anxiety and feeling of weight in the lungs, bloody expectoration, which increases from day to day; faint sound of the voice, and interruption of the speech by frequent paroxysms of cough. In this disease our first remedy is *Aconite*, to be followed at a later period by *Mercurius*, as soon as an aggravation of the symptoms take place.

For a dry and hacking cough, with constrictive sensation in the chest, we give Chamom., and if there is hurried and anxious breathing, *Ipecac.* should be exhibited. *Veratrum* is called for by coldness of the limbs, with great anxiety and constriction of the chest. *Arsen.* is sometimes suitable for such symptoms, especially if the prostration continues to increase. The remedies mentioned in the subsequent paragraphs may likewise be consulted.

The malignant or lentescent form of pneumonia has the following symptoms: Several days before the actual breaking out of the disease the patient begins to complain, without exactly knowing what is the matter. In a few days the patient has a chill, which is followed by shortness of breath and pressure in the chest. These symptoms are accompanied by great heat, cold and clammy sweat, dry and blackish tongue, muttering during sleep. The urine and fæces are passed involuntarily. The debility is increasing, yet the patient does not seem to be conscious of danger. The principal remedies are *Bry., Rhus, Op., Arn., Ars., Verat.*

Favorable signs of a successful termination of pneumonia are: Copious and vaporous perspiration, increased calm of the pulse and the respiratory movements, returning moisture at the nostrils, copious sediments of urates, loose expectoration. The physical exploration of the chest should not be neglected, in order to make sure that these symptomatic indications go hand in hand with the resorption of the effused fluid; the absence of fever is not always a sign that the danger is over.

A bad sign is the extension of the inflammation in both lungs, great anxiety and distress for breath, a frequent and small and finally compressible pulse; heavy, hurried and rattling breathing; breathing exclusively with the abdominal muscles (the pit of the stomach sinking in at the same time during an inspiration); pale and sunken countenance, the patient settles down in bed, lies on his back without being able to help himself, etc.

For the benefit of the reader I here subjoin the symptoms of each particular remedy:

Aconite; chill followed by dry heat, with burning dryness of the skin and violent thirst; anxious breathing, stitches in the chest, dry cough, hurried and full pulse, vertigo on raising the head; bright red, hot urine.

Arnica; pneumonia caused by an injury; stitches in the chest aggravated by coughing.

Belladonna; violent congestion of blood to the head, with flushed and bloated countenance; obscured vision; delirium; burning heat of the whole body; full and hurried pulse; labored, short and anxious breathing; lancinating stitches in the chest, cough with expectoration of bloody mucus; dark or brown-red urine. This medicine may be given after Aconite, if this remedy has no effect.

Bryonia; dry skin, violent thirst; hurried pulse, delirium, anxious, almost subdued breathing, with desire to draw a long breath; stitches in the lungs made worse by coughing and drawing a long breath; cough with expectoration of blood-streaked or rusty-colored mucus; hot urine, dark-red or brown.

Tartarus emeticus; catarrh of the air-passages with copious expectoration of mucus, mucus rale; or great dyspnœa on account of impeded expectoration of mucus, increasing to suffocative distress; incipient œdema of the lungs, with threatening paralysis of the lungs.

China; if the patient had been bled, to be given in alternation with *Aconite,* if the heat continues considerable, and the pulse is hard and quick. This remedy is indicated by a soft and thin pulse, and general debility; painful, short and hurried breathing; rattling in the air-passages, stitches in the chest.

Mercurius; heat in the whole body, violent thirst with desire for icy-cold drinks; fetid night-sweats; hurried pulse, stitches in the chest aggravated by sneezing, breathing, etc.; cough with bloody expectoration; dark, red or brown urine.

Nux vomica; pneumonia of drunkards, or after sudden suppression of hæmorrhoids, to be alternated every fonr hours with *Aconite;* also indicated by obstinate constipation.

Phosphorus; heat with anxiety; pulse hurried, hard and wiry; anxious breathing, oppression on the chest as from a load; stitches in the chest; cough with rusty sputa; the urine is dark and soon becomes turbid.

Pulsatilla; pneumonia after menstrual suppression, to to be alternated with *Aconite.* The patient moans, feels anxious and listless; the pulse is quick and soft, rattling breathing, stitches in the lungs, cough with expectoration of coagulated masses, erratic rheumatic pains in the extremities.

Rhus tox.; the ordinary symptoms of pneumonia are complicated with dryness of the mouth and intense thirst; cloudiness of the brain, excessive anxiety, lameness of the limbs and small of the back; rigidity of the joints.

Sulphur; pneumonia after suppression of some cutaneous eruption, when the disease is still imperfectly developed. It may be given in alternation with *Aconite,* especially if the following symptoms are present: Hard, quick and full pulse; difficulty of drawing a long breath; weight on the chest, stitches in the chest, dry cough with sensation in the chest as if little vesicles were breaking; cough with blood-streaked expectoration; dark urine.

If some trouble in the chest remains after the disease seems cured, a few doses of *Lycopodium* may suffice to remove the whole of it.

If pneumonia should take the form of typhus or phthisis, the remedies which have been recommended for these diseases, have to be consulted.

Inflammation of the Pleura. (Pleuro-pneumonia, pleuritis, pleurisy.)

This disease runs a course somewhat similar to that of pneumonia. These two diseases sometimes co-exist, in which case their respective symptoms form one common series. Pleurisy is characterised by a violent stinging which is felt in the walls of the thorax rather than in the interior of the chest. In some cases this pain extends to the spine, is made worse by sneezing, drawing a long breath, etc. The parts between the ribs feel sore when pressed upon. The cough is dry or accompanied by scanty expectoration of mucus, or by expectoration of blood and mucus, if the pulmonary pleura is inflamed. The breathing is short, but the expired air is not hot. The pulse is hard and hurried, but not intermittent or irregular. The skin feels hot all over, the thirst is intense. The patient feels most comfortable when lying on his back.

Aconite, a few spoonfuls of a solution of six pellets in

a cupful of water, is sometimes sufficient to cure this severe disorder; if it should not yield to Aconite, this remedy may be alternated with *Bryonia* an alternate dose every two hours; in more protracted cases, a dose of *Sulphur* may be interpolated every now and then.

If the disease sets in after heavy lifting or other severe labor, *Acon.* and *Rhus* may be given in alternation every two hours.

There is a spurious pleurisy which sometimes creeps along in a very insidious manner. The disease is sometimes preceded by lassitude and heaviness of the limbs, until the patient complains of aching, stitching and burning pains in the chest, which are considerably aggravated by going up stairs and by other exertions. The cough is generally dry, but frequently very racking as though head and chest should fly to pieces. There is very little if any fever, and the general health of the patient is pretty fair. A leading remedy against this disease is *Arnica,* to be given in water every four hours. In some cases *Bryonia* is preferable, if the patient is restless and feels feverish.

Inflammation of the Air-passages. (Bronchitis.)

The same causes which may bring on an inflammation of the lungs, may likwise result in inflammation of the air-passages.

The patients complain of a stinging and burning pain under the sternum, or of a feeling of anxiety and oppression. This is accompanied by cough which is at first dry, but afterwards is attended with expectoration of bloody mucus. The breathing is exceedingly labored, and the patient has no ease except when sitting up. The face looks pale, the skin is dry, the pulse hard and hurried, the tongue has a coating of a gray or yellowish mucus, the urine is red and scanty.

If the disease is not arrested in this stage, a general prostration of strength supervenes. The dyspnœa becomes excessive, the lips look purplish, the pulse becomes less hard but more accelerated, the skin feels cool and moist, the forehead and chin are covered with cold perspiration. The expectoration decreases in quantity, and finally ceases altogether, after which death takes place by suffocation, either because the air-tubes become closed by spasm or by exuded lymph, or else because the intensity of the inflammation results in paralysis.

If the disease is correctly diagnosed and managed from the very commencement, the dyspnœa soon ceases, the constriction across the chest abates, the cough becomes loose and is attended with a copious, thick expectoration. The pulse and skin become more natural, and the patient is very speedily out of danger.

In the case of children, acute bronchitis is still more dangerous than if full-grown persons are attacked with this disease. In the case of children the disease is characterised by the following symptoms: The breathing is more accelerated than usual, and a sort of panting murmur is heard during the inspiration; the breathing, however, does not seem much impeded, nor does the child seem to obtain much relief by sitting up. The attack seems to resemble a violent catarrh and may very readily be mistaken for it. The cough is not very marked, nor is it accompanied by expectoration. In some patients the tongue is coated, in others it is quite clean; the proffered nourishment is very seldom refused by the little patients. In many cases the fever is inconsiderable. A striking symptom is the *pale complexion* which is observed at the very onset of the disease. In most cases the pulse which is at first hard, becomes soft, but remains hurried.

In the course of the disease the breathing sometimes becomes so easy that it seems as though the child was in full tide of recovery; but suddenly the dyspnœa again becomes so violent that the patient seems threatened with suffocation. The attack passes off, but another similar attack soon takes place, and the whole course of the disease is marked by a continuance of such paroxysms. Between the paroxysms the child generally dozes, and is not much troubled with cough. If the disease increases in intensity, the dyspnœa becomes more violent and the remissions are much less frequent. Sopor supervenes; the lips assume a slightly blackish-yellow hue, which is likewise seen to some extent on the cheeks. Not infrequently we observe spasmodic twitchings of the limbs, especially on one side of the body. Even at this stage signs of recovery sometimes deceive the anxious parent; but suddenly the child dies in a fit of suffocation.

The disease runs a course of five to seven days; acute cases may end in a few hours.

It is difficult, and not always possible to distinguish bronchitis from pneumonia; the following characteristic distinctions may be kept in view. In bronchitis the *face is generally pale*, in pneumonia it is otherwise. In acute bronchitis the dyspnœa is much more marked than in pneumonia; hence the anxiety is much greater in the former than in the latter. The panting murmur which almost always exists during an inspiration in bronchitis, is seldom heard in pneumonia. The pulse is accelerated, but it is less hard and tense than in pneumonia. A physician will always be able by means of he physical signs to obtain a correct diagnosis.

The leading remedy is likewise *Aconite* which is given in the same manner as in pneumonia, in water, a spoonful every fifteen minutes. If no improvement sets in in a few hours, we alternate it with *Bryonia* in water. This remedy is particularly indicated, if the patient has to sit up in order to obtain relief. In the case of scrofulous individuals, and of persons who are subject to chronic affections of the respiratory organs, and to frequent attacks of catarrh of the air-passages, these two remedies are not sufficient; in such cases we may have to give *Phosphorus* every hour, until an improvement sets in. Other remedies may likewise be indicated, the symptoms of which I here subjoin.

Aconite is given at the commencement of the disease, if the pulse is hard and quick, the skin hot and dry, the cough dry and short, and the breathing hurried, moaning and anxious. Scanty and fiery urine.

Bryonia; for the same symptoms as those which have been indicated in pneumonia, especially if the patient has to set up to obtain relief.

Phosphorus; pale face, hard and hurried, or else feeble and quick pulse; loud, panting breathing; dry cough, with expectoration of bloody mucus.

Arsenicum; small, hurried pulse; pale face; dry cough, with expectoration of blood-streaked mucus; burning sensation under the sternum; suffocative dysp nœa, prostration.

Carbo veget.; pale or sallow complexion, dry cough, dyspnœa not relieved by sitting up.

Drosera; bronchitis after measles.

Hepar sulph.; cough with a barking sound, if the upper portion of the air-passages is affected.

Chronic bronchitis may moreover require the use of *Calc. carb.; Caust.; Iodine*; *Nitric ac.; Puls.; Senega; Spongia; Stann.; Sulph.* Compare laryngeal phthisis.

In all cases of disease of the respiratory organs the air which the patients inhale, should be very pure. The patient should not be exposed to the fumes of tobacco, to perfumes or strong odors of any kind.

Sore throat, quinsy. (Angina faucium.)

By sore throat unprofessional people generally mean an inflammation of the fauces, velum tonsils and uvula. As far as the treatment is concerned, it is immaterial what part is inflamed; if we desire to find this out, all we have to do is to press down the tongue with the handle of a spoon, and to look into the cavity by turning the patient's face towards the light.

Generally such patients complain of dryness of the throat, stinging and burning pains in the throat; deglutition is impeded, and some fever is always present.

If the fever is considerable, with dry heat, restlessness, full pulse, etc., we give *Aconite* in water, a spoonful every half hour. This treatment is sometimes sufficient to arrest the disease; if we should not succeed in this, we may then resort to one of the following remedies, which may either be given alone or in alternation with Aconite.

Mercurius; swelling and burning in the fauces, as if a

hot vapor were rising from the pharynx; violent thirst; painful dryness or else copious ptyalism; stinging pains when swallowing, with constant urging to swallow; stinging in the tonsils and submaxillary glands; sensation as if something were sticking in the throat, which has to be detached.

Bellad.; stitches in the throat, shooting as far as the ear, with constant urging to swallow; spasmodic constriction of the fauces, with inability to swallow any thing; liquids return by the nose.

Chamomilla; sore throat with swelling of the parotids, hoarseness, pain on swallowing as if a plug were sticking in the throat; excellent in the catarrhal sore throat of children.

Pulsatilla; feeling of swelling and contraction of the throat during deglutition; dryness of the throat after midnight, with tenacious mucus in the morning.

Hepar sulph.; stitches in the throat, when drawing breath or turning the neck.

Ignatia; feeling as of a lump in the throat between the acts of deglutition, or soreness during deglutition; stitches in the throat, almost always between the acts of swallowing, or passing off by continued swallowing.

Bry., Rhus, Cocculus, Lachesis, Sulphur, China may have to be used in exceptional cases.

An inflammation of the œsophagus scarcely ever occurs except as a consequence of injuries; it is not visible in the throat, the pain is felt lower down and posteriorly near the spine. *Arnica* may be required together with the above named remedies.

A chronic disposition to sore throat may be extirpated by *Mercurius* and *Sepia,* and in scrofulous individuals, *Sulphur.* A dose of the appropriate remedy may be taken morning and night for four or five days. A strict diet has to be observed.

In all cases of chronic sore throat compare the remedies recommended for laryngeal phthisis.

In acute angina the patient may drink much warm milk, or slimy decoctions. Gruel, farina, rice, etc., may be used as nourishment. The sick-room should be ventilated several times a day, of course with the required precaution, in order to avoid exposure.

Mumps. (Parotitis.)

This is a swelling and inflammation of the parotid gland under the ear. Sometimes the whole cheek and neck are involved in the swelling, so that the patient is unable to chew or swallow, and a little tepid milk has to be introduced by means of a small spoon, goose-quill, etc.

This affection is not dangerous, unless it should shift to the private parts, to which it is disposed. Hence it is necessary to keep the patient warm and to protect him from exposure. The swollen parts may be covered with a simple strip of linen.

A great remedy in this affection is *Mercurius* in water, a spoonful every two to four hours.

If the inflammation assumes an erysipelatous character, and the patient becomes delirious and lapses into sopor, *Bellad.* may be administered; and if the jaws are spasmodically locked, *Hyoscyam.* should be given, sometimes in alternation with *Merc.;* if there is much fever, heat, we give *Aconite.*

If much Calomel had been administered, or if the swelling becomes hard, and a slow fever sets in, *Carbo veg.* should be resorted to.

If the submaxillary glands are swollen, *Calc. carb.* may be given.

If the disease shifts to the scrotum, we may give *Pulsatilla*, sometimes *Nux vom.*

The following remedies may likewise have to be considered: *Aur.*, *Cham.*, *Conium*, *Dulc.*, *Hepar s.*, *Rhus tox.*

Inflammation of the bowels. (Enteritis.)

Acute enteritis is readily confounded with other diseases, according as one or the other portion of the bowels is the seat of the disease. It is a most dangerous affection, and may readily terminate in gangrene in the hands of a careless or ignorant practitioner.

The disease announces itself with the following symptoms: violent burning, cutting or stitching pain in the abdomen; proceeding from a given point, it spreads over the whole abdomen, is continuous, increasing from time to time, but never ceasing entirely like colic. The abdomen is hot, distended, and extremely sensitive to the least contact. The pains increase after eating or drinking ever so little. These symptoms are accompanied by almost unceasing eructations, frequent vomiting of a green fluid, sometimes even vomiting of fæces, and singultus. Most generally the patients complain of constipation, but sometimes a greenish diarrhœa sets in, with anxiety in the abdomen, violent urging to stool, retention of urine which is voided only in drops and has a fiery redness. The patient is tormented by the presence of an intense, continuous and increasing fever, with internal heat, a small, soft, frequent, intermittent, and but rarely full and hard pulse, dry tongue, intense thirst, excessive anxiety, restlessness and sleeplessness. Very speedily delirium supervenes, with wild looks, spasmodic twitchings of the facial muscles, contraction of the pupils, obscuration of sight, supor stupor, coldness of the extremities, violent burning in the bowels, rapid prostration, fainting fits, etc.

If the inflammation has its seat in the lesser intestines, where it is most frequently located, *pains are then most violent in the umbilical region,* accompanied with fever, nausea, restlessness, vomiting, dry tongue, intense thirst, singultus. If the pain commences below the umbilicus, invading this region of the bowels at a later period, we may assume that the larger bowels are primarily attacked by the inflammation. In cases where the symptoms are chiefly located in the hypochondria, assuming the form of pleuritis or hepatitis, the colon or cœcum is the chief seat of the affection. If the pain is felt deep in the groin, the patient experiences frequent urging to stool, passing only some tenacious mucus, the rectum is the locality where the inflammatory process has taken up its abode.

If typhoid symptoms are present, the diagnosis of the disease is much obscured. The phenomena of typhoid enteritis are much less marked than those of the simple acute form of this disease; not infrequently the existence of the disease is only fully and satisfactorily revealed by a post-mortem examination. The pulse is very small and quick, sometimes rather soft than hard and contracted, the features sunken and altered, the eyes dim, the abdomen puffed. Soon the extremities become paralyzed, stool and urine are passed involuntarily, the power of speech and deglutition becomes extinct. If the disease is consequent upon the sudden suppression of a flow of blood from the uterus or bowels, the symptoms assume at once a most dangerous character; the pains and vomiting are excessive, the pulse is small, contracted, wiry and nervous. Violent deliruim and spasms are generally present.

By contrasting the symptoms of enteritis with the symptoms of maladies with which it might possibly be confounded, we shall be enabled to establish a correct diagnosis of the disease. Its characteristic symptoms are: More or less intense pain in some portion of the abdomen, aggravated by mere contact, and considerably so by pressure; distention of the abdomen; coldness of the extremities, sudden prostration, altered features, small and irregular pulse; obstinate constipation.

The disease may run its course in three days, and seldom lasts longer than nine days; slight cases may last a fortnight; in its most acute form it may terminate fatally in a day.

Enteritis may be superinduced by a variety of causes: abuse of cathartics and stimulants; mechanical injuries inflicted upon the bowels by the introduction of some deleterious substance, acids, pointed bodies, etc.; cold drinking while the body is over-heated; violent suppression of diarrhœa or habitual losses of blood; lifting heavy weights; exposure of the bowels and feet to taking cold; suppression of existing cutaneous eruptions; gout, rheumatism; mechanical injuries of the the abdomen; childbed; inflammation of neighboring organs; incarceration of hernia, etc. Season and climate, and the changes of temperature incidental to locality, have likewise much to do with the development of enteritis. The small intestines are more frequently invaded in spring and summer; the larger bowels more frequently at the beginning of fall.

We commence the treatment with *Aconite*, six pellets

in a cupful of water, a dessertspoonful every hour, until the patient feels more comfortable.

If given at the very commencement of the attack, *Aconite* will suffice in many cases to control the disease; but if the exhibition of this agent is delayed, one of the following remedies may afterwards have to be resorted to.

Arsenicum; cutting, tearing, burning pains in the bowels; restlessness and anxiety; vomiting, sunken features; coldness of the extremities; small, quick, intermittent pulse; bloody stool.

Belladonna; the ordinary symptoms of enteritis are accompanied by delirium or spasms, (may be alternated with *Arsen.* every half hour in water.)

Bryonia; after Aconite, if the fever is less, but the abdominal integuments continue very sore and sensitive, the pains are aggravated by the least motion, or if a typhoid character develops itself. It may be repeated every three or four hours.

Chamomilla; enteritis of children during dentition, with foul diarrhœa, slimy or watery (in alternation with *Acon.* every half hour.)

Mercurius; cutting and burning in the bowels, sensitiveness to pressure, quick pulse, rheumatic pains in the limbs. Chiefly indicated in the fall, when dysentery, violent colics or rheumatic pains in the extremities prevail.

Nux vomica; enteritis from sudden suppression of hæmorrhoids, with stinging, tension and burning in the bowels, also with eructations, and disposition to vomit.

It is especially useful, if drunkards are attacked with the disease, in which case *Nux* and *Acon.* may be given in alternation every hour.

Pulsatilla; enteritis after menstrual suppression, with tearing pains in the bowels, coming on in paroxysms and being attended with chilly creepings (in alternation *Acon.*, and afterwards alone.)

Rhus tox.; pressure, stinging, tearing, burning in the bowels, worse after drinking; the disease is caused by keeping on wet clothes after exposure to rain; it may assume a typhoid type, and partial paralysis may set in.

Sulphur; if the disease is caused by suppression of cutaneous eruptions (in alternation with *Acon.*)

Most cases of enteritis have yielded in my hands to the alternate use of *Ars.* and *Puls.*, preceded by *Acon.*

If the pains are worse every other day, or if much weakness remains, after the inflammation is subdued, *China* may be given.

Old-school physicians have been in the habit of using cathartics and drastics in this disease; on the contrary, constipation is a much more favorable symptom than diarrhœa, and will always yield to adequate constitutional treatment.

Patients may drink moderate quantities of fresh water; their chief drink should be mucilaginous decoctions. Rest is absolutely required for the restoration of the patient.

Cramp of the Stomach. (Cardialgia, Gastralgia, Heartburn, Pyrosis, Eructations, Waterbrash.)

These various expressions refer to well-known derangements which either occur singly or all together, frequently are very painful, and even incurable under Old-school treatment.

Homœopathy not only cures these affections, if

recent, without any difficulty, but extirpates even the least trace thereof in inveterate cases.

These derangements may result from various causes, immoderate eating and drinking, abuse of coffee oı ardent spirits; emotions, such as anxiety, chagrin, grief, fright; they may also have a catarrhal origin, by getting the feet wet or cold drinking when the body is over-heated.

By neglecting these derangements, serious disorders may often result from them, such as cancer of the stomach, consumption. Hence it is advisable to at once employ proper treatment, and institute a careful comparison of the subjoined remedies, six pellets of one of which may be dissolved in a cupful of water, of which solution the patient should take a small spoonful morning and night for four days, after which no medicine need be taken for some weeks or even months, even if a momentary aggravation should take place after first taking the drug.

If one remedy does not seem sufficient, two may be given in alternation; if *Nux* is indicated by local symptoms, and the patient has been afflicted with an eruption for which *Sulphur* would have been a specific remedy, these two medicines may be given in alternation; or if, in the case of a nursing female, much debility had been caused by nursing, *Nux* and *China* may be given.

In giving a list of the most important remedies for this disease, I have mentioned the most important ones first.

Nux vomica; suitable to drunkards and lovers of coffee; also a remedy for the consequences of an excessive use of Chamomilla. Violent contractive, pressing, crampy, tearing sensations in the stomach, with sensation as if the clothes were too tight, or as if flatulence had become incarcerated under the ribs; bloating of the pit of the stomach, feeling of oppression on the chest, extending to the small of the back, and between the scapulæ; nausea, flow of clear water in the mouth, or gulping up of a sour or bitter fluid, with burning in the œsophagus, heartburn, sour or foul eructations and vomiting; constipation; frontal headache, or headache in the temples or occiput; palpitation of the heart, anxiety. The pains are worse in the morning, after eating, drinking coffee or using acid things; the patient feels better during rest. This medicine is especially adapted to persons who lead a sedentary life, with irritable dispositions; also to females, if the menses are too copious and premature.

Chamomilla; cardialgia from chagrin, painful pressure at the stomach as from a stone; painful bloating of the pit of the stomach, with shortness of breath, anxiety, throbbing headache. Nocturnal aggravations; relieved by bending double, and by taking coffee, (Nux vom. is indicated, if the attack is caused by coffee.)

Belladonna; pressure and cramp in the stomach, returning every day at dinner, also at night, with trembling and even with loss of consciousness on account of the intensity of the pain, which is relieved by stretching the trunk backwards and holding one's breath. Obscuration of vision when stooping; vertigo; vomiting of bile or mucus; intense thirst, the pains are made worse by drinking.

Pulsatilla, stinging and pressure in the stomach, after the use of fat food, pastry, warm bread (heartburn) with thin or papescent stool, vomiting of bile; bitter taste, absence of thirst; flatulence, aggravation in the evening and during motion, especially when making a wrong step; is especially adapted to females having a pale complexion, with gentle, desponding dispositions, scanty or suppressed menses.

Carbo veget.; painful pressure and cramp in the stomach, with burning, after the use of fat and flatulent food; heartburn, with sour and acrid rising from the stomach; the pain compels the patient to bend double; aggravation in a lying position, or after a fright, cold; the mere thought of food excites nausea and vomiting.

Ignatia; the distress is caused by care and grief; feeling of weakness and qualmishness in the pit of the stomach; feeling of emptiness, pricking sensation in this region.

China; oppression of the stomach after eating ever so little; bitter eructations, tasting of the ingesta; the disease sets in after great loss of animal fluids, by depletion, sexual excesses, nursing, abuse of cathartics, etc.; the pains are worse when the patient lies on the side, and relieved when he turns on his back, or rises from his seat; the patient feels most comfortable before breakfast.

Cocculus; constrictive pains in the abdomen, relieved by emission of flatulence, and flow of water in the mouth; hard stool, peevish mood.

Arnica; spasmodic cardialgia, with digging in the pit of the stomach, as if a fall were winding up; bitter and foul eructions; the attack is caused by lifting heavy weights or doing hard work.

Sulphur; cardialgia with sour and empty eructations, regurgitation of food, heartburn; especially suitable if the patient had been or is afflicted with chronic eruptions; it may be given in alternation with some other remedy.

These are the most important remedies for cardialgia; here follow some other remedies which are less frequently called for.

Bryonia; oppression after eating, soreness, stitch when when making a wrong step.

Ipecac.; intense distress in the pit of the stomach, vomiting of quantities of mucus which looks green and gelatinous.

Stannum; cardialgia with retching, griping in the stomach, short breathing, vomiting of blood.

Graphites; cardialgia with scanty menses.

Sepia; pressure in the stomach as from a stone, with stinging and burning, especially at the critical age when the menses are scanty or intermittent.

Calc. carb.; cardialgia, with loss of appetite, especially suitable to fat people.

Staphysagria; pressure in the stomach as from a load, made worse by eating.

Indigestion.

A main remedy, if the stomach is overloaded, with taste of food or eructations tasting of the ingesta, loss of appetite, aversion to food, nausea and vomiting, is *Antim. cr.*, six pellets in a cupful of water, a spoonful four times a day.

Pulsatilla, after eating fat, pastry, rancid butter, fruit, etc.

Carbo veget.; when similar causes prevail, with burning in the stomach, and extreme sensitiveness to external pressure; also after salt food.

Nux vomica; suitable to persons who indulge in the excessive use of spirits, coffee, and are subject to constipation of the bowels; the effects of a late supper or an unusual imbibition of spirits may be kept off by a dose of Nux before retiring to bed.

Arsen.; chilling the stomach by ice, or cooling drinks when over-heated; watery diarrhœa.

China; derangement of the stomach caused by bad fish or meat; if caused by sausage-poison or smoked meat, consult the article "Poisoning" by sausage-poisoning.

In the spring and fall the stomach, especially among persons who inhabit marshy districts, often show signs of derangement, such as loss of appetite, eructation, vomiting of undigested food, feeling of debility, restless sleep, etc.; these symptoms often constitute the precursors of an attack of fever and ague. *China* is an excellent remedy under these circumstances.

Ipecacuanha; the derangement cannot be traced to a definite cause; the patient complains of excessive nausea, qualmishness, disposition to vomit, vomiting of the ingesta, diarrhœa, gagging with vomiting of mucus and bile. (A spoonful every two to four hours.)

The diet should be simple, light soups are best, for they will afford the stomach time to recruit; gradually more substantial food may be used, until the ordinary diet can be resumed.

Persons who are subject to attacks of indigestion, should always partake of every kind of nourishment in moderate quantities, lest habitual attacks of indigestion should finally develope some organic disorder.

Weak Stomach. (Dyspepsia.)

In this condition of the stomach, the lightest kind of nourishment is no longer digested; it remains undigested in the stomach, and finally passes off in this form.

The causes of dyspepsia may be general bodily weakness, chronic diseases, loss of blood, etc.; spirituous drinks, emetics and cathartics, prescribed in the old fashion, may cause dyspepsia; immoderate eating, the excessive use of sweet things, sugar-plums, candies, preserves, may likewise cause it.

Persons with weak stomachs should carefully abstain from tonic bitters, orange-peel, ginger, etc.; for all such artificial stimulants and tonics tend to increase the weakness.

The first thing to be done, in treating dyspepsia, is to regulate the diet. Newly-baked bread, fat, drawn-butter, things baked and fried in butter, flatulent food, should be avoided.

Milk fresh from the cow is generally very agreeable to such patients; stale bread should be used that is at least a day old. At dinner light meat-broth, and boiled or roast meat with vegetables. No veal, because it is indigestible; fowl may be allowed.

If all this kind of food is still too heavy for the patient, he may confine himself for some time to dry bread, without any liquids; this will soon quiet the stomach, as experience has shown. The chief therapeutic agents are *China*, *Hepar*, *Sulphur*, and the remedies which I have recommended for cardialgia and indigestion. The remedies should only be given at long intervals, giving of each single remedy a teaspoonful of a watery solution morning and evening for five days.

Inflammation of the Stomach. (Gastritis.)

This disease is either acute or chronic.

1. The acute form sets in suddenly, and is generally attended with violent symptoms. The patients complain of burning, stinging, lancinating or tensive and constrictive pains in the region of the stomach, which continue without intermission; are aggravated by contact, motion, coughing, sneezing, swallowing, and often spread over the whole abdomen and back. The region of the stomach is distended, bloated, hot and hard. These symptoms are accompanied with great anxiety, frequent and violent vomiting, first of the food contained in the stomach, and afterwards of mucus or a grass-green fluid, and finally even of blood. The vomiting is renewed if the least nourishment is introduced into the stomach, but it affords no relief. If the vomiting stops, a violent, long-lasting hiccoughing frequently sets in, with bitter and foul eructations, or a torturing feeling of constriction in the throat. The tongue is generally red, especially at the tip, in some cases it has a thick coating; stool and urine are retained. All these symptoms are accompanied by an intense fever, with hurried pulse which is very frequently hard and full, but in some cases small, spasmodically contracted and intermittent. Unless the disease is arrested at the onset, it soon reaches its acme, when it is characterised by the following symptoms: The pulse is soft and wiry; the trunk, especially the region of the stomach, is hot, the extremities are icy-cold; the face is pale,

sunken, the features very much altered. Headache, delirium, labored breathing, spasms of the œsophagus, fainting fits and hydrophobic symptoms likewise supervene.

The causes which may induce an attack of gastritis, are quite numerous; a successful treatment of this disease renders a knowledge of its causes absolutely necessary An inquiry into the cause of the existing symptoms should never be omitted. The disease may have been caused by poison, and the poison would have to be removed, unless this should have taken place previously; in accordance with the rules laid down under the head "Poisoning." Gastritis may likewise be caused by swallowing ice when the body is over-heated, by the use of acrid spices, spirits, the introduction of pins, glass-splinters, fish-bones and other pointed bodies into the stomach, violent concussion of the region of the stomach by blows, etc., suppression of existing cutaneous diseases by external means, suppression of habitual losses of blood, such as hæmorrhoids, menses, lochia, etc. In investigating the causes of gastritis, we should never suffer ourselves to be misled by a speculative theory; if the cause cannot be ascertained with positive correctness, the symptoms alone can guide us in selecting a proper remedy.

If there is much heat, and the pulse is full, hard and bounding, *Aconite* should be given in water, a small spoonful every fifteen minutes. If violent vomiting is present, which does not afford the patient any relief; if the features are altered and the extremities cold, *Arsen.* should be administered as the most perfectly corresponding homœopathic specific. Six pellets may be dissolved in a cupful of water, of which the patient may take a dessertspoonful every thirty minutes. If the patient cannot keep the water on his stomach, a pellet may be placed upon his tongue every half hour.

Other medicines may likewise be required, especially if the inflammation invades neighboring organs. Among these we distinguish:

Nux vom., gastritis of drunkards; burning, especially at the pyloric orifice.

Belladonna; burning pains in the stomach, with delirium, dread of liquids.

Bryonia; burning in the stomach aggravated by motion, the vomiting sets in after drinking.

Cantharides; stinging or burning pains in the stomach, with pains in the bowels, kidneys or bladder.

Hyoscyamus; vomiting of blood, dread of liquids; spasms after drinking.

Phosphorus; if Arsen. is not sufficient, and the following symptoms are present: burning in the stomach with violent thirst, anxiety, altered features, spasms in the facial muscles, coldness of the extremities, feeble pulse.

If gastritis is caused by vegetable poisons, the antidotal treatment recommended in the article on "Poisoning" should first be resorted to, after which a few drops of the spirits of Camphor may be given every five minutes on a lump of sugar, or in a small spoonful of tepid water.

Beside the medicinal treatment the patient should pursue the strictest diet. He should only drink small portions of slimy drinks, and never unless he experiences a desire for drink. In order to quench his burning thirst, he may swallow every now and then a spoonful of fresh water. Great relief is likewise afforded by frequently rinsing the mouth with fresh water. The if fever is present, *Aconite* in alternation with the other medicines.

As soon as a stagnation of milk takes place, we give *Bellad.* and *Bryon.* in alternation, every hour or two hours, and if fever is present, *Aconite.* Sometimes *Rhus tox.* may be useful, and if the delirium continues, we may give *Bellad.* or *Acon.* in alternation with *Apis.*

11. Continued pains in the interior of the breast or in the back, also a painful drawing and tension in the nape of the neck, or violent toothache, show that the nursing wears upon the mother; if this is the case, we give *China*, six pellets in a cupful of water, a spoonful four times a day, and if a change does not speedily take place, *Bellad.* in alternation. If the pains recur, nevertheless, we give the same medicine to the child if the pains do not cease in a few weeks, the child has to be weaned. Before resorting to this extreme measure, it may be well to first try Nux vom. in water, a spoonful morning and night, for four days; the dorsal ablutions with cold water should never be omitted; moreover they should be performed by a person in good health and of a robust frame.

12. Constipation will take care of itself, and does not require any medicine; if the bowels have been weakened by cathartics, and the patient is inconvenienced by this state of the bowels, *China* may be given, s pellets in water, a spoonful every two hours, or *Nux vom.* and *Bryon* in alternation, a spoonful watery solution of six pellets every four hours. A injection of oat-meal mucilage beaten up with a little sweet-oil, may likewise be administered. But unless constipation cause or inconvenience, nothing nee be done for it in the of therapeutic treatment.

13. *Retention of urine, spasm of the bladder.* During the passage of the child's head out of the uterus, it is sometimes pressed against the neck of the bladder with so much force, that it causes an irritation and inflammation of this organ. This condition is attended with retention of urine, spasm of the bladder. The best remedy is *Arnica.* Next to Arnica, we have *Nux vom.* or *Canth.*, a dose every half hour, especially if the urine passes off drop by drop, and the discharge causes pain. It may likewise be well to steam the parts, for the warm vapors have a relaxing power. If the urethra is closed to such an extent that no urine can pass, a catheter has to be introduced.

·1⁴ *Puerperal miliaria* generally sets in with fever, ı ɜness, heat, and the body, or a portion of the body, is covered with red little tips. We first give *Acon.*, six pellets in water, a spoonful every hour or two, also in alternation with *Bry.;* and if diarrhœa, colic, fainting fits are present, *Ipecac.* For miliaria alba we give *Arsenic.* if it is characterised by burning itching. If the miliaria suddenly recedes, we give *Bry.* every two hours, in alternation with *Bell.*, if the patient is delirious. Of course, she should be be kept warm.

15. Dietetic transgressions, a cold, a violent emotion, ıy cause inflammation of the womb (metritis). It is ·icated by a pain in the region of the uterus, especi- when touching it, or when touching the uterus through the vagina; this last-named organ feels hot and dry, since the lochial discharge generally ceases; the patient complains of fever, ·· irst, loss of appetite. t the first outbreak of this d· , we give *Acon.* and 'l. in alternation every half ..our; this will be suffi

www.ingramcontent.com/pod-product-compliance
Lightning Source LLC
LaVergne TN
LVHW010234110826
845151LV00004B/1295

* 9 7 8 1 4 2 5 5 2 4 7 3 9 *

HER MAJESTY'S TOWER.

BY

WILLIAM HEPWORTH DIXON,

EDITOR OF THE "ATHENÆUM," AND AUTHOR OF "NEW AMERICA," "SPIRITUAL WIVES," "THE HOLY LAND," ETC.

SECOND SERIES.

PHILADELPHIA:
J. B. LIPPINCOTT & CO.
1869.

PREFACE.

This volume contains the story of the Anglo-Spanish Conspiracy; a story which has not yet been told, except in patches, and only then without the connecting bands.

I have already noted these Studies as a work of identification. Among other things now made out in the Tower, may be named: the situation of our early Court of King's Bench and Court of Common Pleas,—the connection of St. Thomas of Canterbury with the Water Gate,—the lodgings of Lady Jane Grey,—the crypt of Sir Thomas Wyat and the Men of Kent,—the chamber of Archbishop Cranmer,—the apartments of Bishop Leslie,—the various towers in which Raleigh lodged,—the two prisons of Lord Grey,—the dungeon of Guy Fawkes and Father Fisher,—the locality of the conferences of Father Garnet with Father Oldcorne,—the home of the Wizard Earl and the three Magi,—the tower from which Seymour escaped,—the room in which Overbury was poisoned,—and the lodgings in which the Earl and Countess of Somerset lived. The new facts will enter into a good deal of our history and biography.

But the interest of this volume (it may be hoped) is general rather than local; lying mainly in the new lights under which recent research permits a student to tell the great story of our national life.

In making these Studies—the occasional labor of my pen for more than twenty years—I have received much help from Sir THOMAS D. HARDY, Deputy-Keeper of the Public Records, and from Lieut.-Colonel F. C. WHIMPER, Major of the Tower. J. E. GARDNER, Esq., has opened to me his unrivaled Collection of Old Prints and Drawings; and A. KINGSTON, Esq., has lent me his critical eye and ready hand in reading and copying the State Papers in Fetter Lane. I tender them my warmest thanks.

6 ST. JAMES'S TERRACE,
Regent's Park.

CONTENTS.

HER MAJESTY'S TOWER.

CHAPTER I.

THE ANGLO-SPANISH PLOT.

During the fourteen years through which Raleigh wrote in the Bloody tower and lit his fires in the Garden house, a line of prisoners, more or less closely linked with his fortunes, passed into the Tower; some of them to spend within these vaults a week of doubt and pain; others to die in them a daily death for years; this man to baffle his keeper and slip his chain; that man to fret out his soul against bolt and bar; while most of their fellows in mishap were only too glad to escape from damp and gloom, from wheel and cord, by way of either the hangman's rope or the headsman's axe.

The first of these prisoners, in point of time, was Thomas, Lord Grey of Wilton Castle, who lived nine years in the Brick tower on the northern wall. With Grey came William Watson and William Clarke, two Secular priests, the alleged companions of his crime. These men were followed by Guy Fawkes and his companions, who were thrown into the dungeons of the Keep; by Fathers Garnet and Oldcorne, who were lodged in the lower rooms of the Bloody tower; by Father Fisher, who has left his name on a door-post in the White tower; by the Earl of Northumberland, "the Wizard Earl," who lay in the Martin tower; by Lady Arabella Stuart, who lived and died in the Belfry and the Lieutenant's house; by her husband, William Seymour, who escaped from the Water gate; by the Countess of Shrewsbury, who occupied the Queen's lodgings; by Sir Thomas Overbury, who was poisoned in the Bloody tower; and on the morrow of Raleigh's liberation, by Lord and Lady Somerset, who lived and quarreled in the Bloody tower and the Garden house. All these prisoners may be called the Raleigh group.

The story of this group of prisoners is that of the rise and fall of a great conspiracy, the Anglo-Spanish Plot. This conspiracy endured through many years, survived various chiefs, and put on divers shapes. It had a foreign birth and a foreign end, though it was conducted on the English soil by English hands. Conceived in the cabinet of King Philip, it was prepared in the English Colleges of Douai and Valladolid, and put into action in our London suburbs and our midland shires. The men who began it were Jesuits and the pupils of Jesuits; the men who continued it were Councilors and Peers; but whether the work was done by Persons and Garnet, or by Cecil, Suffolk, and Northampton, the purpose kept in view at Madrid was ever the same—the subordination of our national life to that of Spain.

While the Jesuits held the reins, the motive power was religious zeal; when the Councilors held the reins, the motive power was gold. Though trained in a foreign school, the Jesuits could only be persuaded to serve the King of Spain so long as they felt that in serving him they were doing their duty to God and Holy Church. The Peers who succeeded to their office as "Friends of Spain," allowed no such scruples to stay their course. Having a country to sell, they made their infamous bargains with the Spanish ambassador, and built such palaces as those of Hatfield and Charing Cross on the wages of their shame.

This Anglo-Spanish Plot was the mother of many treasons. The Essex rising, the Priests' Plot, the Main and the Bye, the Seymour Escape, and the Powder Poisoning, were but details springing from a common source.

The chief of this plot for many years was Henry Garnet, Prefect of the English Jesuits.

The Prefect, a square, bluff man, of middle age, much worn by care if not by drink, and looking ten years older than he was, had a string of different names. In Flanders he was known as Father Greene, Father Whalley, and Father Roberts. In England he passed under the priestly names of Father Garnet, Father Darcy, and Father Walley, under the lay names of Mr. Farmer and Mr. Mese. He had as many homes as names; not to speak of the houses of his penitents and pupils, which were to him as homes. He had a house called White Webbs, in Enfield Chase; a lodging in Thames Street, near Queenhithe; a secluded residence on Wandsworth Common; an old manor at Erith, which he used for the coming and going of his agents by the Thames.

This man of many names and domiciles is said to have kept a merry table. He was accused of a fondness for female society which ill became a priest, and the name of Helen Brooksby was coupled with this hint of frailty, even more than that of her sister Ann Vaux. These hints of an undue fondness for wine and women rest not on the words of his Protestant enemies, but on those of his Catholic friends—most of all, on the words of his fellow-confessors.

It would be unfair to urge against Garnet all that

was said of him, even by his fellows, after he had played his game and lost his life; for the whole body of the Secular clergy hated him as an upstart and intruder in their Church, while many of his brethren in the Society, blessed with more patient tempers and more moderate hopes, disliked his memory as that of a man who had brought discredit on their craft. From neither side had Garnet much in the way of mercy to expect; a balance must be struck between the words which were spoken and the facts which were proved.

The Prefect was a fine linguist, a subtle reasoner, a good divine; but no one who knows the story of his time will say that he lived a perfectly blameless life. When a lad at Winchester school, he was flogged for offenses which have no name; and the conditions under which he resided as a grown man in Italian cloisters, in Flemish camps, and in English country-houses, were in high degree unfavorable to personal virtue. Most of his days and nights were spent in evading spies, in studying tricks and masks, in passing under false colors, in conducting spurious business. One day he was a rich merchant from the City, next day a poor soldier from the wars; here a married man, there a single one; now a tavern-ruffler, with rapier ready on his thigh; anon a starving curate, full of ardor for his queen. Each day was to him a fight for liberty and life. The fate of his old companions weighed upon his mind. Southwell had been hung. Weston still lingered in the Clink—a daily warning that if he meant to live and labor for his Church he must put on every disguise that natural craft and wide experience could suggest as a cover for what he was. Short of this masking, he would fail at once. Yet while it would be harsh to urge against Garnet that his changes of name and dress were in themselves immoral, as tending to deceive, it would be idle not to see that a life so spent implies a vast deal of lying, and that lying, for whatever purpose it may be done, is utterly corrosive to heart and soul. A saint could not live a daily lie.

That Father Garnet loved good wine and plenty of it, we know from the highest source—himself. Claret was his table-drink, and he liked to wind up his repast with sack. Sometimes he drank so freely that his servants had to put him to bed. Now and then he got drunk. But there is no reason to believe, with Bishop Abbott, that he was a constant sot; the very life he led being evidence against such a calumny. That he was fond of female society, and indulged his weakness to the point of public scandal, there can be no doubt. The ladies living under his roof may have thought themselves the Martha and Mary of a new reign of grace; but the Prefect knew that the world would not judge their conduct in this pious vein. The world condemned them. The Church condemned them. In the writings of the Secular priests, this weakness of the Jesuit Prefect was denounced in terms which leave no room for doubt as to what was meant.

The rival and destroyer of Father Garnet was his successor as chief of the Anglo-Spanish Plot in the second phase. This man was Lord Henry Howard, better known as Earl of Northampton, the title which he bore in the reign of James the First.

Northampton was the second son of Lord Surrey, singer of the Songs and Sonnets, lover of the Fair Geraldine. An Italian soothsayer promised the poet that his child would pass through a youth of want and trouble, a manhood of honor, an old age of wealth. The noble poet may have smiled at such auguries for a son of the ducal house of Howard; but these words of the Italian wizard were called to mind when the poet had fallen beneath the axe and his son was an outcast and a beggar in a foreign land. A dark Greek fate appeared to pursue Northampton's race; his father, the poet, had perished on the block—his brother, Duke Thomas, the lover of Mary, had perished on the block—his nephew, Philip the Confessor, had died in the Tower. A pauper in the land of his birth, an exile in Italy and France, the future patron of learning was unable to buy a new book, and the designer of Audley End was forced to seek shelter in a barn. Is it strange that miseries which few men could have borne at all, should have unstrung in the poet's son a mind that was quick and fertile, rather than great and strong? He had lived in Rome, where his life was gracious, but not pure. In Rome he became a Catholic—a Catholic of Italian rather than of English type. From the Tiber he passed to the Arno, where he studied art in the Pitti Palace and morals in the Piazza dei Signori. In Florence he left behind him that best companion and guide of genius, a loyal and manly heart; for in the court of Cosmo de Medici he learned the art of changing sides with the time, of urging and denying with the same soft speech, of seeming to be all things to all men; a Prelatist in the company of bishops, a Reformer in that of Puritans, a Catholic in that of priests, a Royalist in that of kings. With one lesson learned from the Tower, corrected by a second lesson learned from the Lateran, he lost his faith in creeds, in councils, and in men. Religion, Country, Virtue, were to him but words; words sounding in his ears like the idle wind. Place, Power, and Money, he could understand; and after these things had been won, he could taste the delights of pomp and rank. His taste was fine and his learning wide. He loved to build great mansions, to buy fine pictures, to store up costly jewels, to collect rare books. All these things cost large sums, and money was to him a need, like his daily bread.

Bent on building up once more the fallen house of Howard, he never paused to debate the means. Show him a road that led to place, he took it; show him a road that led to gold, he took it; never stopping to inquire if the path were such as an honest man could take. The brother of a duke who had lost his title and estates, how could Northampton afford to be an honest man? A little was gained on the coming in of James; he was made Earl of Northampton; his nephew Thomas was made Earl of Suffolk; his grand-nephew, the son of Philip, restored in blood, was created Earl of Arundel and Surrey. But the family was poor, and the ducal coronet of his race was lost.

Northampton, now growing old, and fretted by a foul disease, was still stout in purpose and stanch in brain. No sense of shame ever checked his tongue. If a man could help him to get on, he was willing to serve that man in ways which would have degraded the vilest slave. While Cecil reigned, he pandered to that sly and secret voluptuary by putting in his way the Countess of Suffolk, his lovely and venal niece; just as, some years later, he encouraged her still more beautiful and profligate daughter, Lady Essex, to violate her nuptial vows with Carr.

This hoary sinner, having a keen sense of the value of virtue as an article of trade, kept a large assortment of moralities on sale. No lord of the court could make a finer speech. His maxims were always noble; his words were always chaste. He never sold a niece for money without boasting of his honor, and never hung a priest without protesting his devotion to his Church.

The first part of this Anglo-Spanish conspiracy ended with the executions following on the Powder Plot; the second part, with the executions following on the Powder Poisoning. Garnet, the master-spirit of part the first, was hung in St. Paul's Churchyard; Northampton, the master-spirit of part the second, escaped the penalty of his crimes by dying on the eve of his arrest.

CHAPTER II.

FACTIONS AT COURT.

While the Queen's ashes were yet warm at Richmond, a schism broke out in her council at Whitehall, not only in words which pass, but in acts which live. A part of her council was for making terms with the King of Scots, now known to be her heir; such terms as their fathers had often made with uncrowned kings; such terms as their sons had afterward to impose on William the Third. Lord Grey was one of those who urged that James should be asked for pledges to respect our English rights and to follow our English laws. Sir John Fortescue supported the views of Grey; while Cecil and the two Howards (soon to be known as the Earls of Suffolk and Northampton) contended that all such things could wait, that subjects must not make conditions, and that the wisest course would be to trust their King.

Cecil knew too well in what he placed his trust. For three years past he had employed Lord Henry in a secret correspondence with the Scottish court, from which he had learned enough of Jamès to see his drift and gauge his strength. The Scottish prince, he found, was bent on peace; peace with the Austrian Cardinal, peace with the Spanish court, peace on every side and on any terms; even though it might have to be the "King of Hungary's peace." This policy suited Cecil, who felt that in case of war the public power would pass away from clerks and secretaries into the hands of warriors, such as Raleigh, Nottingham, and Grey.

The war party wished to shape the policy of James so as to give him glory abroad and peace at home; a government that should be a living force, a people who should be content and free. The way to these ends, they said, was to raise the siege of Ostend, to drive the Jesuit missionaries out of London, to unite the English people in defense of public liberty and public law. The peace party wished to leave the question of policy to the King; well knowing that he spoke of the Dutch as rebels, that he wished the Cardinal success, and that, in reference to the treaties which bound him to aid his allies, he openly announced his intention not to be tied by the contracts of a woman and a fool.

Thus, in the gardens of Whitehall, on the day of the Queen's death, before the King of Scots was yet proclaimed, two parties were in line; an English party, having an English platform, on which stood Raleigh, Fortescue, and Grey; a Spanish party, having a Spanish platform, on which stood Cecil and his friends. The first party wanted liberty and war, and the cry of their partisans in the streets was, "Down with the Austrian! Ho for the Dutch!" The second party wanted peace and place; they had no public cry, for they had no partisans in the street; but their purpose was to become the "Friends of Spain."

These factions fell into a strife, which raged until the King arrived at the Tower and made known his will. James wanted money and quiet; neither of which he could receive so long as the guns were booming over Dover Straits. Cecil promised him money and quiet in return for place and power; blessings which he persuaded James no other man could give. The King could not know, in that early time, that his Secretary of State would sell his secrets and his services for Spanish gold; and, had he known the truth, he might only have chuckled in his sleeve, sworn a coarse oath, and begged some portion of the spoil. Anyway, the new King gave his confidence to that smooth and serpentine clerk, so that Cecil, in any war he might have to wage against Grey and Raleigh, would have the crown, the army, and the judges at his back.

The King came in without terms; in fact, these terms were not made until the times of his son and of his son's son.

People in the Strand and Cheape, who heard that their young Prince was bent on forsaking the Holy War, could not believe it. How, they cried, betray the Dutch! How could we betray them and not ourselves? Was not the war of the Armada burning? Had not Mountjoy just smitten the Spaniards at Kinsale? Was not Vere at Ostend? Had we not thousands of troops in the Netherlands? Were not Flushing, Rammekins, and Briel in our power? Were we not bound by treaties? Were we not fighting our enemies on a friendly soil, in lieu of having to fight them on our own?

Such was the view then taken by every one, except the King's friends and those who wished to be thought his friends. So strong and wide was this popular feeling for the Dutch, that James could not help seeing that to recall his troops from Ostend and Flushing might be fatal to his peace, if not perilous to his crown. The change must be wrought out step by step. Ere such a course could be safely taken, the war must have lost its charm for the public mind, and the fighting generals must have been tarnished by some dubious charge. Could Vere be starved out of Ostend? Could Raleigh and Grey be compromised with the partisans of war? The first was easy, the second not so easy. Vere had only to be dropped; his letters to be left unread, his prayers unnoticed, his supplies unsent. A cold intelligence, working in a chamber at Whitehall, could count the very hours of Vere. One day the height of human daring would be reached. Brave hands would faint through famine, stout hearts would fail in force, the city would fall into the Austrian's power, and James could affect a sorrow which he would not feel. But neither Grey nor Raleigh could be ruined by leaving him alone. If Grey was to be got out of Cecil's way, he must be lodged in the Tower.

Now, Cecil was a perfect master in the art of snaring men into suspicion; yet he could hardly have succeeded in so short a time in meshing his powerful rivals, had he not been aided in his work by an unexpected group of spies. These spies were the Jesuit missionaries whom Grey and his Puritan friends proposed to harry from the land.

For many years past, a few cautious Jesuits, under their Prefect, Garnet, had been hiding in the country, chiefly in the London suburbs and in the midland shires; but on the Queen's death becoming known abroad, a larger body came over sea from Flanders and Castile, to aid in promoting the peace with Spain. In crossing the Straits, they knew they were breaking the English law, since no member of their Order could then reside on English soil; but they reckoned, not without cause, on the Secretary of State being purposely blind to their coming over, since their object was to promote the King's most ardent wish. In Cecil these Jesuits met their match. The men who moved the Order were no strangers to him; some of them were in his pay, still more of them were in his power. A list of the fathers lay in his desk; a list giving their true names and their false, with an account of the houses in which they lodged, and of the persons who helped them to come and go. He knew something of Father Fisher, otherwise Percy, otherwise Fairfax, who lived in Sir Everard Digby's house. He was acquainted with Father Oldcorne, the confessor of Mrs. Abington of Hendlip Hall. Garnet was his neighbor, and might almost be called his chum. Father Creswell wrote to him from Valladolid, Father Persons from Rome. By these and other means he held the threads of their purpose in his grasp, and felt that should the day for a tussle with the Order ever come, he would be strong enough to drag them down.

The fathers were allowed to land and spread themselves through the London suburbs and the country districts; but they were not suffered to come and go unwatched. The Secretary had his agents on the quay of every port and the deck of every ship. The jovial skipper who gave the fathers a passage in his bark, and who seemed to them the pink of good fellows, was his spy. The bland old priest, who welcomed them on shore and gave them such wise counsels, was in his pay. One band of Jesuits came over in the Golden Lion, Francis Burnell commander. Fresh from Antwerp, where the Austrian Cardinal and the Spanish Infanta had been proclaimed King and Queen of England, these fathers were hot with zeal, and, finding the skipper a man of their own mind, they were free in talk about the King of Scots. They said the

King was doomed, and talked of the speedy destruction of all his house. Before they were put on shore, Captain Burnell had reported their words to one of Cecil's spies in Harwich, who sent a copy of their speeches to Whitehall.

The spy who watched the coming and going of these fathers in Harwich was Francis Tilletson, a priest.

A part of Cecil's craft in dealing with political rivals, lay in the adroit advantage which he took of the bitter feuds then raging in the ancient Church; so as to gain from each party in that Church the means of crushing the other, when a policy of repression happened to serve his turn. Blood ran so high between sections of the Catholic clergy—between the Secular priests and the Jesuit missionaries—that each was ready to betray the other into his hands. Tilletson was not more eager to denounce the Jesuits in Harwich, than Garnet was to destroy the Seculars in London. Each rejoiced when his rival fell. If Jesuits and Seculars were both opposed in theory to the crown, they opposed it in a different spirit, and sought their ends by a different path. Each had a purpose and a plot; and the purpose dearest to each was to betray his fellow-priest to the law.

From his neighbors of Enfield Chase, Cecil got the clew to a wild, spent plot, in which two members of the Secular priesthood, who had made themselves hateful to the Fathers, were much concerned. The plot had failed, the plotters had dispersed. Some ale had been drunk in Carter Lane, a gang of rufflers called the Damned Crew had been raised, and two or three secret conferences had been held between persons of still higher rank; but the dream was past, and the design would have been shrouded in a spy's report, and laid in the grave of all dead things, had not one of the names, which incidentally occurred in the papers, been that of Grey.

A Priests' Plot—there was a name to strike the public ear! A charge was wanted against Grey, the Puritan peer, the enemy of Philip, the advocate of war. Now, Grey was said to have given two or three private meetings to Sir Griffin Markham, a notorious Papist, and an agent for the priests. What more could men like Cecil and Northampton ask?

CHAPTER III.

LORD GREY OF WILTON.

Among the young men of high rank who strove in the later years of Gloriana's reign to make a true religion of their daily lives—to be at once brave soldiers, faithful citizens, and pious sons—to live in the world, yet also live to God,—and the roll of these high and noble men was not a short one,—the most eminent for his birth, his genius, and his misery was Thomas Grey, the sixteenth baron of his line; in whom was to expire, in a cell of that Water gate which Henry the Third had built, the last male heir of a house which that same Henry the Third had summoned to his side.

Grey was nursed under a mother's eye. Until he was ten years old, he lived at Whaddon Hall in Bucks, the family seat, where he was taught to read the word of God, as well as to ride and fence, to leap the barriers and to run the ring. As he grew in size, the playmate of a tiny sister, Bridget, and of a baby-brother, who was taken from him at an early day, his mother Sibyl saw with pride and love that he was growing rich not only in the arts which adorn high rank, but in that spiritual grace which she prized in her son above all the accomplishments of earth. At ten he was called a man and sent into the world. The Greys had always been men of war, and a Grey of Wilton Castle could have no other home than a camp. His chair was to be a saddle, his coat a corselet, his cap a casque of steel. But Lady Grey was anxious that her boy should be a faithful soldier of Jesus Christ, no less than a stout defender of his Queen; and she lived to see him all that she hoped he would become.

Grey was happy in both his parents. Arthur Grey, his father, that renowned Lord Deputy of Ireland who was the patron of Gascoyne and the friend of Spenser, is known to lovers of great books as Artegal, the Knight of Justice, in the Faery Queen; a princely figure, noble as it is spotless; not more true to the poetic art than to the human life.

In court and camp young Grey was ever at his father's side, often in the thickest of bloody fields.

> "For Arthur's son
> Held Arthur's spirit."

Once, when he was hardly twelve years old, in a sudden fight, some English horsemen giving way before a swarm of kernes, the Lord Deputy, who had seen the waving line, pricked up, the lad at his heels, and, shouting, "Grey and his heir for the Queen!" dashed in among the foe and cut them through. That Irish camp was a terrible school of arms; for a gang of reckless devils, the sweepings of Italian bagnios and Spanish jails, had been flung into Connaught, where they had built a fortress, called the Fort Del Oro. Roaming through Galway and parts of Kerry, these gangs had ravaged two counties before the Lord Deputy could move against them; but when Artegal leaped to horse it was to strike a blow that men should not be able to forget. Never, since the Lion of Judah went forth to battle, had a sterner spirit ruled a camp than he who led the English force against Del Oro. Grey asked no quarter, and he gave none. The fort was taken, and the enemy destroyed.

It was in this action under Grey that Raleigh, then a young captain, won his first red laurels in the field.

From this fierce school of war the boy was sent to Oxford. Robert Marston, who wrote a life of Grey in verse, declares that now

"Arms entered into league with arts;"

but the young soldier was too busy with his work to stay over-long at college. Like his father, and like his comrade Raleigh, he vowed his sword to the Good Old Cause; and while he was yet in his teens he crossed into the Low Countries, to finish his education in the trench and field. The Dutch received him with open arms; and in the front of every charge, his countrymen saw with pride the trail of his crimson plume. Grey brought into the patriots' camp not only a soldier's sword, but a statesman's thought; not only a dauntless eye, but a clear and resolute mind. He knew not merely how to fight, but how to turn the tide of battle to a righteous end. He saw what should be done, and how it should be done. Nursed on the passions which breathe in the Faery Queen, the legend of his house, he loathed Grantorto with all his soul, and spurned the Idol as he would have spurned the nether fiend.

Loving his Queen and country as he loved his

mother and his sister Bridget, Grey was with the foremost in every enterprise by land and sea. He served against the Irish rebels; he sailed on the Island Voyage; he fought on Nieuport sands.

On his return from camp to court, he found the Earl of Essex, his old companion of the Island Voyage, commencing that evil course which was to bring him, in a few mad months, to the Devereux tower and to St. Peter's Church. Grey warned his friend, and heard his warning received with gibes. Less vexed than pained by his rebuff, he stood apart in silence, until he saw that Essex was falling away from all his English friends and taking hold of an Anglo-Spanish crew; giving up Bacon and Raleigh for the pupils of Father Garnet,—for men like Monteagle, Father Wright, and Captain Lea. Then he spake to the Earl once more. But all was vain: the Earl having entered on a course from which neither love nor fear could draw him back. Grey told these faithless peers and tavern-plotters to count him in future as a foe.

Lord Southampton, a young fellow like himself, but weak and fitful, heard this warning with open scorn, and put such words on Grey as a soldier could not bear. Grey stopped him and beat him in the public street. This quarrel of the young peers so stirred her court, that the Queen had to send Lord Grey to the Prince of Orange, who was lying in front of Grave, until the storm passed by.

The mettle of the young man having now been proved, he was courted by the chiefs of every side. He joined the party of Raleigh, Nottingham, and Cecil, against the Earl of Essex. He went over to Dublin in command of a regiment of horse to watch the plotters, and when Essex swept back to London, Grey was quickly in his front. When the Earl's folly maddened into crime, the pious young soldier was commissioned by the Queen as her General of the Horse.

Grey's heart was thrown into these courtly broils only so far as they formed a part of that war which his country had to wage against the King of Spain. Not against Essex the courtier, not even against Essex the politician, would he have drawn his sword. The foe whom he smote in the guise of Essex was Grantorto; the Earl, who had fought by his side, having gone over to the enemy, making a companion of Robert Catesby and a counselor of Father Wright. When the court was purged of factions, Grey turned his eyes once more toward the fields in which his country's battles were being fought on a foreign soil. Most of all, he strained his vision toward Ostend.

For in those last days of the Queen, a roar of guns was booming above the Straits, which spoke to the heart of England as no other crash of earth's artillery could speak. An Austrian Cardinal, married to the Infanta, Clara Isabel, "heiress of France and England," lay with a mighty host before Ostend, the last rampart of the Reformed religion in Flanders; the lines of which were held by a garrison of Dutch and English troops, commanded by Sir Francis Vere.

Lying low in the sands, behind a wall of mud, with narrow streets, stone houses, and a place of arms, Ostend was a fishing port and village of barely three thousand souls. The town itself was nothing; but this speck of coast was strong in the dikes and sand-hills, in the line of sea, and in the thews of a gallant race. The folk were Protestant, eager to be free; and the people, both in London and the Hague, were conscious that the battle of their freedom was being fought, and might haply be decided, in the trenches of Ostend.

The strength of Spain was planted before this village

in the sands, and month after month went by without giving her the prize. Assaults were made with a vigor which has rarely been seen in war, and never except in a religious war. Yet the town stood out. A rash vow, made by the Infanta, had been kept by her, but kept in a fashion to become the by-word of every land. Looking over the low roofs and simple works, Clara Isabel, on the day of her arrival, swore by her saints that she would enter the place before she changed her chemise; and that chemise had grown from white to yellow, and from yellow to black, yet Isabel had not entered into the place yet. The Cardinal Archduke's lines were daily creeping closer to the town, and at length a front of batteries built along the coast swept all the outlets to the sea, and cut off succors from the Dutch and English fleets. One day, a whisper ran through the galleries at Whitehall that the port of Ostend was closed, and that news from the beleaguered city must be got by roundabout and unsafe roads.

In this stress of evil, Grey undertook to force the passage with a single ship, and show the troopers in Ostend that they were not cut off. The ship was found and the passage forced. A hundred cannon from the sand-hills opened on his flag, but Grey shot into port, unscathed by the Austrian fire, and, landing in the town, amid the shouts and thanks of the besieged, he brought to the brave defenders not only much needful succor, but the congratulations of his country and his Queen.

Grey was not simply a man of war. Like his father, he was a friend of poets; like his mother, he was a friend of preachers. In his religious views he was a pupil of Reynolds and Cartwright, and the strong party of the Puritans looked upon him as a chief. Yet Grey was the reverse of a bigot. Law and policy were as much his study as divinity and soldiership, and he is known to have held some views on the civil power going far beyond the science of his age. Young, noble, rich, illustrious, what gifts might not fortune be supposed to hold in store for such a man!

Some people thought the highest state of all was not too high for one so gifted and so good. Shrewd wits were heard to guess that Grey would wed the Lady Arabella Stuart; in which case he might be called, in his partner's right, to ascend Elizabeth's throne.

No one who watched the young General of her Majesty's Horse prancing past Charing Cross, in the closing months of her reign, could have dreamt that his course was already run; that one short year would find him a prisoner in the Tower; that a flagitious charge, a splendid defense, a theatrical reprieve, a lingering imprisonment, and an early death, were all that remained on earth to that dashing peer, the heir of so many glories, the object of so much love.

CHAPTER IV.

OLD ENGLISH CATHOLICS.

The plot in which Cecil was to entangle Grey was not a conspiracy of worldly and wicked men, so much as a fantastic dream on the part of two dull and excited priests.

To see how this plot arose, to understand why the Jesuits betrayed it, and to follow the chain which binds it to the Powder plot, one should recall to mind the exact relation in which the two chief sections of the

Catholic clergy stood toward each other in the opening years of James the First. A few words will suffice.

When the great Queen had come to her crown, one body, and only one body, calling themselves Catholic, existed in her realm. During her reign a second body, calling themselves Catholic, sprang into life. The first were the English Catholics, the second were the Roman Catholics; and in the opening year of James's reign these two sections stood, not simply apart, but in hostile array.

To the first party belonged the thousands on thousands of families, in every shire, who had clung, through good and evil, to the ancient rite. These families clung to that rite because it was old and venerable, because it was the rite of their fathers, because it was woven into the texture of their social and moral life. These people never thought of their Church as a thing apart from their country. How could they have done so? The English Church was just as old as the English name. Their sires had been members of a free Church; and they could boast, with cause, that in all their efforts after freedom that Church had borne her part. "The English Church shall be free," was the very first clause set down in the charter won from John. To tell these English families that their creed was a foreign creed, to be kept by them for the benefit of a foreign priest and a foreign king, was to speak to them in an unknown tongue. They reverenced Rome, as the oldest of Latin sees; but they thought of her as a sister, not as a mistress; and, while they gave to Pope Clement the highest honor, they denied his right to meddle in their courts of law. Submitting to his will in spiritual things, they refused his briefs and declined his authority in worldly things. Even as to church order they had ways of their own which were not as the

Roman ways. They had their own feasts and vigils, their own policy and method, which an Italian could hardly understand, and in which he could have no share. Their country was what Rome had once proudly called her, an island of the saints. In one word, the old English Church was to these stanch Catholics a national Church.

To the second party belonged the new men, few in number and fierce in spirit, who had been drawn away by Jesuits from the reformed English Church. They were converts; converts of a recent date and a malignant type; accused of having gone over to the enemy less from religious heat than from political passion, and even from family pique. The times were apt to such desertions from the Church. Apostasy was a protest, a form of going into what is now called "opposition." When a man failed at court, like Philip Howard, the ready way to insult his sovereign was to change his creed. When a man quarreled with his father, like William Parker, the surest way to worry that father was to send for a priest. When a man wasted his fortune, like Thomas Percy, the quickest way to escape reproaches from his friends was to be seen attending mass. From Robert Catesby down to Thomas Winter, the motive for desertion seems in almost every case to have been either personal or political discontent.

Each of these parties had their own priests,—the first party being led by the Secular clergy, the second party by the Jesuits.

The old English priests were for the most part learned, tolerant, timid men, who gave their thoughts to spiritual things, and wished to leave politics to Kings and Queens. Their duty lay in the care of souls. Their hope was to live in peace, to say their office, to watch their flocks, and leave the results of their patient toil in the hands of God. When the law left them alone,—and, on the whole, they were wisely left alone,—they were content. Striving to do good, in the belief that what they taught and wrought was best for their country, they paid scant heed to what was considered the best for Spain.

On the other side, the Jesuits were men of the world, with worldly purposes in view. They were the servants of Philip, whom he had sent into England to do his work. That prince, having received them into Spain, having given them money and power, having placed the colleges of Seville and Castile in their hands, having espoused their quarrels in Flanders and in Rome, had led them to see that his glory would be their glory, and that in him they would find not only a powerful master but an indulgent friend.

The old Catholics, a slow and sober folk, who tried to keep their fingers out of fire, esteemed it no less a sin to kill a King than to kill a Pope. The new Catholics, hot of blood and bold of speech, contended that a good cause might justify foul deeds, and that the highest cause on earth was that which they professed,—the cause of a single empire and a single Church.

No outward sign, no inward motive, separated the English Catholics from their neighbors of the countryside. In all invasions, and in all threatened invasions, they were prompt to march. Loving their native land as other men loved it, they were stung to frenzy by reports that a foreigner meant to profane their soil; and, moving into line with the first, they struck the foe, not caring to inquire under what flag he fought. The best of the old Catholic peers and gentry were out in the Armada year.

The new Catholics were strangers in the land. While Lord Montagu, born a Catholic, was riding down to Tilbury Fort, with his son, his grandson, and his tenants in his wake, all armed to defend their country, Lord Arundel, the son of a Protestant duke, was saying clandestine mass and uttering a traitor's prayer in the Beauchamp tower. English but in name, the Jesuits had taught their lay disciples to accept a foreign purpose and a foreign prince. Spain was to be their country, and they were to seek her glory in a way from which their neighbors would be likely to recoil, not only with aversion, but with scorn. They were to consider their native land as lost to God, their neighbors as the heirs of everlasting death. They were to treat their prince as an outlaw, and to hold his judges as accursed of Heaven. The converts were not suffered to feel proud of their English birth, but rather to bow their heads into the dust for shame. They were to have no part in the common weal. "I am become a stranger to my brethren," cried their oracle, Father Persons, "an alien to the sons of my mother." Spain was to be their only country, Philip their only King.

These two bodies were of unequal force.

The English Catholics were half the population, if they were not more. One-third of the peers, one-half the country gentlemen, two-thirds of the hedgers and ditchers, were Catholic. A change of faith is not to be made in a year, not in a hundred years; in England the change had been a work of time, and the work was still going on. Among the county magistrates every second man was still a Catholic. The Reformed religion had its seat in the great towns; but even in these great towns the opposite opinions were held in strength.

The Roman Catholics were few in number, and scattered through distant shires. It is doubtful whether the Jesuits could at any time have rallied a thousand voices to support them against the ancient clergy of their Church. The secret of the influence wielded by Garnet and his helpers lay in the wonder and fear inspired by the great Order to which they belonged.

CHAPTER V.

THE ENGLISH JESUITS.

The form in which the English branch of the Society of Jesus presented itself to a statesman's notice was that of an Anglo-Spanish plot,—whether he judged them by their personal bearing or by their public acts.

In all countries, the members of this Order mixed with the world, which they affected to despise and studied how to rule. They were great in colleges, greater still in courts. They made tools of women, and dupes of men who were the slaves of women. They affected to know strange secrets, to possess indefinite funds, to govern by inscrutable means. They could change their names, their costumes, their nationalities, at will. A priest could wear a beard, a monk could deny his shaven crown. They could put on plain stuff, they could sparkle in satin and gold. In making war on the powers of darkness, they had a right to seize all weapons of war, to employ all arts of deception. Doing Heaven's will on earth, they were free from all scruples which might impede their work.

But what was dubious in the conduct of Jesuits in other lands was carried to the farthest reach by the English branch. Claudius Aquaviva had no disciples so unruly as his English pupils. All Jesuits were inclined by habit to subject the interests of religion to those of politics; the English brethren made that subjection unconditional and complete. As men of the world, they took the extremest views of what is permitted; classing conspiracy with love and war, in which everything is said to be fair. They justified treachery; they justified rebellion; they justified public murder. In the schools which their patron, Philip of Spain, had caused to be placed under their control, they bound their pupils by an oath to go back when their course was finished to their native land, and strive by fair means and by foul to win it for the Church of Rome and the King of Spain. Inured to danger, these pupils of the Jesuits crossed the sea, prepared in mind for trouble, and wearing in their fancies the martyr's crown. But they were taught to make the best of a good cause, and not to throw away their lives. Provided with masks and money, served by their own agents, fed by their own converts, they were able to preach and teach with but little risk. They had means for landing in the ports, for evading spies, for slipping through the nets of justice. Living in what they called "a strange land," they mapped off the country in shires and hundreds, and on these small charts they marked each lonely beach on which a boat was kept, each country-house in which they had a secret room. A Jesuit's business being to go about the world unseen, he had a dozen garbs, a dozen professions, and a dozen names. He had the jargon of many arts and the patter of many tongues. A confessor of women, he learned from them the secrets which he turned against their lords, and through these secrets he could sometimes reach at persons whom he dared not openly address.

This permanent conspiracy on the English soil in

favor of a foreign prince was offensive not only to the old Catholics, who wished to live in peace, but to politicians like Cecil and Northampton, who meant to become the chiefs of a new Spanish party in the state.

For the moment, these politicians were willing to use the Jesuits; but, even while using them, they hoped to compromise and destroy them as a political power.

The Jesuits had not been twenty-three years in London; Persons, the first English Prefect, had not been thirty years a Jesuit; so that the men whom they had trained to act in this foreign spirit were none of them yet beyond middle age. Robert Persons and Edmund Campion had come over sea in 1580,—come over against the wishes of the English Catholics, since they came in defiance of the law, and meaning to be a cause of strife, "creating disturbances," as Persons had frankly said, "in places where everything till that time was tranquil." Being then at peace, the Catholics wished to remain at peace; but this smooth state of things, if good for the clergy and their flocks, had been the reverse of good for Philip, who would gladly have seen the Catholics driven mad with misery, in order that his generals might count on finding a partisan under every roof. The Prefect had come over with two sets of instructions, one of which he had kept in reserve. He was to stir up lawless passions, so as to sting the civil power into a severer course; and he was to put down the native fasts, and substitute those of the Italian Church.

When Persons returned to Rome, leaving Father Weston with the rank of Prefect, he could boast of having made converts of Sir Thomas Tresham of Rushton Hall, Sir William Catesby of Lapworth, and their sons Francis and Robert, then boys of a tender age.

Campion, who stayed behind to carry on his work, wrote a letter to the Privy Council, in which he said, ". . . Be it known to you that we have made a league; all the Jesuits in the world, whose succession and multitude must overreach the practices of England; for bearing the curse that you shall lay upon us; and never to despair of your recovery while we have a man left to enjoy your Tyburns, or to be racked by your torments, or to be consumed within your prisons. Expenses are reckoned; the enterprise is begun. It is of God; it cannot be resisted; so the faith was founded; so it must be restored." This challenge was answered by a stricter law. Father Weston was locked in the Clink Prison, in spite of Lady Arundel's tears and gold; and the luckless Jesuit who defied his country was flung into the Tower, convicted of high treason, and put to death.

Robert Southwell and Henry Garnet were sent from Rome by Persons, to fill the dangerous posts. Southwell took up Weston's place in Lady Arundel's household, while Garnet became Prefect of the English mission. Even the poet showed that in his foreign schools he had lost the human and tender sense of home. "We have sung the Canticles in a strange land," he wrote; and that "strange land" was the country of his birth! In due time he followed Campion to the Tower, and, after three years of waiting, was tried and hung; leaving his more cautious and unscrupulous friend, the new Prefect, to continue and complete his task.

Philip found no trustier servants than these English priests, who spread themselves not only over England, but over Europe, in order to do his will. They stood by the side of Kings, and the ministers and mistresses of Kings. Robert Persons was near the Pope; Joseph Creswell was in Madrid, the Spanish capital; Henry

Fludd in Lisbon, then the principal Spanish port. William Baldwin followed Spinola's banner on the Rhine. John Jones lived at Douai. Hugh Owen, the most active and most unscrupulous of these fathers, was in the Cardinal's camp. One of Father Owen's closest friends was Sir William Stanley; one of his nearest followers was Guy Fawkes.

A crime of the rarest kind and the darkest dye had covered the name of Sir William Stanley with an odium which has hardly any mate. This knight had given up the city of Deventer to the enemy, while commanding an English and native garrison in his sovereign's name. The Jesuits owned his work, praising him for doing what he felt to be right, in face of the adverse verdicts of the world. A medal, commemorative of his treason, was struck in Rome. The rage and shame with which the news of this treachery was received in England cannot be expressed in words. Men said it was the Jesuits' doing; and when they afterward spoke of Jesuit morals, they mentioned the betrayal of Deventer as one of those facts from which there is no appeal.

A soldier hated and reviled as Stanley was drew all the desperate spirits who left their country to his side, and a regiment of English renegades was formed by him in the Cardinal's camp, which he fondly hoped to have a chance of one day leading against his Queen.

Garnet fixed his quarters near London, so as to be within easy reach of his lay supporters, and able to direct the many coadjutors who came over from Spain and Flanders to help in putting England beneath the yoke.

The chief of these helpers were Father Fisher, Father Gerard, and Father Greenway, whom he sent into the midland shires, with orders to attach themselves to ardent women and discontented men. They were to treat the country as a missionary land, to regard their Church as a missionary Church. England being lost to the faith of Christ, their business was to convert it back,—that portion of it which claimed to be Catholic, no less than that which avowed itself Reformed. All were gone astray from Rome, they said, and all must be brought into the fold, out of which there was no salvation from death and hell.

The head-quarters of this conspiracy were planted in Enfield Chase.

CHAPTER VI.

WHITE WEBBS.

On the edge of Enfield Chase, about ten miles from Paul's Cross, stood—in the days of James the First—a large and lonely house of the Tudor sort; a house in a narrow lane, so screened by trees that a few paces off it could be hardly seen. It had many rooms, a big garden, and a high fence. The place was a maze of ins and outs, with passages by which visitors might come and go, with traps in the oaken floors, and secret chambers in the chimney-stacks and dividing-walls. Deep vaults lay below, while a conduit led to the dams and waters of the Lea. This house was called White Webbs, and from its situation and its size it might have been built as a hiding-place for priests and a rendezvous for plots.

Like the whole of Enfield Chase, White Webbs belonged to the Crown. Some thirty years before that time the Queen had granted it to Robert Hewick, her physician-in-ordinary; and this Robert Hewick had afterward let it to Rowland Watson, Clerk of the Crown, whose wife still held it on a lease.

One day—about the time when Essex was beginning to court the foreign Catholics, to consort with Catesby and Tresham, to consult with Father Wright—a man of middle age, thick-set, with rather jovial manner, came to see the place. He gave the name of Mese, the address of Berks. He wore a coat of fustian stuff, and looked like a grazier of the better class. He had a sister, he said,—one Mrs. Perkins, a lady of good means, who wanted to hire a house near London, where she could live in quiet, yet see her friends from town. The Queen's physician saw no reason to suspect his guest; and, when the terms were settled between them, Mr. Mese became the tenant of White Webbs.

Robert Skinner, who passed for Mrs. Perkins's butler, took possession and prepared the rooms, putting James Johnson, a servant whom he hired, in charge of this house, while he rode over to Enfield, and engaged one Lewis, a carrier, to go with his team to London and fetch in goods. One room was set apart as a chapel; all the things necessary in performing mass were bought; and the chambers were furnished with books and relics as well as with household stuff.

Three months elapsed before Mrs. Perkins came. She was a lady in the prime of life, and seemingly of ample means. Skinner and his wife waited on her; but she had other servants, both male and female, in her train, including Will Shepherd, her coachman, and Bess, that coachman's wife. In fact, the lady's establishment was framed on a large and costly scale.

She was a Catholic, and her people were also Catholic.

Mr. Mese, of Berkshire, followed his sister to White

Webbs, and, when he came, he brought his man-servant, a cunning fellow, who was known as Little John. By-and-by, a Mr. Perkins came to White Webbs,—a lean man, with a long face, brown hair, and yellow beard. He had a serving-man with him, called George, whose full name was George Chambers. In what relation Mr. Perkins stood to Mrs. Perkins no one seemed to know. Skinner could have told, no doubt, but Skinner never spoke. He might be taken for her husband, since he came to her very often, and stayed with her very long. In fact, although he went away on business from time to time, he never failed to come back to White Webbs as to his proper home. Mr. Mese also spent much of his time in the Chase, many gentlemen riding down from London to see him, some of whom sat up late at night talking business in his room. These strangers put up their horses, had beds prepared for them, and sometimes stayed in the house for two or three days; on which occasions much venison would be sent for, and much claret drank.

Once, when Mr. Mese went away from White Webbs on business, he came back in a new name. He was now called Mr. Farmer, and the servants were told to speak of him as such. Shortly afterward, these servants heard him addressed by some of his friends as Father Walley; and then they knew, if they had not previously suspected, that the homely personage in the fustian coat was a priest. James Johnson, the hired domestic, kept his eyes and ears open; and, after a little waiting, he found reason to believe that his mistress was not what she seemed,—was not named Perkins, was neither wife nor widow, but a single woman, the daughter of a peer. But James was clever enough to keep his secret and his place.

In no long time a second lady came to White Webbs,

and took up her abode there. She gave the name of Mrs. Jennings, and the people about the house were told that her husband was a merchant of the City, a good deal away from home. Mrs. Jennings was said to be a sister of "Mrs. Perkins," in which case she would be a sister of "Mr. Mese." That a warm affection bound the lady and gentleman to each other, any one might see. Now and then a small creature, with a red beard and a bald pate, made his appearance at White Webbs, who called himself Thomas Jennings and claimed Mr. Mese's sister as his wife.

None of these people were what they seemed. The homely man in fustian stuff was Father Garnet, Prefect of the English mission. The serving-man called Little John was Nick Owen, a lay Jesuit, of singular skill in devising places for concealment. "Mr. Perkins" was Father Oldcorne; and his serving-man, George, was also a lay Jesuit, in attendance on his chief. The two ladies, passing under the names of Mrs. Perkins and Mrs. Jennings, were Ann and Helen, daughters of William, third Lord Vaux of Harrowden. Ann was a single woman, Helen a wedded wife. "Mrs. Perkins" had no other relation to "Mr. Perkins" than that of a penitent to her priest. No ties of blood connected the ladies with "Mr. Mese." Helen was not Mrs. Jennings; nor was the small creature who called himself Jennings a merchant from the City. The bald pate belonged to Bartholomew Brooksby, a country gentleman of good estate and of little wit, who had given himself body and soul to work out the Prefect's will. He was allowed to pay most of the rent for White Webbs.

Lord Vaux, the father of these two ladies, had been a grievous sufferer for conscience' sake. No small part of his life had been spent in jails, and no small part of his fortune had been lost in fines. For more than two years he had lodged in the Fleet prison, in company with Sir Thomas Tresham, whose sister he married on his first wife's death. He had seen his family broken up, and the honors of his line renounced. For his eldest son, Henry Vaux, had been persuaded by the Jesuits to lay down his name and title, to assume the higher mission of the cross. This heir to a noble name and good estate had thrown away all his worldly advantages to enter a foreign cell and to die a monk. Nor was this all that he had to bear. His second son, George Vaux, now heir to his honors, had almost broken his heart by marrying against his wish, and family strife had embittered his later days. Lord Vaux outlived his sons, he quarreled with his connections, and, when he died, he left the honors of his house to a child not seven years old, the son of a woman whom he could not bear. Ann Vaux and Helen Brooksby were the aunts to this young peer.

White Webbs was called a seraglio; a child was born there,—Helen Brooksby's child; and when Sir Edward Coke got the papers into his hands, he made coarse allusion to the paternity of this child. Garnet confessed that he was the christener; Coke demanded to be told whether he was not the father. The baby was said to have a bald head; Coke requested to know whether it had not a "shaven crown." From these impertinences it is easier to defend the Prefect than from the accusations of Father Floyd. Griffith Floyd, a Jesuit agent, was sent to England by his superiors to inquire into the life which Garnet had been leading at White Webbs, especially as to his love of dainty food, and his alleged familiarities with Mistress Ann. He told his masters that he had "found too much." The words are somewhat vague; they were meant to damage Garnet; but we must not follow them from what they describe to what they merely hint. No proof exists of an immoral intimacy. If Garnet felt a love for either Ann Vaux or Helen Brooksby beyond what is allowed to a priest for every soul committed to his care, he never put that love into written words. But, while he may be acquitted of criminal passion for his fair penitents, he must be held responsible for all the scandals piled upon their names. He led them into a false position, and he kept them in that false position before the world. They were not nuns. They had taken no vows. They lay under no female rule. One of them was a married woman. In living under the same roof with two single men, in passing under false names, in pretending to a near relationship of blood, and in assuming a condition to which they had no right, they laid themselves open to jests and sneers from which they ought to have been saved by more prudent friends. Garnet had not the grace to act a more manly part. He loved the soft ways of these high-born women, and rather than forego the pleasure of their company he was willing to darken and blight their fame.

To this lonely house in the royal demesne came other Jesuits besides Oldcorne, other laymen besides Bartholomew Brooksby. Father Fisher, Father Gerard, and Father Greenway were often there,—coming in a score of varying names and garbs. Besides the lay characters which they assumed, each Jesuit had three or four priestly names, so as to be known to the servants of different houses as different persons. Fisher was called Father Percy in one place, Father Fairfax in a second. Gerard was known as Father Standish, Father Brooke, and Father Lee; Greenway, as Father Greenwell, and Father Tesmond. All these emissaries moved about the country, passing from house to house, saying mass in secret, raking up the fires of discontent, and keeping alive in their scholars the prospect of a change.

Lay visitors came to the lonely house.

After the death of Essex on Tower Hill, the men who were out with him in the streets, and were afterward pardoned by the Queen, came over to consult the Jesuits as to what should be done. The first of these lay visitors were Robert Catesby and a companion whom he called Tom. Catesby was a young gentleman, tall, handsome, well bred, with a presence which took the eye; his blood being gentle, and his bearing that of a prince. Early converted from his Church, early united to a Protestant wife, early left a widower with an infant son, early engaged in treason to his Queen, he had passed through many lives and was a worn-out sage before he was thirty years old. The companion whom he called Tom, and who addressed him in reply as Sir, was a dumpy little fellow of middle age, with person and manner exceedingly unlike those of his handsome friend. They asked for Mr. Mese.

The dumpy fellow had just come back from Rome, to which city he had been sent by the Fathers on a secret errand; and, having conversed with persons at the English college, he could explain to the company at White Webbs the latest views of the political exiles at the Roman court.

Other visitors came; not in crowds, but in twos and threes, so as to pass unnoticed in the Chase. Catesby was strict in his own coming and going; riding out either alone or with his dumpy friend. As a rule, the callers gave no names; they wanted Mr. Mese; and they were shown by Skinner into Mr. Mese's room.

CHAPTER VII.

THE PRIESTS' PLOT.

THE men of his own Church whom Garnet, as chief of the Anglo-Spanish party, had most cause to fear, were two priests, William Watson and William Clarke, who were loud supporters of the old Catholic party against the new; writers of books on the Jesuits, and warm denouncers of the foreign school.

Having taught their flocks the duty of defending the soil, the freedom, and the sovereign of their native land, these priests were scouted by Father Persons as pedants and fools. To this attack Father Watson replied in a book called "Ten Quodlibetical Questions;" from which title he got the droll nickname of "Quodlibets," by which he has ever since been known. Of a good family, holding high office in the Church and State,—a kinsman of that Thomas Watson who was Queen Mary's Bishop of Lincoln,—he regarded the new ideas preached by Persons and Garnet with the contempt of a Catholic of ancient lineage and unswerving faith. How, he asked himself, could these converts understand his Church? What had they done, save vex the people and alarm the government? Loathing their creed, he felt no pity for the fate of Campion and Southwell; and he told the Catholics of Europe, in many a stinging phrase, that the Jesuits who were hung in London suffered, not because they were servants of their Church, but because they were traitors to their Queen. This view was the English view. In that luscious and ornate style which the clergy learned from the poets, Father Watson denounced the ambition of King Garnet and the turbulence of Emperor Persons, asserting that the angel faces, the flower of England's youth, the beauty of Britain's ocean, should never be appalled—nor the vermilion blush of English virgins, the modesty of married wives, and the matronhood of widows, put to shame—either by Spanish plots or Spanish force. Persons replied to the Secular priest in his "Manifestation," a book disfigured by much bad English and much fierce invective; in which the Jesuit, in place of covering the nakedness of his fellow-priests, accused them of living in a state of drunkenness and uncleanness; nay, he went so far in vituperation as to charge some of these reverend fathers with dicing, and others with stealing pewter pots.

Father Clarke, a man of higher gifts than Watson, answered this "Manifestation," in a "Reply" of some reach and vigor; charging home upon the Jesuits, whom he accused of a design to overthrow all liberty of thought and action, even that of the Pope himself. It would have been well for the old Catholic clergy if Father Clarke had been content with this victory of the pen; but, unfortunately for many besides himself, he conceived the idea of proving to Pope Clement that the old English clergy were a match for these vaunting Jesuits in political craft no less than they were in literary power.

His friend Watson, one of the few priests of their party who had talked with James while he was yet in Scotland, pledged his word that Catholics would be favored by the King. For saying so much in public, he was seized by Bancroft, Bishop of London; though the prelate changed his mind and set his prisoner free. When James came in, and day after day went by, and gave no sign, the priest began to think he had been duped. On his asking for a fresh audience, the King replied, "Since all the Protestants are for me, I have no need for the Papists." Father Watson thought the King mistaken in that view, the Catholic hosts being like the summer stars for multitude; and he said the King must be made aware of a fact which he did not seem to know.

Taking Father Clarke into his councils, he found they were of one mind as to the policy of proving, by an open effort, how strong the Catholics were. Two advantages would grow out of such a course:—(1) the King would be frightened into doing right; and (2) the Jesuits, who fancied themselves the only plotters in the world, would be put to open shame. The second of these results would seem to have been regarded by the priests as much more precious than the first.

They meant the King no harm, except a little fright, and their project was to be carried out in the blaze of noon. A Catholic host was to be raised in London and the nearer shires; they were to ride good horses, to show their quality; they were to go forth and meet their King. They were to break upon him like an army in line of battle, to offer their petition of grievances, and, in a frenzy of loyal ardor, to sweep him to the Tower. Surrounded in his palace by a court of Catholic peers, he would be only too willing to dismiss his Secretary, to dissolve his Council, to call new men into office, and openly return to the Church in which he had been baptized. The English Catholics would form his guard, while the Jesuits would be routed from the country as the enemies of God and man.

Such was the dream of these simple priests. But, when they came to talk with their sober and conservative flock, they found that such a display of numbers could not be made. Here and there some reckless spirit might be tempted by the hope of plunder to join their ranks; but the busy farmers and fearful citizens were averse to public action of any sort. They wanted to live in peace. They saw no reason to believe the King was with them. They had much to lose by plots, and were slavishly devoted to the maintenance of public law. Not yet reading the moral of their failure, the two priests turned elsewhere for aid, and in these new walks their feet began to slide.

Dining with Duke Humphrey in St. Paul's, rousing in the taverns of Carter Lane, were hosts of stout fellows, who might be willing to mount a good horse on the chance of getting a fat purse, not to speak of such tempting baits as a place at court. One such fellow was Sir Griffin Markham, of Beskwood Park, a knight who had smelt powder in the Low-Country camps, but, having lost his commission, was now dawdling away his time between the confessional, the tavern, and the stews. For the moment he was much excited against Lord Rutland, the young kinsman of Essex, from whom he had suffered some slight; and Father Watson, finding him in a sullen mood, suggested that the nearest way to his revenge upon that proud young spark was through the chances offered by this plot. Markham snapped at the golden bait; but this broken hero bargained for substantial favor; and before he pledged his sword to Watson he stipulated that, on a Catholic ministry being formed by the King, *he* was to have the Secretary's place!

The next fellow to be gained was Anthony Copley, a kinsman of Southwell. At fifteen years of age Copley had left England for Rome, where he accepted a bed and platter in the Jesuits' college, with a pension of ten crowns a year from the Pope. From Rome he passed into Flanders, where Father Owen obtained for him a pension of twenty crowns from the Prince of Parma, in whose service he remained fighting against his Queen, until he sickened of the Jesuits, when he returned to London and procured a pardon from Burghley on expressing his eagerness for instruction in a better creed. From that time he had been much abused by Persons, though he had never ceased to be a member of his Church. Hating the men at White Webbs, Copley came into Watson's plans, on the simple promise that those Jesuit intriguers were to be put to open shame.

In his first confession Copley boasted that those Jesuits were kept in ignorance of his plot; Watson thought the same; but this impression was a great mistake. A dozen members had not been told of their purpose, before Garnet, jealous and amused, had placed an agent at their board to learn their object and betray them to the law. That agent was Brooksby, whom Garnet set to watch the priests, while his wife Helen remained in her false name and false character beneath the Jesuit's roof.

The parts in this comedy of intrigue being cast, the comedians met in a tavern behind Paul's Churchyard, to wrangle, over pots of ale, about the strength of parties in the court. High names were mentioned in these pot-house meetings,—the names of Raleigh, Nottingham, Windsor; but no one spoke of intercourse with these great persons, since no one in the room pretended to know them, except by sight. The scheme for a great display of Catholic strength not only failed, but failed at once; for not a single lay Catholic of name and weight could be induced to join.

The comedy was played out, when Father Watson one day met in the street George Brooke, a man of birth, a brother of Lord Cobham, a brother-in-law of Cecil, having friends among those Puritan and patriotic gentry who were anxious to relieve Ostend. Brooke knew Lord Grey. A disappointed man, ill used by Cecil, Brooke lay open to the tempter's voice; and as he listened to Father Watson's talk he fancied that he saw some chance of crossing Cecil by this plan of waylaying and frightening James, if only Grey and some others could be got to help. Father Watson begged him to see what could be done.

Calling at Grey's house, on the pretense of mourning with him over the ruin of God's cause in London as well as on the Flemish coast, Brooke hinted that James had been deceived by Cecil as to the facts of public opinion, and asked whether it might not be well for some gentlemen of birth to lay a humble statement of the case before the King. Grey thought it would be well. James was at Greenwich. Such a statement, Brooke suggested, might be offered to the King, as he rode from that place to Windsor Castle,—but offered to him openly, in the light of noon, so that all the world might see how many gentlemen of rank and fortune held their views. For such a purpose, Grey said he could muster a hundred gentlemen of the best blood in England in a single day. Secure so far, Brooke asked whether Grey saw any objection to the old Catholic gentry, who had fought with them a common battle against the Jesuits, offering a petition of their own. Grey saw none.

A few days later, Brooke called on Grey again, bringing with him Markham, as one of those Catholic gentlemen who wished to have their grievances made known. These men had other plans, which they could not explain to Grey. They hoped to change the government; in order to change the government they must seize the King; and they could only seize the King by fighting with his guard. Alone, they could not venture on such a fight. Could Grey and his friends be tempted into offering them the chances of a fray? If swords were drawn, no man could tell where the broil might end. In a sudden tumult, every one could strike for himself, and on a cry being raised of "To the Tower!" the whole body of riders might be swept along, in a panic of fear, under the guidance of a few strong spirits who knew their minds. Could Grey be tempted?

Brooke, who seemed as though he had only come for instructions, asked the young general what must be done in case the King's guard set on them. Grey only smiled; the guard was not likely to attack a body of gentlemen in holiday attire. Still, urged Brooke, they might draw their swords in error and in panic. Suppose they drew: must the gentlemen stand on their defense? "No," answered Grey, at once; under no alarm could he suffer his friends to draw on the royal escort.

Such an answer left the dreamers without a hope; but Watson, falling deeper into treason every hour, thought otherwise. He saw his way, and felt his ground. If Grey would raise his friends and meet the King, that fact should be enough. A new plan could be built upon the old; for the priest could now speak to his loyal and conservative flock in a voice which they would understand.

Fired with his new purpose, he ran to the house of Sir Edward Parham, a strict old Somersetshire Catholic, whose sword was keen as his wit was dull. "Quodlibets" told this gentleman, as a secret, that the new King was more than half converted to their faith, that many of his councilors heard mass, and that Pope

Clement enjoined his children to guard their prince. Guard him from what? Then Watson whispered in his ear the still more perilous secret that Lord Grey and a gang of Puritan wretches were about to waylay their King, to seize his royal person, and to separate him from the devoted servants of his Church. Out of pure affection he offered to Parham a golden chance. If he could silently and swiftly raise his Catholic friends,—who would promptly arm in such a cause,—he might be able to win such favor and fortune as Ramsay had won in Gowrie house; for when those Puritan rascals pricked up in the Surrey lane, he could rush upon them, rescue his prince from danger, and carry him to his palace in the Tower. All that being promptly done, they could then fall at his Majesty's feet and ask him to do them religious justice. What grace could the King refuse to men who had saved his life?

Parham, burning to become a hero of the court like Ramsay, pledged his help. Yet the plot was hardly now complete. To give Parham his cue, there must be some appearance of attack. How could a scuffle be brought about? Could Grey be induced to admit Markham, Copley, and a few other Catholics in his train? If so, all would be well; for a kick of Copley's horse might raise a dust, a snap of Markham's pistol might raise a cry, the King would be sure to faint, the guards would probably charge, and the Puritan gentry might be trusted to draw their swords. Then, and then only, would be Parham's time.

Markham went down with Brooke to Lord Grey's house; but Grey would not listen to his prayer. If the Catholics wished to speak, let them do so, he said, another time in another place. Sir Griffin hinted that the Catholic gentlemen might go to meet the King, whether Grey approved their course or not. In that case, Grey announced that he should not go at all. The conference then broke up; and, seeing that for the present no good was to be done at court, Grey crossed the sea to Sluys, in the hope of either finding his way into Ostend or doing some better service to the Dutch.

This departure of Grey from London killed the comedy and brought the curtain down. James rode in peace from Greenwich to Windsor Castle; and then the Jesuits, after hearing a full report from Brooksby of what had been said and done by the plotters, sent Father Barneby, a creature whom they made their tool, to the house of Richard Bancroft, Bishop of London, to denounce the plot and to say where Copley might be seized.

CHAPTER VIII.

WILTON COURT.

A PLOT in the air,—a dream in the cloister,—a comedy in the tap-room,—a scheme which, dying in the throes of birth, could have no public history,—was no bad stuff for men like Cecil and Northampton to recast and shape. The secrecy and folly were in their favor. Grey had been consulted; and among the names which had been bandied about in Carter Lane was that of Raleigh. Striking for place and power, the subtle minister and his hoary pander had many motives, personal and political, for pushing their advantage to the last. White Webbs would laugh at the trouble of Watson and Clarke; the English college in Rome rejoice over the ruin of Copley; the Cardinal Archduke give thanks for the arrest of Grey. George Brooke was the brother and heir of Cobham; these two lives were all that stood between William Cecil, now Lord Cranborne, and a vast estate; and Cranborne was already promised in marriage to Northampton's niece. They put the case into the hands of Coke.

On Copley's first confession, Markham, Watson, Clarke, and Brooke were thrown into the Tower. Parham the dupe, and Brooksby the spy, were lodged in the Gate house, near Cecil's lodgings in Whitehall. Barneby, the priestly informer, having nothing more to tell, was hidden in the Clink. Not many days elapsed before it was rumored at Paul's Cross that Grey was in close arrest at Sluys, and not many more went by before the young Puritan peer was brought in a war-ship to the Tower.

Coke's brief against the prisoners was a work of legal art. Out of Barneby's report and Copley's confession he wove an appearance of three plots, which he proposed to call—

I. The Spanish Treason.
II. The Surprising Treason.
III. The Priests' Treason.

For the trial of these conspiracies he proposed to have separate courts, so as to give each trial its due importance in the public eye. In the Spanish Treason he indicted Count Aremberg, the Archduke's minister, together with Raleigh, Cobham, Grey, and Brooke, on a charge of plotting to deprive the King, and to raise his royal cousin, the Lady Arabella Stuart, to his throne. In the Surprising Treason he indicted Grey and Brooke, on a charge of conspiring to waylay and surprise the King as he rode from Greenwich to Windsor Castle. In the Priests' Treason he indicted Markham,

Copley, Parham, Watson, Clarke, and Brooke, on a charge of conspiring to change the government by force. Much was withheld from Coke. Nothing was said to him about the peace with Spain; but enough was hinted to tell him that Brooke must die. Hence the luckless uncle of Cecil's son was included as a principal in every charge.

Cecil spoke, though in vague, suspicious phrase, of the whole affair as the Arabella Plot, and his creature Coke tried hard to include Lord Grey in a second charge. It had been often bruited through the town that Grey would marry the Lady Arabella; and if Coke could show that Grey had ever entertained this project, he could lay him open to proceedings under the Royal Marriage Act. Cobham, who was said to have recommended such a match, was questioned in the Tower; but his examination ended without supplying evidence fit to be adduced in court.

While these prisoners lay in the Tower, awaiting trial, Don Juan de Taxis, Conde de Villa Medina, arrived from Spain. Don Juan's master wanted peace. Peace was worth to him more than a hundred thousand crowns a year, and this great sum of money his agent was empowered to spend in corrupting James's court. The wealth of two Indies flowed from the Ambassador's bounteous palm. Gems, feathers, perfumes, rained upon councilors' wives and on women who were thought to be more charming than their wives. In a month, Don Juan was the rage. Every one courted him, every one swore by him. Fine ladies, rustling in the silks of Seville and pale with the pearls of Margarita, voted him the most perfect gallant they had ever met. The Countess of Suffolk, as Cecil's most confidential friend, was the prime object of Don Juan's courtesies. The great house, then rising at

Charing Cross, was said, in reference to these gifts, to be plated with King Philip's gold.

Much of Don Juan's money passed into Cecil's pocket; for the minister knew the worth of peace to Spain, and when he sold his country to a foreigner his pride compelled him to sell her at a noble rate. Don Juan could not dispute his terms. "Buy others cheap; pay Cecil all he asks," was the substance, though not the form, of Don Juan's daily message from Madrid. Cecil named his price,—a king's ransom down in gold, and a yearly pension to be paid for life.

Northampton and Suffolk also obtained the most princely sums. When the terms of peace had been settled, Coke received an order from the Council to unmake his plots and cast his materials into other shapes. The charge against Aremberg must be withdrawn, and the Spanish Treason must disappear. Coke must have been deeply hurt, for the brief which he had drawn was a triumph of legal art. When he began afresh, he remembered Cecil's phrase of the Arabella plot, and he cast his confessions into a shape that would support the theory of such a conspiracy. But, as neither Copley nor the priests had mentioned this lady's name, he was told even now, at the ninth hour, to drop her name, and to divide the plot into two new parts. When his brief was drawn, the plot consisted of the Main and the Bye. Raleigh was in the Main, Grey was in the Bye, Brooke was in both the Main and the Bye. One was a conspiracy to raise Arabella to the throne, the other was a conspiracy to change the government by force.

For reasons which can only now be guessed, the name of Grey was dropped at the last moment from the article charging Raleigh and Cobham with the Arabella Treason. Brooksby, not being sent to the

Tower, expected to escape a trial; but unseen influences worked against the spy, who was carried down to Winchester like the rest, leaving his fair young wife at the Jesuits' lodgings at White Webbs.

The King rode down to Wilton Court, to be near the scene of trial; and in the quaint old house where Mary Sydney lived, and under the solemn cedars that her brother loved, gay pages fluttered and wily courtiers mused; while the hardier gentlemen of the chamber leaped to horse and dashed into the neighboring town.

Popham and Coke made very short work with the smaller fry of prisoners. A few hours sufficed for them to bully and condemn Brooke, Watson, Copley, Markham, and Clarke. Parham was spared. Brooksby, though pleading that he joined the conspirators only to betray them, was condemned to die. Clarke alone showed genuine courage. Having played his game and lost, his only trouble appeared to be that he, a man of order and of letters, should leave behind him a traitor's name.

Raleigh came up next; after Raleigh came up Cobham; and after Cobham, Grey. Grey was tried by his peers, some of them his personal enemies,—one of them that Lord Southampton whom he had beaten in the public street. Dudley Carleton says that Southampton "was mute before his face," but spoke much against him when the lords "retired to consult among themselves." Lord Grey's defense was simple. If the thought of presenting a petition was high treason, he was guilty; if it were lawful, he was not guilty. To the charge of conspiring with Brooke and Markham to surprise the King, he offered his proud denial and defied the proof. Only thrice had he seen these men, and on the first suggestion of force being used he had peremptorily declined all further talk with them. The peers condemned him to die a traitor's death.

When asked if he had anything to urge why sentence of death should not be passed upon him, he answered, "Nothing." The court was awed into deep, pathetic silence. After a pause, he added, "Yet, a word of Tacitus comes into my mind:—*Non eadem omnibus decora.* The house of Wilton have spent many lives in their prince's service. Grey cannot beg his life."

Raleigh himself never passed that height; and the proud refusal of this young soldier of twenty-five to ask a pardon from the King amazed and fascinated James.

When Brooke was fallen by the axe, and the two priests were hung and quartered, the King made a fidgety secret as to whether he would go on or pause. Under the green trees and by the limpid streams of Wilton House two parties were contending night and day; the gentlemen who were fumbling the edge of Don Juan's gold defending the verdicts passed and clamoring for what they called traitors' blood; while those who had kept their fingers free were crying out against the sentence as infamous, the witnesses as perjured, the peers as corrupt. The ladies were on the side of mercy; and all the prisoners were willing to ask for mercy, excepting Grey.

Pembroke sent to London for the Globe comedians, in order that the Teacher of his Age might help to infuse some mirth and tenderness into the royal councils; and William Shakspeare's troop rode down to Wilton on this gracious errand. One play was given before the court; and there is reason to believe that play was "Measure for Measure." The play was new; composed that very fall, as the many allusions to events then passing prove,—to the plague, to the war, to the expected peace, to the proclamation, to the revival of obsolete laws, to the razing of a certain class of houses in the suburbs. Such an expression as "Heaven grant us its peace, but not the King of Hungary's!" might have been heard in every street that summer; and the characters of Angelo and the Duke are but highly-colored and flattering pictures of Cecil and the King. The play may have been written for the Wilton stage. That it was first produced before a courtly audience is clear from the text; not only from the passage on ladies' masks, but from the many allusions in it to James's easy nature and his great dislike to crowds. It may be safely gathered from the story of this play that the noble lines,—

> "Not the King's crown, nor the deputed sword,
> The marshal's truncheon, nor the judge's robe,
> Becomes them with one-half so good a grace
> As mercy does!"

were addressed from the stage of Wilton House to James.

The King, who had no poetry in his soul to be touched by noble phrases, caused the warrants to be drawn out and passed under the Great Seal, for the execution of Markham, Cobham, and Grey; and Tichborne, Governor of the Castle, received instructions to prepare a scaffold in Castle yard, and strike off the conspirators' heads on Friday morning before ten o'clock. The Duke of Vienna could hardly have devised a vainer plot.

Friday morning came, and the party of clemency was in despair. The Wilton lawns were drenched with rain; the air was chill and raw; yet thousands of people swarmed from an early hour into the Saxon city, rolling over Castle Hill, choking up the city gates, spotting every balcony and roof with black,—yeomen from the Sussex downs, gentry from the glebes and parks, pages and courtiers from Wilton House, possibly the Globe comedians, and the Globe poet himself. James was to prove himself that day a greater comedian than any in that famous troop.

Sitting in his room at Wilton House, the King called to his side a lad named John Gibbs, then raw from Scotland, barely able to make himself understood in English speech. The lad's face was unknown to Tichborne; that was the point of the King's joke,—the fact out of which was to leap his great surprise. James put a paper into his hand, and bade him ride over to Winchester Castle, where he was to watch the proceedings until the axe was being raised to strike, when he was to rush into the ring, draw Tichborne aside, and show him the royal mandate. When the lad was gone, the King remembered that in his haste he had forgotten to sign his name. Riders flew after Gibbs, and brought him back, and, the fault being mended, the Scotch lad dashed over the downs to Winchester, where he found the Castle yard crowded with Tichborne's men. These fellows pushed him back into the crowd, deaf to his cries, impatient of his Scottish twang; so that, while the headsman was getting ready, Gibbs had to hang about the gate, fretting at the pikemen, and hoping that some one would arrive who would know his face and understand his tale.

Markham was brought out first to die; and, after saying a short prayer, he was bending his neck to the stroke, when a quick cry from the crowd caught the sheriff's ear. Gibbs had found Sir James Hay, who cut a path for him to Tichborne's side. In a moment the seal was broken, and Tichborne learned, under the

King's own hand, that the prisoners were to be put—as it were—to the axe, but only in sport, and, when they had been frightened to death, were to be told that the King had been graciously pleased to spare their lives. Having read these strange commands, the sheriff told Markham to stand aside.

Grey came out next,—his footfall firm, his eye elate, his expression proud and gentle; for he had supped as well and slept as softly as he could have done at Whaddon Hall. A band of youthful nobles, few of them younger, none of them nobler, than himself, marched with him from his cell to the Castle yard. Gay in his attire as though the block to which he was going were a bridal board, his countenance bright with unearthly joy, he passed through the kneeling lines,—the only man, perhaps, whose pulse beat calmly in all that quivering throng. Dropping softly at the headsman's feet, he poured out his soul in prayer; and, when he had made his peace with God, he confessed his sins in the face of man, admitting his many offenses, but haughtily putting away from him the stain of crime. The rain fell fast; but the crowd stood sadly in the Castle yard. From his prison-window Raleigh was looking on. Grey made his sign; for the pang of death was past; and he laid his neck for the lifted steel. Then Tichborne broke upon his peace. An error, said the sheriff, had crept in on their proceedings; Cobham must die first, and Grey must abide for an hour in the hall.

When the ghastly comedy was played out, the three prisoners were ranked in the Castle yard, face to face; Tichborne read the King's letter of reprieve; and the people threw up their caps and cried, "Well done!"

CHAPTER IX.

LAST OF A NOBLE LINE.

THE prisoners spared at Winchester were brought in time to the Tower; but only the three great ones were confined beyond the year. Within a few weeks Copley and Brooksby were pardoned and restored in blood. Markham was set free, on the sole condition of his going to live abroad; and Barneby was paid his wages and sent away. Raleigh and Cobham were left in the Tower, that Philip might be easy in his mind, and that Cecil might receive the rents from a large estate.

On his first return to the Tower, Lord Grey was miserably housed by the Lieutenant, Sir George Harvey, a man suspected by the court, and eager to regain the Secretary's good opinion. Grey complained to Cecil, who still professed to wish him well, and who was never harsh, like Northampton, beyond his need. Cecil stood his friend so far; and on a hint from court that, though Grey must be kept in safety, he need not be kept in torment, Harvey remembered that he had an empty room in the Brick tower, Sir George Carew's official apartment,—a tower which had been Raleigh's first prison, and was afterward to be his last. This house stood on the northern wall, above the ditch. It was high and cold. As Sir George Carew was never in residence, the rooms were empty and unused; and Harvey, fearing that Grey would still object, informed his master that prisoners had been put into that tower in Peyton's time. Hither, then, Lord Grey was brought; and in this gloomy tower he spent the next nine years of his feverish life.

Eight pounds a week were allowed him out of his great estate. He was suffered to write to his mother and sister, and his servants were allowed in ordinary times to wait upon him. But his condition changed with the seasons and lieutenants. Generally his imprisonment was close and his treatment harsh. One likes to know the effect of gloom and chains, of damp and silence, on so proud a spirit. The old, old story comes up again:—they broke his health; and when they had ruined his health they easily broke his heart. The man who could not be induced to beg for life was worn into begging fretfully for such poor freedom as the liberties of the Tower!

Yet there was nothing mean in Grey from first to last. If his life in the Brick tower had not the beauty of Raleigh's life in the Garden house, it had a nobleness all his own. In his younger days he had amused his leisure by translating St. Cyprian's tract on "Patience," and when he found himself a prisoner in the Tower he sent to his mother for his book, and asked that his boy might come to him and read for him. Cecil moved the King to grant him so much favor; but the King was in no mood to comply. "I beseech you," Grey wrote again, "to move the King for my scholar, who will yield me much comfort." When the request was granted, it was only on condition that the reader should occupy the same room with his lord, and should never leave it.

In his letters to his mother, Grey seemed more anxious to remove any lurking seeds of suspicion about his loyalty from her mind, than to engage her in efforts for his worldly good. "Madam," he writes, "be not dismayed. I am in the Tower, but neither for thought nor deed against King and country." Again he writes to her, "I fear not evil. My heart is fixed. I trust in the Lord."

Grey found it hard to be patient in the Brick tower, while Ostend was calling to him, as he thought, for help. The peace with Spain was a sore trial to his spirit, though he fancied that the terms of that peace would allow him to take service in the patriotic army. Markham had been suffered to serve under the Archduke, and he counted on the same indulgence in his own relations with the Prince of Orange. Then came the fall of Ostend.

While his old commander, Vere, remained in the Low Countries, he hoped against hope; but when that veteran was recalled by James, his big heart almost burst with rage. "No one accident," he wrote to his friend Winwood, a Puritan like himself, a partisan of the Dutch like himself, "hath so much grieved me as this of Vere, that he should forsake the Low-Country employment, when my misfortune hath made me so unavailable."

There lay the core of his offense. Grey longed to be in the field, fighting against the enemies of his country and his faith; and the courtiers at Whitehall were earning pensions by preventing men like himself from offering their swords to the insurgent Dutch. Like Raleigh, Grey was the prisoner of Spain.

Years dragged on; but, the pensions of Cecil and Northampton being duly paid, the prisoner lay in his lonely tower above the ditch.

At length the war itself wore out; the Dutch republic was acknowledged; the twelve years' truce was signed; and the cause of their savage watch on Grey was in some degree removed. Yet year on year went by without a change. At length Northampton affected to remember Grey. He went down to the Tower, and saw his comrade of the court. The prisoner asked for leave to walk on the terrace under the Ordnance house, for the benefit of his health; a liberty which Sir Walter Raleigh and the Earl of Northumberland then enjoyed. This indulgence was refused, but a change was made in his lodgings, from the gloomy Brick tower on the northern wall, to the cheery Water gate on the Thames. Grey fancied that Northampton had become his friend, after being for so many years his foe. The Earl was never to be feared so much as when he appeared to be doing good.

William Seymour (afterward Duke of Somerset) had just escaped from the Water gate; and his wife, the Lady Arabella, had been ordered to the Tower. Thus the Lady who had been Grey's unwitting demon was once more brought within his range; and, through the treacherous courtesies of Northampton, the evil of his younger time repeated itself in his desolate cell. The royal lady lay in the Belfry and the Lieutenant's house; their prisons were therefore near each other. One of Arabella's women contrived to see Grey in the Water gate, and his lordship was accused of sending love-messages to the royal lady. Grey denied it, turning the affair into an act of innocent flirting with her maid; but the rumor served Northampton's purpose; for the King became alarmed at what he supposed to be a new intrigue; the chance of pardon for the lady vanished, and Grey was ordered into close confinement in his tower.

This rank injustice broke his spirit.

In this Water gate the last Lord Grey of Wilton died, in the summer of 1614, eleven years after his first arrest in Sluys; leaving a mother, who quickly followed her noble and gallant son, and a sister, from whom descend the Grey-Egertons, now the sole representatives of Arthur and Sibyl Grey.

> "Inexorable Death in this sole stroke
> Had lopped the laurel and hewn down the oak."

Yet, brief as were his days in the Tower, Grey long outlived the Jesuit schemer of White Webbs.

CHAPTER X.

POWDER-PLOT ROOM.

ONE chamber in the Lieutenant's house has a life apart from the rest; a chamber on the upper tier, built on the old wall, with oaken panels, and a window opening on the Thames. In a house of no great size this room looks large, and the window in it is high and wide. No one could mistake it for a prisoner's cell; yet this chamber on the old wall is almost as famous in English story as the Belfry and the Bloody tower. The mantle-piece shows a royal bust; the wall is plated with records from a royal pen. Round the cornice are the shields of some of our noblest families,—Howards, Somersets, Cecils, Humes, and Blounts. The bust, though stained to look like bronze, is carved in wood; while the panels are laden with much Latinity and many historic lies.

The wooden head is that of James the First, the lying record is that of the Powder Plot.

James used to speak of the Powder Plot as his master-piece; a term which might be taken to hint that the King had worked it out from his own fancy, much as Cecil had worked out the Arabella Plot. But this could not have been his meaning. James had neither the wit to conceive, nor the steadiness to control, such a scheme of political vengeance. The plot was an actual plot, with living agents and a settled plan. Yet the dreamers who ascribe this plot, in general terms, to the Catholic clergy and laity, go further astray from fact than the dreamers who ascribe it to King James.

The plot was not a Catholic plot.

This wild project of political murder was the work of a few converts from the English Church, conducted by a gang of outlaws and fanatics, not only against the conscience, but against the interest, of every Catholic in the realm. The Pope condemned it. The Arch-priest condemned it. All the Secular priests and all their sober flocks condemned it. What these children of St. Edward and St. Thomas had to do with the Powder Plot, was to bear, during many reigns, under protests which were seldom heard; the social odium and political penalty of a crime which they abhorred.

Nor was this project properly a Jesuit crime. It found some friends in the Order of Jesus, beyond a doubt; but these friends of the Powder Plot were of no high standing in the body, and the society, as a society, gave them no support. Not one, but many, of the more eminent fathers fought against the scheme. The General, Claudius Aquaviva, set his face against the plotters, when he could only guess their purpose; and when the details reached him, just as he was entering on the festival of Christmas, the noble old man was smitten to the heart.

Those who throw the blame on Catholics miss the great moral of the crime.

The men who contrived, the men who prepared, the

men who sanctioned, this scheme of assassination were, one and all, of Protestant birth. Father Persons was Protestant born. Father Owen and Father Garnet were Protestants born. From what is known of Winter's early life, it may be assumed that he was a Protestant. Catesby and Wright had been Protestant boys. Guy Fawkes had been a Protestant, Percy had been a Protestant. The minor persons were like their chiefs,—apostates from their early faith, with the moody weakness which is an apostate's inspiration and his curse. Tresham was a convert—Monteagle was a convert—Digby was a convert. Thomas Morgan, Robert Kay, and Kit Wright were all converts. The five gentlemen who dug the mine in Palace-yard were all of English blood and of Protestant birth. But they were converts and fanatics, observing no law save that of their own passions; men of whom it should be said, in justice to all religions, that they no more disgraced the Church which they entered than that which they had left.

The plot was the main clerical effort of that Spanish conspiracy against English law which the converted Jesuits had been trained to conduct; a political conflict in which these English Jesuits appealed to the sword and perished by the sword.

The first panel on the wall, a pious prayer, pagan in form, yet far from classical in style, sets forth the virtues and dignities of those who were to have suffered in the explosion:

JACOBVS MAGNVS MAGNÆ BRITAÑIÆ
REX, PIETATE, JVSTITIA, PRVDENTIA, DOCTRINA, FORTITVDINE, CLEMENTIA, CETERISQ. VIRTVTIBVS REGIIS CLARISS'; CHRISTIANÆ FIDEI, SALVTIS PUBLICÆ, PACIS VNIVERSALIS PROPVGNATOR, FAVTOR, AVCTOR ACERRIMVS, AVGVSTISS', AVSPICATISS'.

ANNA REGINA FREDERICI 2. DANORV̄ REGIS INVICTISS FILIA SERENISS'.

HENRICVS PRINCEPS, NATVRÆ ORNAMENTIS, DOCTRINÆ PRÆSIDIIS GRATIÆ MVNERIBVS, INSTRVCTISS'; NOBIS & NATVS & A DEO DATVS.

CAROLVS DVX EBORACENSIS DIVINA AD OMNEM VIRTVTEM INDOLE.
ELIZABETHA VTRIVSQ. SOROR GERMANA, VTROQVE PARENTE,
DIGNISSIMA.
HOS, VELVT PVPILLAM OCVLI TENELLAM
PROVIDVS MVNI, PROCVL IMPIORVM
IMPETV ALARVM TVARVM INTREPIDOS
CONDE SVB VMBRA.

No one but James was likely to have penned this invocation; in English thus:

"James the Great, King of Great Britain,

Illustrious for piety, justice, foresight, learning, hardihood, clemency, and the other regal virtues; champion and patron of the Christian faith, of the public safety, and of universal peace; author most subtle, most august, and most auspicious:

"Queen Ann, the most serene daughter of Frederick the Second, invincible King of the Danes:

"Prince Henry, ornament of nature, strengthened with learning, blest with grace, born and given to us from God:

"Charles, Duke of York, divinely disposed to every virtue:

"Elizabeth, full sister of both; most worthy of her parents:

"Do Thou, all-seeing, protect these as the apple of the eye, and guard them without fear from wicked men beneath the shadow of Thy wings."

Then comes a list of Lords Commissioners, followed by the chief panel of the series, in more pretentious and much worse Latin than the first. This panel, the work of Sir William Waad, contains the following votive offering from the King's Lieutenant of the Tower:

DEO OPT: MAX: TRIVNO, SUSPITATORI, & TANTÆ, TAM ATROCIS, TAMQ. INCREDIBILIS IN REGEM LEMENTISS; IN REGINAM SERENISS': IN DIVINÆ INDOLIS & OPTIMÆ SPEI PRINCIPEM, CÆTERAMQ. PROGENIEM REGIAM, ET IN OMNEM OMNIUM ORDINEM, & NOBILITATIS ANTIQUÆ, & FORTITUDINIS AVITÆ ET PIETATIS CASTISSIMÆ, & JUSTITIÆ SANCTISSIMÆ FLOREM PRÆCIPVUM, CONJURATIONIS EXEQUENDÆ NITROSI PULVERIS SVBJECTI INFLAMMATIONE, CHRISTIANÆ VERÆQ. RELIGIONIS EXTINGVENDÆ FVRIOSA LIBIDINE, ET REGNI STIRPITUS EVERTENDI NEFARIA CVPIDITATE, A JESUITIS ROMANENSIBUS PERFIDÆ CATHOLICÆ & IMPIETATIS VIPERINÆ AVTORIBUS & ASSERTORIBUS, ALIISQ. EJUSDEM AMENTIÆ SCELERISQ. PATRATORIBUS & SOCIIS SVSCEPTÆ & IN IPSO PESTIS DEREPENTÆ INFERENDÆ ARTICULO (SALUTIS ANNO + 1605 + MENSIS NOVEMBRIS DIE QUINTO) TAM PRÆTER SPEM, QUAM SUPRA FIDEM MIRIFICE ET DIVINITUS DETECTÆ AVERRVNCO, ET VINDICI, GRATES QUANTAS ANIMI CAPERE POSSENT MAXIMAS ET IMMORTALES. A NOBIS OMNIBUS, ET POSTERIS NOSTRIS HABERE ET AGI GVLIELMUS WAADE MILES TVRRI A DOMINO REGE PRÆFECTUS, POSITO PERPETUO HOC MONUMENTO VOLVIT, DIE NONO MENSIS OCTB. ANNO REGNI JACOBI PRIME SEXTO AÑO DÑI 1608.

In English thus:

"To Almighty God, the guardian, arrester, and avenger,—who has punished this great and incredible conspiracy against our most merciful lord the King, our most serene lady the Queen, our divinely-disposed Prince, and the rest of our royal house, and against all persons of quality, our ancient nobility, our soldiers, prelates, and judges; the authors and advocates of which conspiracy, Romanized Jesuits, of perfidious, Catholic, and serpent-like ungodliness, with others equally criminal and insane, were moved by the furious desire of destroying the true Christian religion, and by the treasonous hope of overthrowing the kingdom, root and branch; and which was suddenly, wonderfully, and divinely detected, at the very moment when the ruin was impending, on the fifth day of November, in the year of grace, 1605,—William Waad, whom the King has appointed his Lieutenant of the Tower, returns, on the ninth of October, in the sixth year of the reign of James the First, 1608, his great and everlasting thanks."

After this panel comes a third, containing a list of

the conspirators' names, both clerical and lay, with tags of pious verse and foolish appeals to gods and men.

These panels on the wall record a series of noticeable scenes.

About the hour of noon, on a dark November day, in the year 1605, a very high company came down from Whitehall Palace to the Tower; men in whose sleepless eyes and troubled haste of speech a drama of unusual tension might be read. Sir William Waad, then new in office, met them by the gate; but the greeting which these great ones deigned to give their humble tool was scant. A small bent man, past middle age, with shuffling gait and furtive eyes, passed in, going quickly through the arch of that Bloody tower in which Raleigh was then confined, and straight across the Green to the new Lieutenant's house. The small bent man and three gallant personages who followed him had each a George upon his breast.

They met in this poor chamber on the wall to examine a prisoner then in the Tower, on a matter which would cause the place in which they sat to be called in all future times the Powder-Plot Room.

Who these persons were may be read on these panels,—their names, their titles, and the offices they held,—names which are familiar still, not by the Thames only, but in every zone of the earth in which our English speech is heard. In the chair sat Robert Cecil, Earl of Salisbury, Secretary of State; and near him were Charles Howard, Earl of Nottingham, Lord High Admiral; Charles Blount, Earl of Devon, Lord Lieutenant of Ireland; and Henry Howard, Earl of Northampton, Lord Privy Seal. Is it too much to say that, high as were the offices filled by these Knights of the Garter, the men had higher claims to notice than their official rank? Cecil was a son of Lord Burghley, a cousin of Sir Francis Bacon; Nottingham disputed with Raleigh the foremost place at sea; Mountjoy was hardly more renowned as the Pacificator of Ireland than as the friend of Sydney and the lover of Lady Rich; Northampton, the second and favorite son of Surrey, was a scholar, a writer, a speaker of the highest class.

Cecil laid before the lords a paper, drawn that very day (Tuesday, November 6), and written from first to last by the King's own pen. This paper, addressed to the Lords Commissioners for the Plot, directed certain peers and gentlemen, in quaint old Scottish phrase, to question a prisoner then in the Tower, and to make him tell the truth by gentle means, if gentle means would serve; if not, by slinging him to the hook and binding him on the rack.

The man to be examined had been seized on the previous night, on the door-steps of a house in Parliament Place, under circumstances to excite the wildest terror. Dragged by armed men to Whitehall, and brought into the King's presence, he had been questioned by James himself, as to who he was and what he meant to do; to which questions he had answered, with reckless devilry, that he was a poor serving-man, and that he meant to slay, by a sudden burst of powder, laid in a vault beneath the throne, the King and Queen, the young prince, the royal councilors and judges, with the principal persons of the court. Pressed still more, he had given his own name as John Johnson and his master's name as Thomas Percy, one of the King's Gentlemen Pensioners, a kinsman of the great northern Earl. Bandying jokes with the guard, this fellow had shown a savage scorn of life which all-but fascinated James.

After he had left the presence, a letter had been found in his clothes; a letter written in French, and by a lady's pen. This letter, found upon him open, was signed Elizabeth Vaux (the lady of Harrowden), and was addressed to him as Guido Fawkes.

At a sign from Cecil, Waad brought in his prisoner. Some of the lords, not all, had seen that face before,—seen it for an hour, under the glare of fitful lamps, in the midst of scared, inquisitive eyes, when, roused from their beds, and hurried to Whitehall at midnight, they had heard from the royal lips a tale, the like of which courtiers have seldom been called to hear in the dead of night from kings. They had seen the black brow beetling over those fiery orbs, now sullen with rampant rage, now rippling with low, fierce laughter, as the King, seated on the edge of his bed, forced out in gasps and screams his version of the powder and the mine; and now, in the fog of a November noon, they looked on that face again.

CHAPTER XI.

GUY FAWKES.

A MAN to study with a curious art was the stiff, bronzed fellow, with sandy beard and fell of auburn hair, now standing in this Tudor room, before judges of such high fame and power, and answering these lords of war and masters of law as lightly as though the inquiry were some tavern jest; giving the false name of Johnson, the false description of a serving-man; and only laughing roughly when they found him out.

Tall, strongly built, and thirty-five years old, he stood before them in the prime of all his powers. His face was good, in some of its aspects fine. His tones were those of gentle life; his words, though few, were choice; and his bearing spoke of both the cloister and the camp. Despite the grime upon his hands, the grime of coal and powder, he was evidently a man of birth. Mountjoy could see that he had been a soldier; Northampton found him an adept in the schools. Even Cecil, who knew a good deal more about him than he liked to say, was smitten by his jaunty air.

"He is no more dismayed," wrote the Secretary of State, "than if he were taken for a poor robbery on the highway." Not a dozen hours had yet passed by since he was seized in Parliament Place; seized in the very fact, with matches in his pocket, with a lantern behind the door, and in such guise and manner as made his conviction sure. All that could have happened to cross his purpose and crush his spirit had come to pass. His plans had failed, his friends were scattered, his cause was lost. Behind him lay the wreck of a life; before him lowered the jail, the rack, the gibbet, and the yelling crowd. All that he could call his own on earth was a day of feverish pain, an infamous and cruel death, a memory laden with a lasting curse. Yet the man was rock. The lords had spent a sleepless night, and he had slumbered like a child. They had been tossing on beds of down, while he had been sleeping on a plait of straw. They had sought for rest in vain under painted ceilings, and he had been dreaming lightly in the darkest dungeon of the Tower. The Lieutenant, coming early to his cell, had found him sleeping "as a man void of trouble."

Not that he was cold and strong; still less that he was dark and subtle. The man was open, and even frank. He told the truth so far as he meant to speak, at once. When he told a lie he told it of fixed design, and rather to screen some brother in misfortune than to save himself. He was neither mercenary, nor inscrutable, nor heroic; he was simply a fanatic, with the vices and virtues which belong to a fanatic. Like nearly all fanatics, he was a convert to his faith, glowing with the zeal which sharpens a fakir's knife and comforts a martyr at the stake. Fasting and observance had helped to drive him mad; until he felt, like many of those familiars of the Holy Office whom he had met in Antwerp and Madrid, that it was his duty to kill men's bodies on the chance of saving souls.

Cecil read the paper which he had received from James, a warrant containing sixteen questions to be put, with a power of compelling answers to these queries in case of need. This quaint old paper of instructions, which the lords must have had some sport in spelling through, may be given in the King's own form:

"This examinate wolde now be maid to ansoure to formall interrogatours.

"1 as quhat he is, for I can neuer yett heare of any man that knowis him.

"2 quhaire he uas borne,

"3 quhat uaire his parents names,

"4 quhat aage is he of,

"5 quhaire he hath liued,

"6 hou he hath liued and by quhat trade of lyfe,

"7 hou he ressaued those woundes in his breste,

"8 if he uas euer in seruice, uith any other before percie, and quhat thay uaire, and hou long,

"9 hou came he in percies seruice, by quhat meanes, and at quhat tyme,

"10 quhat tyme uas this house hyred by his maister,

"11 and hou soone after the possessing of it did he beginne to his deuillishe preparations,

"12 quhen and quhaire lernid he to speake frenshe,

"13 quhat gentle womans lettir it uas that uas founde upon him,

"14 and quhairfor doth she giue him an other name in it then he giues to him self,

"15 if he uas euer a papiste, and if so quho brocht him up in it,

"16 if other wayes, hou uas he conuertid, quhaire, quhen, and by quhom, this course of his lyfe I ame the more desyrouse to know, because I haue dyuers motiues leading me to suspecte that he hath remained long beyonde the seas, and ather is a preiste, or hath long seruid some preiste or fugitiue abroade, for I can yett (as I saide in the beginning heirof) meite with no man that knowis him, the letter found upon him giues him another name, and those that best knowis his meister can neuer remember to haue seene him in his companie, quhair upon it shoulde seeme that he hath bene reccomendit by some personnis to his maisters service only for this use, quhairin only, he hath servid him, and thairfore he uolde also be asked in quhat company and shippe he went out of englande, and the porte he shipped at, and the like quœstions wolde be asked anent the forme of his returne, as for these tromperie waires found upon him, the signification and use of euerie one of thaime wolde be knowin, and quat I have obseruid in thaim, the bearare will show you, nou laste, ye remember of the crewallie uillanouse pasquil that rayled upon me for the name of brittaine, if I remember richt it spake some thing of haruest and prophecied my destruction about that tyme, ye maye thinke of this, for it is like to be the laboure of suche a desperate fellow as this is, if he will not other wayes confesse, the gentler tortours are to be first usid unto him et sic per gradus ad ima tenditur, and so god speede youre goode worke. "JAMES R."

These questions were put by Cecil, and the prisoner's answers were written down. His name was Johnson —he was born in Netherdale—his father was called Thomas, his mother Edith—he was thirty-six years old —he had lived in Yorkshire, Cambridge, and elsewhere —he had a farm of thirty pounds a year—his scars came of a pleurisy—he had served no one but Percy—he had served him since Easter, 1604—his master had hired the house about Midsummer-twelvemonth—at Christmas last he had brought in the powder—he had learnt French in England, but improved it abroad—the letter was from a gentlewoman in Flanders—she called him Fawkes because he used to call himself so —he was brought up a Catholic—he was not a convert. Some of these replies were true; most of them were false.

Next morning, Wednesday, a sharper board of inquisitors came down to the Tower, and sent for Fawkes into the Powder-Plot Room. Northampton occupied the chair, assisted by the Lord Chief Justice Popham and Sir Edward Coke. If England had been raked from end to end, the mates of these three men, in craft of brain, in hardness of heart, could nowhere have been found. Fawkes soon felt that it was one thing to baffle soldiers like Nottingham and Mountjoy, another to fence with lawyers like Popham and Coke.

Northampton pointed to the rack, and told the prisoner to speak the truth, or he would tear it from his heart. To these new judges Fawkes confessed the facts, so far as they touched himself His Christian name was Guy, his surname Fawkes. He was born in York, where his father, Edward Fawkes, had lived; but his father died about thirty years ago, leaving him a small estate, which he had spent. He took service with Percy under the name of Johnson, and by this name he was known in Parliament Place. He had sworn on the Primer never to betray his friends in the plot—he had taken the sacrament with that oath. Five was the original number, but five or six others had come in since. He was now sorry for what he had tried to do, since he saw that God would not suffer it to be done. He was not a priest. He could not name his accomplices on account of his oath, and he would not say where he had sworn that oath. All the five plotters swore the same oath as himself: they swore it a year and a half ago. Some speech had been held among them, that they would free the prisoners from the Tower, that they would marry the King's daughter to a Catholic, and that they would raise her to the throne.

All these confessions made a good day's work, but after Northampton had left the Tower, Waad went down into Fawkes's cell, and, finding him full of talk, began to urge him, as he looked for grace, to set forth all that he knew of the plot from first to last; how the design arose, who were the agents, and what they proposed to do when the King was dead. Fawkes seemed touched in spirit; he had not yet been tortured; but the rack was before his eyes; and unless he gave up all his secrets the morrow would see him stretched. Waad left him that night in the belief that he would yield; but on his return to the cell next day a change had come upon the prisoner's mood. Fawkes would not speak, he would not write. Vexed at his stubborn spirit, the Lieutenant called his men, and bound his prisoner to the rack. Fawkes may have thought that he could bear the pain and not cry out; but after thirty minutes of the cord and pulley, he gasped out faintly that he would tell them all he knew.

A first confession was taken down. The plot, he said, was a religious plot; he heard of it first from an English gentleman in Flanders; and he went on to describe the mine, the powder, and the train. Later in the day he made a more important statement. The pain had quelled his courage, and the man who would have faced a blazing mine could not resist the slow, cold agony of the cord. On the rack he gasped out names, addresses, details of many kinds. So much matter being gained, the Lieutenant spoke with him once more. Why not cleanse his bosom? What had the Jesuits been about? Who had given him the sacrament? Broken in nerve, the strong man yielded; but he could not be persuaded to write his shame. If the Earl of Salisbury would come to him, and come alone, he would tell him everything which it concerned his Majesty to learn. A messenger from Waad soon bore this news to court, and almost as quickly as horses could devour the road between the Strand and the Tower, Cecil was closeted with Fawkes in the Powder-Plot Room, listening to the first words from his lips which could be used in open court against his neighbors of White Webbs.

When these words were written down, the prisoner was asked to sign his name. He took up his pen, and essayed to write, but the quivering flesh refused to obey his will. "Guido," he wrote; the rest of his name he could not write. From that day forward silence on his part was vain; others beside himself were in arrest,—some in the Tower, some in the Gate house, some in the Fleet; and then, in gasps and spasms, the singular facts of the Powder Plot came out.

But the story told in these gasps and spasms may be given with less waste of words, in a closer form, than that of a prisoner's record on the rack.

CHAPTER XII.

ORIGIN OF THE PLOT.

The dumpy man called Tom, who rode so often to White Webbs with Mr. Catesby, was Thomas Winter, a younger brother of Robert Winter, a small Worcestershire squire. A shrewd fellow, who had seen the world, both in courts and camps, this Tom could patter in many tongues, and was familiar with many lands. In his youth he had fought against the King of Spain; but on falling under Jesuit influence he had given up the cause of freedom and the profession of arms, to spend his middle age in the secret service of Lord Monteagle, whose pay he took and whose man he was called. Going hither and thither, from London to Brussels, from Madrid to Rome, he had borne the latest news from Father Persons and Father Creswell to their friends in Flanders and at White Webbs; and generally he had earned his wages by promoting that revolution which the Jesuits told his master would shortly come about.

Catesby and Tom had tried their luck in a street fight, with a royal favorite in their ranks, and, having been crushed, condemned, and fined, were anxiously seeking some safer way to upset their Queen. What could they do? The people were against them. Even the Catholics were against them. While the citizens were loyal and the lords alert, rebellion was clearly a waste of blood. What then? They came for counsel to White Webbs.

"Mr. Mese" had strange news to tell them; for he had just received from Rome, where Persons was then the ruling spirit, two papal breves; one addressed to the Archpriest, George Blackwell, and the Catholic clergy, the other addressed to the nobility and commons, in which breves the children of Rome were enjoined, on their salvation, to admit no prince except such as the Pope should appoint to reign over them. These breves were not to be published until the Queen was dead; but Garnet showed them to Catesby, by whom they were shown to Lord Monteagle and his cousin Frank. Monteagle had a villa near Hoxton, from which he could easily ride over to White Webbs; and Catesby hired a house in the same suburbs, at Moorcroft, under London Wall. These two gentlemen, seeing that such breves could never be enforced without foreign help, agreed with Father Garnet that two secret agents, one a Jesuit, the other a layman, should proceed at once to Madrid, with orders to find their way into the Duke de Lerma's cabinet, to assure that minister of Catholic support, and to urge that a Spanish army should be thrown upon these shores. Father Greenway was chosen by the Jesuits, Tom Winter by the laymen. Tom not only knew the country and spoke the language, but, as a deserter from his flag, was sure of a welcome from the monks and mistresses who governed Spain.

These secret agents were well received. Giving Lerma charts and maps of the English coast, they pointed out Milford Haven as the point where it would be best to land, as the Welsh people were Catholic, and a Spanish general, fortified in Pembroke, would have the friendly Irish at his back. But Lerma, though polite, was cold. The Queen was failing fast; a change must come; and his policy was the waiting game. This answer having been foreseen, Tom Winter had been told to urge upon the Duke that nothing could be done with James, and that the King of Scots must be cut off, he and his progeny, root and branch, so as to open a passage for the Infanta to come in under the Papal breves. But Lerma, pursing his darksome brow, said only that his friends must wait.

Had he by any sign or shrug approved of Tom Winter's hint that James should be cut off? We only know that Tom returned through Flanders, where he spread the latest news from Madrid, and that the policy of cutting off the King of Scots was from that time adopted in the cloister and in the camp. The very first batch of Fathers who came over in the Golden Lion talked openly of the King and all his house being speedily cut off. A priest sent word to Cecil that the duty of killing James was being canvassed in the English colleges of Cleves and Douai, and that two fanatics in holy orders had pledged their souls, if they might have the blessing of Heaven upon their deed, to cross the sea, gain access to his table, and stab him as he sat at meat.

On the day Elizabeth died, Catesby went about the town, watching events and eager for a sign; but in the afternoon he rode over to White Webbs, and told the Prefect that the new King had been proclaimed, that every one was pleased, that the City bells were ringing, and the streets alive with bonfires. When Garnet heard this news, he took the Papal breves from his desk, as things too dangerous to be kept, and threw them on the fire.

In Rome another spirit ruled the hour. Persons told the Pope that now was the time for his children to strike a blow. The day for intrigue was past, the day for action come. The Catholics, he cried, were ready; they only waited for a sign; and at a word from Rome a hundred thousand swords would flash into the air. The King of Scots had forfeited his right, and they must bar his entrance in the name of God and Holy Church. The cry which Persons raised in Rome was echoed by Owen in Brussels, by Garnet in Enfield Chase. But the cry was not taken up, and the Jesuits dared not commit themselves by a publication of the breves. Opinion, too, veered round in the Roman court, where Persons fell into suspicion; and, what was worse for Garnet, Frank Tresham and Lord Monteagle were inclined to act with Northampton in supporting James. A new course had to be fetched, and Catesby, finding a friend in Ambrose Rokewood, a young Suffolk squire, who had been trained in the Jesuits' college at St. Omer, consulted Garnet and Greenway on the policy of seeking in Madrid the support they could no longer find in Rome. Kit Wright, a reckless fellow, who had been out in the streets with Essex, and had narrowly escaped the rope, was chosen to go over; and on his way to Madrid this agent of disorder met Guy Fawkes, who was proceeding from Brussels on the same black errand as himself. As Kit represented Garnet and Catesby, Guy represented Owen and Stanley, in this common appeal from Rome to Spain.

They met with no response; for Philip had neither ships nor men to bury in the Irish seas; and Lerma, who was counting his doubloons and conning his reports, imagined he could buy with gold from Cecil and Northampton far more than he could gain by Garnet's craft and Catesby's zeal.

Rebuffed on every side, the fanatics were in despair. Without a friend in Rome, in London, in Madrid, what could they do?

One course at least lay open. They could kill the King. No foreign help was wanted to "cut off" James, in what was then the commonest form of public assassination. They could blast him with powder, as an engineer blows down a wall. Had not his father, Darnley, been killed in this simple way? The thing was not only easy to do, but safe to do. Darnley had been killed in the Kirk of Field, and no one else had suffered by the shock. That which could be done in the Canongate could also be done in Parliament Place. The House of Lords was larger than the Kirk of Field; but what should prevent them from using a larger blast? Bothwell had employed a dozen sacks of powder; why should not Catesby employ a hundred sacks? Powder was cheap.

The idea was not new, still less could it be called heroic. Every soldier had in those days helped to drive a shaft, and thousands of men who were not soldiers had heard the crash of exploding mines. The war then raging beyond the Straits was a war of engineers; and in the trenches before Ostend whole companies were occasionally blown into the air. Among the visitors at White Webbs, many had seen service in the field; so that the power of cutting off an enemy by a charge of powder was familiar to their minds.

A train had been laid against Farnese in the streets of Antwerp; a second such train had been laid against the Provincial Council at the Hague. Not once, but many times, the great Queen's life had been threatened by a powder-plot. One such attempt was made by Michael Moody; and, in later times, Thomas Morgan, a pupil of Father Owen, had offered to carry out the scheme in which Moody failed.

If any one gave the main idea of the Powder scheme to Catesby, that man was Morgan. There is proof that Morgan told Hugh Owen of his plans, and that Owen explained them to his creature Fawkes.

This Thomas Morgan, otherwise known as Charles Thomas, a brother of Rowland Morgan, seminary priest, and of Harry Morgan, Customer of Cardiff, was one of those dangerous exiles on whom Cecil kept a watchful eye. Himself a spy, his steps were always dogged by spies; and many a merry fellow who roused and drank with him in the Flemish wine-shops lived on the wages of their common shame. A tool of the Jesuits whom they hardly cared to own as friend, he was employed by them in work to which few could stoop,—in following frail women, in tempting soldiers to desert, in watching base intrigues, and following to their source the scandals of a camp. For such foul things Morgan had a natural taste. He had spent his days between the back-stairs of a palace and the black hole in a jail, now playing the part of pimp, anon of lover, and then of spy. After threatening Elizabeth's life, he had blackened Farnese's name; on which the great Italian soldier had flung him into prison, instead of flinging him into the Scheldt. But rogues like Morgan are not easily stamped out. He got away to Spain, where he could show his teeth. One day we find him at Porto Santa Maria, giving secret hints to the Adelantado of Seville, on the way to surprise and capture English ships; and shortly afterward in Madrid, moving heaven and earth to get his contemptuous enemy recalled from those Netherlands which he had saved for the Spanish crown.

The fellow had changed his field, but he had not done with plots. He was now in Paris, in the pay of Mademoiselle Catharine d'Entraigues, Marquise de Verneuil, the King's mistress; deeply engaged in the criminal intrigues which led to the arrest, and nearly to the ruin, of that royal favorite.

Catesby had a lodging on the river-bank at Lambeth, near Horse Ferry, as well as one in Moorcroft, under the city wall. He was living in that village of boatmen and fish-wives with Jack Wright, the elder brother of Kit, a ruined North-Country squire, a great fencer, a pupil of the Jesuits, and a pardoned rebel, whom he housed and fed. The fine gentleman and his needy follower walked by the river, brooding over plans for "cutting off" King James. Before them, across the Thames, rose the majestic front of the House of Lords. Within that pile stood the throne, on which the King would have to sit when he came from Whitehall to open his Parliament, surrounded by his wife, his son, his councilors, and his peers. Would not a train of powder, laid below that throne, destroy them all?

Wanting a fellow with more brains than Jack Wright by his side, Catesby wrote to Huddington, where Tom Winter was staying with his brother Robert, in a very low state of mind. When Tom came up to Lambeth, Catesby explained his project. "This strake at the root," said Winter, musing; "but what if they should fail?" They could not fail, urged Catesby, if they got a man who knew his trade to construct the mine. At once he mentioned the name of Fawkes, with whom Kit Wright had journeyed into Spain.

The two fanatics deferred to Catesby's views; for Catesby was to them not only a man of daring spirit, but a fine gentleman,—the Lord of Lapworth and Ashby St. Leger; while they were only Jack and Tom. But ere they took that step, from which they could never turn back, Tom urged that a last appeal should be made for help on the side of Spain; and Catesby, though he said it would come to naught, was willing to oblige his tools. He had to deal with the weak no less than with the strong. He had to ask what could be done when the blow was struck. He had to satisfy his friends before he could destroy his enemies; and Tom Winter imagined that when the old Catholic families saw how the search for help had been made on every side, and on every side in vain, many of those who would otherwise stand aloof might be induced to join them after the King was killed.

That last appeal could be made without loss of time. A great hidalgo, Juan Fernando de Velasco, Duke de Frias and Constable of Castile, was on his way to London, armed with powers to arrange the terms of peace. Velasco was then at Bergues, in Flanders, a small inland fortress, near Dunkirk, where he was waiting for his final order ere he crossed the Straits into Kent. To him they could send Tom Winter on a last appeal; and if, as they supposed, the Constable was bent on serving his earthly rather than his heavenly master, they could then go forward in their work with the certainty of finding troops who would join them with a conscience free from doubt. But in a mission of so much moment they must have Jesuit counsel and Jesuit help. They rode to White Webbs, and Garnet advised that Tresham and Monteagle should be asked to join in the message to Velasco, in order to give it importance in the Constable's eyes. Monteagle, Tresham, and Catesby held a meeting, at which Winter's instructions were drawn up and signed; but these three gentlemen, painfully aware how little they could pretend to represent the English Catholics, and certain that the Constable would ask their messenger why he had brought no letters from Northumberland, Montagu, and Mordaunt, told Winter to explain that the three gentlemen were of a quality most fit for such an enterprise, since they were not so deeply suspected and closely watched as the great Catholic peers. But the mission was, on Catesby's part, a blind. The true business on which Tom went over sea was to confer with Owen and engage the services of Fawkes.

Winter found Father Owen at Dunkirk, in waiting on Velasco, who was still at Bergues. Owen walked with Tom to Bergues, where they saw Velasco, and learned from the Constable that he had not only received strict commands from his royal master to do good offices to the Catholics, but was bound in his own conscience to do them. As the Jesuit and the conspirator walked back through the marshes to Dunkirk, they canvassed Velasco's words. "Will they help us?" asked Winter. "Not a jot," said Owen: "they seek their own ends, and care nothing about us." Then Winter told the Father what the three men had contrived, and asked him whether Fawkes could be trusted in such a work. Owen said yes; Fawkes was in Brussels, but Owen undertook that he should start for London in a trice.

Then Winter rode to the camp before Ostend to see Sir William Stanley and inquire of Fawkes's "sufficiency in the wars." Stanley spoke well of him; and, while they were talking together, Fawkes came in to salute his captain. "This is the gentleman," said Sir William; and the two men who were to labor in the mine shook hands. "Some good friends of yours," quoth Tom, "desire your company in England; and, if you please to come to me, we will confer on that subject." Two days later, Fawkes rode over to Dunkirk, where they talked the matter over with Father Owen and other Jesuits,—Winter explaining to them Catesby's plan for laying a train of powder below the throne. At last, near Easter term, the talk was over and the bargain made. Fawkes took the name of John Johnson, in which his pass was drawn, and the two conspirators crossed from Gravelines to Greenwich, where they took a pair of oars and pulled for Lambeth, and landed at Horse Ferry, near Catesby's door.

CHAPTER XIII.

VINEGAR HOUSE.

IN Parliament Place, the narrow lane going up from the river stair, then called the Queen's Bridge, stood Vinegar House, a small stone tenement leaning against the Prince's Chamber, which formed a part of the old palace, known as the House of Lords. From the cellars of this small tenement a shaft might be driven through the foundations into the dark passages and vaults below the throne. Catesby supposed that these dark passages and vaults were empty,—ready, in fact, to become the chambers of his mine. Vinegar House was, therefore, his Kirk of Field.

But how was he to gain possession? This tenement, a part of the crown estate, was held on simple lease by John Whynyard, Yeoman of the Wardrobe, whose official residence it was. What chance had a pardoned rebel, a notorious plotter, of getting such a house into his power? Catesby could not go and make inquiries; for, his face being known to Cecil's spies, he could hardly have landed at the Queen's Bridge or strolled up Parliament Place without being watched. Tom Bates, his serving-man, was therefore sent across to see who lived in the house, and learn if it could be hired. Bates brought word to Lambeth that the Yeoman's rooms were under-let to their old Warwickshire neighbor, Henry Ferrers, of Baddesley Clinton, the famous antiquary. Lapworth, in which Catesby was born, is but a mile from the moated old manor in which Ferrers lived. Yet Catesby dared not move one step; for the famous antiquary, though a Catholic, was a Catholic of the English school. In hiring such a place, he must have the use of some free and unstained name. What name? Jack Wright, his chum, was compromised like himself; but Jack had a brother-in-law, in Thomas Percy, who seemed the very man to get Vinegar House from the collector of county pedigrees. Percy was a fine gentleman, of kin to the great Northumbrian Earl. A courtier by birth, a Gentleman Pensioner, in attendance on the King, he would excite no question by pretending that he needed a lodging near the court. This Percy had never been concerned in plots, and his reputation was that of a merry fellow who spent his money in the Cheapside taverns and his health on the Bankside dames. But Wright could answer for a change having come over his sister's spouse. A wasted man of forty-five years, with lanky face and feverish eyes, Percy had been found by Jesuits in the stews, and brought by them to a sense of his abominable life. Once he had cared for nothing but a bottle and a bright eye; now his comfort lay in a daily conflict with the flesh. He had a grievance, too, which might help to serve them; for, in his opinion, the King had used him as a tool and mocked him as a dupe.

Catesby, who knew that Percy was sore in spirit, invited him to the house at Lambeth, in which Wright was living, and to which Winter came. "Well, gentlemen," said the new-comer, "shall we always talk and never do?" That was the key to strike; and Catesby, taking him aside, explained to him the project,—showing him the House of Lords, which they could see from his window, telling him how they would drive the shaft from the cellars of Vinegar House, and giving him the names of those who were already privy to his hope. Percy entered into the design at once, for his hatred of the prince who had deceived and mocked him was at fever-point.

A lodging was taken for Guy Fawkes (Mr. "Johnson") in the house of Widow Herbert, in Butcher Row, an alley behind St. Clement Danes. To this house in Butcher Row came Father Gerard from White Webbs, bringing with him the stuff to decorate an altar, bread and wine for the sacrament, and all the things required by a priest when celebrating mass. An upper room of Widow Herbert's house was turned into a chapel; and when the priest was ready for his part, Catesby, Percy, Tom Winter, Jack Wright, and Fawkes assembled in the house,—a quaint old Tudor pile at the corner of Clement's Lane,—first in the lower room, where they swore each other upon the Primer, and then in the upper room, where they heard Father Gerard say mass, and took from his hands the sacrament on that oath. Each of the five conspirators was sworn upon his knees, with his hand on the Primer, that he would keep the secret, that he would be true to his fellows, that he would be constant in the plot.

The question now arose more sharply, How were they to get possession of Vinegar House? The good old antiquary, it seemed, was seldom in town, and might be persuaded to sell his lease; but, on application being made to Ferrers, they found that he had no power to sell, unless with Whynyard's knowledge and consent,—a thing which it might be hard for them to get. Percy made the task his own. Whynyard was away from town, attending on the court, and when Percy spoke to his wife Susan, the thrifty woman made some ado about it, as she knew that to let an official residence was wrong; but on Percy hinting that he would buy her "good will," her scruples melted into air. Besides the money, she felt that a Gentleman Pensioner might be a good friend to a Yeoman of the Wardrobe. Yet Mrs. Whynyard was prudent enough to ask for references, and she only parted with the key of her house on the pledge of Sir Dudley Carleton and other of the Earl's gentlemen. Percy was to pay twenty pounds to Ferrers for his lease, and four pounds a quarter for his rent.

A small tenement adjoined Vinegar House, in which Gideon Gibbins, the porter, lived. This tenement Percy was to have at any time he pleased; and in the mean while Mrs. Gibbins, the porter's wife, was hired to keep his house.

Vinegar House, like many official lodgings at the court, had only one bedroom; so that when Percy brought Guy Fawkes, in the character of his servant "Johnson," to the house, he had to lie elsewhere himself. Percy made a friend of Mrs. Gibbins as well as of Mrs. Whynyard, so that little was said about his going and coming to Parliament Place. He was said to be at Sion, at Alnwick, at Wressil, at Petworth, busy about the Earl's affairs.

The conspirators had got their cellar, and only a dozen feet of masonry divided them from the passages and vaults below the throne. But the house was too small for a magazine, and stood in a lane too much exposed. They would require a second house, in which to hoard the planks, the powder, and the mining-tools,—a house near the river, and not too far from Parliament Place. On looking round, they saw that Catesby's lodging on the Lambeth side would do; but his housekeeper could not be trusted; and before they could begin to pile up planks and powder they must find some "honest fellow" to keep their store. This "honest fellow" they found in Robert Kay, a reprobate son of Edward Kay, Vicar of Staveley. Kay was starving in the streets, having left the service of Lord Mordaunt, in whose family his wife was an upper nurse. Kay took the oaths, and went to the river-bank, on which Catesby removed to his place in Moorcroft, under the city wall.

In this lonely house by the river-side, Winter and Kay began to collect the tools, to frame the planks, and to prepare the powder, which they afterward boated over in the dead of night, and put on shore in a covered nook of the wharf, near the Queen's Bridge. Except from the river, it was impossible to see their boat, and only then by persons who were close in shore. One autumn night, a servant from the Wardrobe office, coming late to Westminster, and going under the wall of Sir Thomas Parry's garden, saw a strange boat by the wharf, with men going to and fro, through the back door of Percy's house; but, one of these men being Gibbins, the porter, he thought no more about it. Gibbins had been taken into Percy's pay.

Some months elapsed before Fawkes was ready to begin the mine; for, Vinegar House being public property, held by the Yeoman on simple lease, he was subject to interference of many kinds. Once, indeed, Fawkes was thrown into despair by news that the house was wanted by the crown.

Parliament was sitting, busy with fifty committees and conferences, when the King brought forward his great and premature scheme for a legislative union of the two kingdoms. Warm debates took place on this proposal, in which Bacon played the leading part. The judges objected to the change of title from England to Great Britain; sixteen commissioners, of whom the first was Bacon, were appointed to consider the project in all its bearings on policy and law; and, as room for Bacon and his fellows could not be found in the palace proper, the adjoining tenement was ordered to be cleared. In fact, those famous conferences between Bacon and Hamilton, the Lord Advocate of Scotland, which are celebrated in the "Essays" as an example of grave and orderly proceedings in affairs of state, were held in Vinegar House.

Surprised by this bad news, Fawkes sent for Tom Winter, who quickly came in to see what could be done.

The powder, planks, and mining-tools could hardly be taken away unseen. The lesser danger was to leave them; yet the plotters must have left them in despair,—since the chance of a discovery hung on such accidents as that of a servant going down into the vaults. Bacon and Hamilton, with some of the best gentlemen of England and Scotland, met for many weeks to debate the terms of union in a powder-magazine!

At length their work was done, and the commissioners went away, not dreaming of the perils from which they had so narrowly escaped. Then Fawkes returned to arm and strengthen his house, so that he and his fellows might be able, in case of sudden attack, to resist some hours. The four gentlemen who were to be his companions in the mine had all seen service, more or less, and two of them had been regularly trained to arms. Jack Wright was said to be the finest swordsman of his day.

When all was ready for them, the five confederates came to Parliament Place, late in the night, and one by one, unseen, each with his pockets full of baked pies and boiled eggs. They went down into the cellar, carrying with them iron bars, and powder, and holy water, to find that the task on which they were entering was beyond their strength. When wasted and worn by toil, they fetched in Kay from Lambeth, leaving the house locked up, and swore Kit Wright of the brotherhood; but, when all was done, the seven were found to be as weak in presence of the stone foundations as the five. Fawkes, who kept the watch while his fellows toiled in the mine, gave notice of the coming of any one down the lane. Much time was spent in grubbing at the stone before an incident let in a flood of light upon their minds. What did they expect to find on the other side of that solid wall? Large vaults and passages lying below the Prince's Chamber and the House of Lords; but in what state could they expect to find these passages and vaults? What if they were tenanted? A noise was heard in the earth: the miners sprinkled holy water on the ground; but still the noise went on. What could it be? They sent for Fawkes, who listened on the ground with a miner's ear. As he could make no guess as to whence it came, he covered his dress with a porter's frock, and went upstairs into the street. In a closed court, behind the Prince's Chamber, he found a low door open, with men going up and down the steps, which led, as he could plainly see, into the passages and vaults beneath the House of Lords. On prying further, he learned that a sale of coals was going on; for Andrew Bright, distiller of sweet herbs to the court, the tenant of these vaults, was selling off his stock and giving up his lease to one Skinner of King Street, for the purposes of his trade.

When Fawkes returned with this news, the confederates saw that their shaft was a mistake; for what would they gain by driving through a dozen feet of granite to arrive in a magazine of goods? They must get those vaults. They must get them at any cost. But how? Skinner was now their man; but how could they induce him to forego his lease? What lie could they invent, that would not seem a lie? They hit on a device, which Percy was to put in train. Going to Mrs. Whynyard, Percy told that dame that his wife, who was then in the country, wished to come up and see the town. She was to live with him at Vinegar House, to be near the court; but, before she came, he wished to lay in stores of coals and billets, and would therefore like to hire the adjoining vaults. If she could help him with Skinner, he would give her twenty shillings for her trouble, and pay her one year's rent in advance. Skinner's rent was four pounds a year, and Percy offered to pay her five pounds down. This money tempted her, though she felt some qualms; and, going up to King Street, she arranged the business with Mrs. Skinner, who undertook, for a present of forty shillings, to persuade her husband to oblige a gentleman who was not only a kinsman of Northumberland, but a servant of the King.

The place now bought for a year for seven pounds was a long series of passages and vaults, of early English work, with walls of enormous strength, and a roof supported by beams and shafts like those in the White Tower. Being low and dark, the stores brought into them from the street could be easily hidden out of sight. The task of the plotters was therefore done so soon as the boats had ferried the sacks of powder across from the Lambeth side, and Fawkes had covered them over with sticks and stones, with broken glass, and a litter of coals.

Vinegar House being now ready for Mrs. Percy, the gentleman left for the country, telling Mrs. Whynyard that he was going away to fetch his lady up to town.

CHAPTER XIV.

CONSPIRACY AT LARGE.

THE comrades parted company in Parliament Place, each of the seven going off to his several home, conspirators at large.

Giving up his keys to Mrs. Gibbins, Fawkes went back to Flanders, where he had work to do, which could only be done through Father Owen and Sir William Stanley, now recognized in Butcher Row and Enfield Chase as the Foreign Minister and General of the plot. On looking to the moment when the blow was struck, the fanatics saw that two things would be wanted in that hour of need,—an armed force within easy reach of the Tower, and a favorable disposition on the part of foreign courts. The two great men in Flanders could promote these ends. Owen was the most active and experienced agent in court and camp. The exiles would obey his slightest hint, and the statesmen of Europe would listen to him more readily than to any other English priest. Stanley could arm and drill the volunteers whom Owen drew over to their cause, so as to hold a force in hand to cross when the mine was fired and the King was slain. Some doubts were felt as to whether it would be safe to trust these exiles with the secret; but Catesby overcame all doubts by saying it must be done; and Fawkes arrived in Brussels empowered to tell the Jesuit and the General all.

Stanley was then in Spain; but Father Owen received his news with rapture. Yes; they could count on him. Of Stanley he was not so sure. That exile was in Madrid, persuading Lerma to make his peace with James; and he would hardly tie his hands by entering into yet another plot. But Owen, believing he would fail with Lerma, expected him back in Brussels with the bitter heart of a newly disappointed man. The Father undertook to deal with him at the proper time; and he pledged his word to Fawkes that, when the deed was done, Sir William and his regiment should cross the Straits and march upon the Tower.

The Jesuit also took upon himself to prepare the way for them in Rome, where, at the moment, things were looking black for the cause in which they had staked their lives. The Pope seemed more and more inclined toward peace; the English college was in disgrace; and Aquaviva, at the personal request of Clement, had ordered Persons to retire from Rome. The Jesuit was in Naples, fretting his life out in that Spanish city, while the Pope was receiving messages from James with every mark of personal good-will. To have an agent in Rome was now essential; and, with the advice of Catesby, Sir Edmund Baynham was sent by Father Owen into Italy, instructed to prepare the Roman court for what was coming, and to justify it when the crash should come.

Catesby rode down to Lapworth with Jack Wright, whom he left in the old manor, while he rode on to Oxford with Tom Winter, whither he had called two country squires to meet him,—Robert Winter, of Huddington, Tom's elder brother, a slow and rather stupid fellow, and John Grant, of Norbrook, one of those reckless devils who had been out with Essex in the Strand. These squires he meant to draw into his plot.

As the fine gentlemen of the circle, Catesby and Percy had a place and power apart from the other five. Fawkes had been a servant to Lord Montagu. Winter was a servant to Lord Monteagle. Kay had been a servant to Lord Mordaunt. Jack Wright, the fencer, was a ruined man, whom Catesby had to feed and lodge. Kit Wright was poorer than his brother Jack. The money which had gone in hire of houses and in pay of men was either Catesby's money or Percy's money. Large sums were needed to conduct their enterprise; and no one could suggest a way of raising funds except by drawing on the purses of richer men. But where could they find such comrades? Men with money are shy of plots. This Catesby and Percy told their fellows, saying, truly enough, that many a country squire might lend them his money, and even promise them his sword, who would not care to put himself wholly into their power by giving in his name. On this ground, Catesby asked from the five a singular and dangerous power; no less than that he and Percy should be free to communicate their secret to any one they pleased, if it were done in the presence and with the consent of any sworn brother. That power was given up to them; for how could Jack and Tom, Kit and Guy, resist such men?

When Robert Winter heard from Catesby's lips of the design in which his brother Tom had risked his neck, he turned away sullenly, saying the project was too dangerous, and would be sure to fail unless the Catholic powers abroad and the Catholic lords at home should give their aid. John Grant raised no objection to the mine; and, after much debate, the two country squires were sworn into the plot.

Tom Bates, the serving-man, was now brought in, from fear of his idle tongue. Being much about Vinegar House, in waiting on his master, Bates had come to know of the mine and vault; and Catesby knew of no way to shut his mouth except by swearing him on the Primer and making him a party in their perils. Bates had no brains for such a work, and in his very next confession he blabbed out the secret to his priest, whose game it was to have known nothing about the design on foot. The priest was Father Greenway, one of Garnet's circle at White Webbs; and the holy man could not pacify Bates without telling him, in express terms, that the cause was good, that he must keep the secret, and that then only he should have absolution for his sins.

From Oxford, Catesby rode down to Bath, where Percy was drinking the waters for his health. Their work was going on well, yet many things had to be arranged before the blow was struck. The King and Prince being slain, they must get Charles, and his sister Elizabeth, into their keeping, to use as policy should prompt them. Charles, it was hoped, would be in London; Elizabeth was at Combe Abbey, two miles from Coventry. Percy undertook to seize the Prince, Catesby the Princess. As an officer of the household,

Percy could go into the Prince's chamber, and he arranged to be there when the blow was struck. He was to station a dozen men at the palace-doors, to post three mounted gentlemen at the court-gate, and then go in —with a trusty friend—and chat with the Prince until the crash was heard in Parliament Place, when he was to hurry Charles away. Catesby, on his side, was to call his Catholic friends together at Dunchurch, near his seat of Ashby St. Leger, on pretense of a great hunting-party, which he hoped Lord Harrington and the knights in attendance on Elizabeth at Combe would be induced to join; so that the confederates, moving secretly and rapidly from many points on the Abbey, might take the Princess by surprise and all-but alone.

But more was needed than a plan of operations. They needed money, and they needed men; for both of which they saw that they would have to go beyond the narrow circle of converts to their faith. Catesby urged on Percy that many gentlemen would trust him and help him who would not put their lives into the hands of all by taking a formal oath, and Percy, knowing from his own experience that this was true, raised no objection to Catesby's proposal that each of them should have the power, without consulting their comrades, to act—from time to time—in the common cause as in their judgment should seem well. Percy consented to this new and still more dangerous stretch of their separate power.

As the time to act drew near, the man who had most to gain and most to lose began to play with his comrades' lives, but only, as he fancied, for their good, because he knew better than his fellows how far he could go; putting this man on his guard by a hint, taking that man into his confidence by an oath; telling half the truth to one, the whole truth to another, according to the service which he hoped to secure from each. Armed with his new powers, he rode to Huddington, Robert Winter's seat, from which he wrote to Stephen Littleton, of Holbeach, and Humphrey, his younger brother,—members of an old Catholic family, to whom he dared not reveal his plot in full. He told these squires that he was raising a Catholic regiment for the Cardinal Archduke's service, to consist of three hundred horse; and he offered to Stephen the rank of captain in this troop. Stephen, pleased with his prospects, undertook to raise money and men and to hold his company in readiness to march.

Ambrose Rokewood was a man of similar stamp. A great breeder and lover of horses, of which he kept a stud at Coldham Hall more fit for a prince than for a country gentleman, it was of vast importance for Catesby to bring Rokewood in. But the task was not easy; for the Suffolk squire, though educated in a Jesuits' college, and equally attached to Garnet and to Catesby, with whom he had acted in the dangerous affair of Wright's mission to Madrid, was of an ancient Catholic race, not much inclined to adopt such desperate remedies for his wrongs as public murder in the name of God. His love for Catesby was like that of a woman; yet his soul recoiled from the thought of shedding blood, and he told his tempter he could not in conscience join him. Long and subtle were the arguments employed to draw him in. The case, his friend assured him, had been settled by the Catholic divines; a case of conscience having been drawn up, in which the facts set forth would cover their own design. But many persons, urged the squire, would perish in the explosion who had done no harm. They could not help that, Catesby said; and their divines had laid down the rule, that if an action otherwise right could not be done without killing some innocents, it might still be done. Rokewood was not convinced, and even his love for Catesby might have failed to draw him in, had not the persecuting spirit of the times inflicted on his proud nature a bitter sense of personal wrong, in his indictment before the Middlesex magistrates as a notorious Papist and recusant. Full of fear and sore with insult, Rokewood threw himself into his tempter's arms.

The snare was thrown at Sir Everard Digby. Digby, educated in the national Church, had been caught by the Jesuits in his early manhood, and his house of Goathurst, in Bucks, had long been used as a hiding-place for priests. When Catesby spoke to him, Digby started at the news; he could not seize the principle of such a crime; and when Catesby told him it was sanctioned by the Jesuits, he expressed some doubts of such a fact. But on consulting Father Fisher, his confessor, he learned that what Catesby said was true; on which he promised his support, and a contribution of fifteen hundred pounds.

This doubt was also found in his cousin Frank. Frank Tresham had of late kept clear of plots, believing, like Monteagle, that his wiser course would be to make friends at court, and take his chance with Northampton and the Catholic peers, instead of with Garnet and the converts of White Webbs. He was not mad; he shrank with visible dread from the crime of murder; and before the secret oath had passed his lips his friend was troubled with a ghastly fear. Would Frank betray him? Catesby asked himself. More than once he wished he had not spoken. Frank was hot and cold by turns,—suggesting doubts as to what would be said in Rome, proposing questions as to how their brethren could be saved, and generally objecting to the mine and the march on Combe Abbey as sure to fail. Yet, as Frank promised help in money and in men,—in money, two thousand pounds,—his jealous cousin could only take his gold and stick a poniard in his belt; so that on the slightest sign of treason he could plunge the steel into his heart.

Mrs. Vaux of Harrowden, sister-in-law of Ann and Helen, was used by the conspirators without being sworn. This lady, by birth a Roper, was of ancient Catholic stock, and not to be trusted with a knowledge of Catesby's plans. But she was asked to invite such persons to her house as Henry Hurlstone and other squires whom Garnet and Catesby desired to meet,—gentlemen who might be persuaded to join the hunt at Dunchurch, in the hope that when their blood was stirred by news from Parliament Place they could be drawn into marching on Combe Abbey with the rest.

CHAPTER XV.

THE JESUITS MOVE.

THE time was now come for the Jesuits to move, so as to rouse their pupils without committing themselves too openly to the plot.

Good news came in from Rome, to which Persons had returned from Naples, at the call of a new Pope. Clement was dead; and Leo, his successor, was also dead. In thirty days three Popes had reigned in Rome; the last of whom, Paul the Fifth, a man of chilled and fervent passions, gave his ear to the English Jesuits, as counselors who *must* understand their country better than Italian cardinals and Spanish monks. Paul heard nothing from Persons about Catesby's crime; but he listened with zeal to his statements on English affairs, and promised his wily visitor that he would think over his request for help in the task of converting souls to God. Persons was about to send a priest to London, one Father Robarts, to stand by the side of Fawkes. It was of high importance that Robarts should go to England fresh from the Pontiff's presence and with the Pontiff's blessing on his head. Persons obtained for him a special audience and benediction from Paul, and then dispatched him to London, with orders to report himself to Garnet and Catesby and to take up his post where those counselors should suggest.

Good news came in from the Flemish camp, to which Stanley had returned, as Father Owen expected, in bitter mood. He was easily induced to join a plot in which he was to play the most brilliant part. His comrades in London heard with delight that he was raising a brigade of Swiss, Walloons, and Irish, which he would lead in person across the Straits so soon as he received a summons from White Webbs.

Coming back from Flanders, Fawkes took up his abode in Vinegar House, to which Mrs. Percy was said to be coming from her country-seat. He paid the quarter's rent then due, and Mrs. Whynyard observed that his purse was full of gold. But he often went from home and stayed away all night. In fact, he kept his old lodging in Butcher Row, at Widow Herbert's house, as a more convenient place of call for his friends than either the tavern in Carter Lane or the house in Parliament Place. Mrs. Herbert hardly liked her lodger, whose coming and going she could not quite make out, but he paid his rent to the hour, and was much away from Butcher Row,—points in his favor in the landlady's eyes. Often he was at Moorcroft and White Webbs in secret conference with Catesby and Tom. His masters deemed it prudent for him to be rarely seen in Parliament Place.

Early in the year, Father Garnet, Father Oldcorne, and the two ladies left White Webbs for the midland shires, where the chief conspirators were gathering into knots and groups. "Mrs. Perkins" left her servant James in the house.

They began their travels in the double character of laymen and of priests. On the road and at inn-yards, Garnet was "Mr. Mese," Oldcorne was "Mr. Perkins," while in the houses of their penitents they were known as Father Walley and Father Tesmond. The ladies had a similar choice of names. Ann was "Mrs. Perkins" on the road, Mrs. Vaux in the house; Helen was "Mrs. Jennings" on the road, Mrs. Brooksby in the house. Brooksby was sometimes with them, oftener he was far away. They seldom slept on the road, and never when it could be helped, but passed from one Catholic mansion to another, under secret arrangements, which never failed.

In June they came to White Webbs for a week, and left it for a second round of visits, on the close of which they came home again for three or four days.

The time was now come for every one to assume his post. The Fathers held a council, and, when it broke up, the Prefect and his two most trusty brethren separated, never to meet again. Garnet was to go into the midland shires. Oldcorne, under his lay name of "Perkins," was to remain in London. Greenway was to cross over to Flanders. By this arrangement, each knot of the conspirators would have a Jesuit in their midst.

The two ladies were to ride down with Garnet, so as to be at head-quarters; but, ere they rode away, "Mrs. Perkins" called her servant James, and gave him charge of her house, with orders how to act. The house was to be kept open, and the stable ready, to receive her friends. Some gentlemen would call, and beds must be kept for them. He must see to their comforts, and look well after their horses. Then the company rode away for the last time, going straight to Goathurst, Digby's seat in Bucks, where they found the knight and his lady, Father Fisher their confessor, Ambrose Rokewood and his wife, with a company of some thirty squires and dames.

The Prefect had arranged a picturesque and striking scene as prelude to the tragedy in Parliament Place,— a pilgrimage to some holy well, in which the men and women could equally have their part. He chose St. Winifred's Well, in Flintshire, as the term of their journey; and, after a mass of special meaning had been said at Goathurst, the whole company mounted and rode away, with Father Garnet and Father Fisher in their midst. The first resting-place of the cavalcade was Norbrook, where Grant received them, and Garnet said mass; the second, Huddington, where Winter received them, and Garnet again said mass. From Huddington they rode to Holt, where the ladies left their horses, and, putting off shoes and socks, walked barefooted to the Well. A special mass was said once more; after which the party spent a night in the open air, with the Flintshire saint. When daylight came, the penitents walked back to Holt, put on their shoes and socks, and returned the way they had come, through Huddington and Norbrook, to Digby's house, where the company dispersed to their several homes, all the guests going away except Garnet, Mrs. Brooksby, and Ann Vaux.

Lapworth, Catesby's house, near Warwick, was the natural center of the plot; but Lapworth was too small a place; and, on the advice of Catesby, Sir Everard Digby moved to Coughton, Thomas Throckmorton's seat, near Alcaster, a central station and convenient house. Rokewood also, on the same suggestion, hired Clopton, near Stratford-on-Avon, from Lord Carew. Jack Wright was at Lapworth; Thomas Morgan, the assassin, was at Norbrook with a female companion of dubious fame. Stephen Littleton was at Hagley, waiting for his summons to mount and march.

When all was ready for the blow in London, Father Garnet and the two ladies rode over from Goathurst to Coughton, where the Prefect lodged in the midst of his unruly scholars until he heard from Digby that the plot had failed.

CHAPTER XVI.

IN LONDON.

In spite of his haughty bearing, Catesby was much perplexed in mind.

He feared that his cousin Frank was false, that his enterprise would fail, that his neck was forfeit to the law. The last ten days of his London life were spent, with intervals, at the lonely house in Enfield Chase.

Coming up from the shires, in company with Guy Fawkes, he stopped on Friday, October 25, at White Webbs, to which house he called Tom Winter from Montagu Close. Reports had reached him that Prince Henry would not attend his father in the House of

Lords; in which case all their plans in seizing the Princess Elizabeth at Combe Abbey, and the Duke of York in Whitehall Palace, would be thrown away. The father killed, his son would be King. Could Winter say whether these reports were true? Yes, Winter had heard this news. "Then we must have our horses beyond the water," cried his chief; "and a company to surprise the Prince, and leave the Duke alone." They sent word to Percy, then in the north, to ride up to London with his utmost speed.

What lay with Catesby had been done. The mine was laid; the torch was ready; and the man was sure. A boat was lying near the Queen's Bridge, by which it was hoped that Fawkes could push into the stream, so as to avoid the shock and ruin of the mine. Lower down the river lay a vessel, ready to set sail, by which he could escape to a foreign port, with news of the King's death, and a message for Stanley to cross, with his Swiss and Irish companies, into the Thames. Parliament was to meet on Tuesday, November 5,—a day, as Catesby thought, to be ever glorious in the calendar of his Church. Excepting Percy, the chiefs were now in London, waiting for that Tuesday to arrive. Father Robarts had been stationed in Vinegar House, under the care of Mrs. Gibbins. Catesby was at White Webbs. Fawkes returned to Butcher Row for two or three nights. Tom Winter was in Montagu Close. Jack Wright was at the Horse Ferry, Lambeth. Cousin Frank was in Clerkenwell. Rokewood, Kay, and Kit Wright were lodging at St. Giles's Fields, in the house of Mrs. More. When Percy came to town, he was to stay with his friends Rokewood and Kay, in their lodgings at Mrs. More's. Fawkes, who was now become the nearest of Catesby's comrades, spent most of his time secreted at Enfield Chase. All things were prepared,—and all things, down to the inscriptions on their swords, in what the conspirators conceived to be a religious spirit. Rokewood had employed a cutler named Cradock to make three sword-hilts, on each of which he was to engrave the Passion of Christ. These swords were for himself, Kit Wright, and Kay. Their chief, though he ordered no such hilt for himself, was so much interested in the work that he called very often at Cradock's shop to see what progress he had made.

A fancy sword was not the thing of which Catesby stood in most pressing need. He wanted money, and he wanted men. The absence of Prince Henry crossed his plans; and the means of seizing that Prince at the moment of explosion were now beyond their reach. His scheme was falling into chaos. Cousin Frank, too, was suspected by him more and more. Frank had not yet supplied the whole of his two thousand pounds, and his general conduct had been so strange of late that Catesby, though he loved him dearly, had more than once thought of soothing his jealous rage by plunging the dagger into his heart.

In truth, the Frank Tresham who had played with him as a boy, and who had sworn the oath to keep his secret, was not the Mr. Tresham with whom he had now to deal. A serious change had come. His sworn companion was not the rich Northampton squire, for his father, Sir Thomas, had been then alive; but while the penitents were walking bare-legged to St. Winifred's Well, Sir Thomas had passed away, and Frank had been left the master of Rushton Hall, with one of the best estates in the midland shires. Then only he saw the error of his way, for what he had done in taking the oath of secrecy put this large estate in peril, and Mr. Tresham was suspected by his desperate kinsman of a design to undo what Cousin Frank had done.

This task of undoing what he had done was not easy for Mr. Tresham; since the payments which he had made under his first rash promise had put him equally into Catesby's power and into Cecil's power. As a conspirator, guilty of compassing the King's death, his life and fortune were at stake, and one word from his disdainful cousin would send him, a ruined traitor, to the Tower. How far Cecil and Northampton were acquainted with the plot he shrewdly guessed; for any man who watched the Secretary's action, with the clew in his hand, could hardly help seeing that the government knew as much as they cared to learn.

A man must have been ignorant of Cecil and Northampton in no common measure who could have dreamed that a secret which was known to a hundred persons in Douai, Madrid, and Rome—that a design which had been nursed at White Webbs and carried out in Parliament Place—could have escaped the greatest masters of intrigue alive. Many of the court papers have been burnt, yet enough remains to show that the Council were informed of the plot in almost every stage. Tilletson had told them of the design to cut off the King and his progeny. Southwick, one of their priestly spies in France, had sent them news of everything done by the Jesuits, and the name of every Jesuit who crossed the sea into Kent. Wilson wrote to them from Valladolid, that the Jesuits were to try once more what they had tried in the Queen's time, and that the King and Prince were to be killed. The matter was so far known as to be made a subject of negotiation with the Papal Nuncio in Paris, who proposed to guarantee the King's personal safety on condition of his suspending the penal laws and granting freedom of the mass. A sorcerer named Wright, a spy named Williams, an informer named Coe, sent warnings to Cecil, whose agents were in Enfield Chase, in Warwick, in Stratford, in Dunchurch,—following the Jesuits from mass to funeral, from pilgrimage to hunt, counting their numbers, marking their proselytes, mapping out their haunts.

It was no part of Cecil's policy to step in one hour before the dramatic time. He knew the value of a plot too well to sacrifice the chances which Garnet and Catesby were throwing into his path. A sudden surprise, a chase of malefactors, an arrest of Catholic peers, with a state trial, and an execution of Jesuits, would make his peace with a patriotic House of Commons, and secure to him the confidence and gratitude of James. The King was vain enough to think that he was personally a favorite of Heaven, and he wished the world to see that he was really protected from above. He wanted a day to be set apart in the calendar to his glory; and he had tried to get his Council to adopt the fifth of August, the date of the Gowrie Plot, as his sacred day. The thing could not be done; for the Council knew that the King's escape from Ruthven had produced only a slight—and not in any sense a dramatic—shock of the public mind. The Scots themselves made a comedy of the day in Perth; and even those among his courtiers who thought he had been in danger smiled at the affair as a personal feud in a provincial town. But a conspiracy in London, managed by the Jesuits, and threatening a hundred lives, would serve his weakness well, if it could be only watched and turned so as to keep the actual peril far from his throat and crown. If all went well, the King might write his name in the calendar on a day to be called his own.

But Cecil and Northampton had other purposes in view. They had to convince the Duke de Lerma that they and their party in the Council were the only agents at the English court whom it would be worth his while to employ in carrying out the policy of Spain. Philip, a fanatic in creed, was still inclined to trust the Jesuits; and it was necessary that these Jesuits should be swept away.

Measures of precaution had been taken long ago, and nothing less than the blindness which afflicts all criminals could have hidden from Catesby and Percy the movements made to defeat their game. During the summer and autumn months sharp eyes would have noticed an unusual stir among the train-bands. The musters had been called, the companies strengthened, and the arms inspected in every shire. The Lord Lieutenants of counties had been asked to see after this great work in person; while in the shires which had no such officers, the most able member of the Privy Council had been charged with the task. If Spinola had been menacing Kent, the preparations could hardly have been more complete. Much and wise attention had been given to the bands in Warwickshire,—Lord Compton, the King's Lieutenant, receiving sharp commands from Whitehall to hold reviews of men and arms, and to see for himself that both were in readiness to take the field. Edmund Nicholson, the famous armorer, was sent from London with a supply of guns and pikes for these Warwickshire bands, some of whom were then being drilled in the fields near Norbrook. Father Southwick was sent for out of France, to help in hunting down the Jesuits; and Cecil, remembering the Essex rising and the Blackfriars play, shut up the theaters, and confined the comedians to their homes.

On the very day of Catesby's arrival at White Webbs,

Father Southwick was in consultation with Cecil's secretary, Levinus Munck.

The incidents through which the plot was brought to light bear traces throughout of Cecil's art.

On Saturday afternoon, October 26, Monteagle, who lived in Montagu Close, near the Globe Theater, sent a messenger to his place in Hoxton (probably Brooke House), with orders to prepare his supper, as he meant to come out with a friend that night. The friend who rode out with him to Hoxton was Thomas Ward, a gentleman of his household, who was also a friend of Winter, and an unsworn member of the plot. As the peer and his man were sitting down to sup, a page came into the room with a letter in his hand, which had been given to him, he said, by a strange man in the lane, who bade him give it to his lord and to no one else. Monteagle broke the seal, and tossed the paper to Ward, who read it out aloud. The words were vague enough, but they warned Monteagle, as he tendered his life, to go into the country instead of going to the Parliament house, as God and man had concurred to punish the wickedness of the times by a "terrible blow." Pages, servants, all his household, heard these menacing words, which Monteagle's conduct made more menacing still. He rose from the table, called for his horse, and rode away to town.

About ten o'clock that Saturday night, he dashed into Whitehall Yard, and ran up-stairs into Cecil's private room, where he found a curious group for him to meet by chance on such a night; four Catholic Earls, whom James had now taken into his Council, Nottingham, Northampton, Suffolk, and Worcester; all of whom had come into Cecil's room to sup. Ten-o'clock suppers were rather late; but the five lords were in no hurry; and the letter which had been left at Monteagle's door in Hoxton, by the unknown man, was read aloud to them ere they sat down to eat. At table they agreed to keep their secret, as the King, who was hunting deer at Royston, was daily expected back in town.

On Sunday morning the game was wholly in Cecil's hands, but the player was too crafty to show his cards. One of Catesby's crazes was that Cecil was a fool; and Cecil, taking care that his victims should not be alarmed one hour too soon, so veiled his action that Catesby could neither carry out his plan nor save himself by flight. Levinus Munck, his private secretary, sent for Father Southwick, who was to take horse and ride down into the country, where he was to say little and to see much, running the Jesuit agents to their holes, and marking the cover, so that Munck could issue the warrants and throw them into jail whenever his master pleased. Northampton sent for Sir Thomas Knyvet, a connection of Lady Suffolk, and a man whom he could trust. Knyvet, Warder of the Mint, and a justice of the peace for Westminster, was to prepare for a sudden and secret service to the crown, for which in time he might expect to receive a great reward. He was to make a search and seizure for the King, which could be more conveniently made by a justice of the peace than by a captain of the Guard.

Monteagle, having interests in the plot beyond those of Cecil, to whom it was a work of political art and not a personal peril, was of all things anxious that Catesby should escape unhurt. But he could not act in person. Though his peace was made with Cecil, it would never do for him to be known as giving a conspirator the advice and the means to fly. He spoke to Ward, of whom he had a great conceit; and on Sunday night, as Winter lay in bed, Ward went to his bedside and told him all,—describing the letter left in the Hoxton lane, the public reading in the hall, the ride to London, the interview of Monteagle with the five lords, and urging him, as he loved Catesby, to ride over in the morning to White Webbs and force him to take the boat for France.

At dawn on Monday, Winter left Montagu Close in search of Father Oldcorne and Jack Wright; and when he found them in their lodgings, they rode together to White Webbs with their doleful news. Catesby reeled beneath the blow, but his spirits soon leaped proudly up. Tom begged him to save himself, since he could no longer hope to serve his God. But Catesby would not hear of flight. He could not think their secret was betrayed. A fancy seized him that the news sent down by Ward was all a trick devised by his cousin Frank to drive him off. He would look farther into things than Tom saw need. The mine should be examined; for, if Cecil had received such a letter from Monteagle, his very first care must have been to inspect the vault. Fawkes should go up to town and see. Winter urged the peril; to which Catesby answered that the vault was Fawkes's post, and that they need not tell him why he was sent in. Tuesday was spent in these debates, during which the servant James was told to look after their geldings and buy what was wanted in Enfield town,—anything to keep him from the house.

On Wednesday morning Fawkes rode up to town, and, opening the door into the vaults, found everything as he had left it, down to the private mark which he had placed to show whether any one had passed the door. That night he rode back to Enfield Chase, where the conspirators received his tidings with gladsome hearts. On Thursday, Winter rode in to town in search of Tresham, and, finding him in Clerkenwell, proposed, in Catesby's name, that they should meet next day in Barnet to confer upon their course. Catesby, who knew his cousin capable of trick, could not believe him capable of treachery; but he had so far steeled his heart against him that, if they found him false, he told Tom Winter, they must stab him on the spot.

CHAPTER XVII.

NOVEMBER, 1605.

On Friday, November 1, Catesby and Tom rode over to Barnet, where Tresham came out from Clerkenwell to meet them. Catesby bluntly accused his cousin of having broken his oath and betrayed the secret. "How?" asked Frank, in an injured tone. By writing that letter which was left by the unknown messenger at Monteagle's door. It was a critical moment for Cousin Frank. If he had paused in his reply, the daggers of his comrades would have passed into his flesh; but he denied the charge with so much heat and scorn that they were staggered and knew not how to treat him. Tresham was a pupil of the Jesuits; he held that lying and deceit were lawful in a good cause, and Garnet's treatise on Equivocation was known to be his favorite book; but they could not bring themselves to believe that he would palter with an oath on the Primer, especially when that oath had been sworn for ends which his Jesuit teachers had at heart.

Frank made no secret of his opinion that the plot had failed, that everything was known to Cecil and Northampton, that his cousin was in peril and ought to fly; but he was not the less ready, in Catesby's presence and under the spell of his haughty spirit, to pledge his soul that, if his cousin elected to stand his ground and wait events, he would live and die at Catesby's side. Perplexed in soul, the proud young squire could not consent to desert his post. Percy was still in the north, collecting rents on the Earl's estate; and Catesby would not hear of any change being made in their plans until that gentleman arrived in town. But, if he could not fly, how could he leave his suspicious friend at large? A test of Frank's sincerity occurred to him: he asked his cousin for two hundred pounds, to be spent in buying horses, arms, and powder. If Frank had made his peace with Cecil, he would not dare to compromise himself afresh; he would refuse to pay the money; and then they would know with whom they had to deal. A poniard-thrust would make him safe. If he paid the two hundred pounds, he would be with them for life and death.

Frank promised them at once. He did so, as he afterward declared, in the hope that when Catesby got the money he would leave the country. He appointed to meet Tom Winter that very night in Clerkenwell, and put the gold into his hand.

Tom went to Clerkenwell, where Tresham paid him a hundred pounds,—perhaps thinking that, if Catesby meant to go away, that sum was quite enough; but Tom was urgent for the balance; and Tresham, though he hoped to see no more of Tom, arranged to meet him the very next night in Lincoln's Inn Walk, whither he would bring the second of his two hundred pounds.

Catesby spent the Saturday (November 2) in buying arms. In the evening, Winter was at his post near Lincoln's Inn; to which Tresham came in the dark, with a very sore spirit and a bag of gold containing ninety pounds, the largest sum that he could raise in so short a time. Winter took his money and heard his speeches. More than ever, Frank felt certain that the plot was known; and once again he urged on Tom that Catesby should escape into France. He had a yacht in the river, and this vessel he was willing to lend them if they would only fly.

On Sunday morning (November 3) Ward paid another visit to Winter's room. The news he brought was graver, in his own opinion, than the first. The King, he said, was come to town, and, having seen the Monteagle letter, was deeply moved by it; though he had urged the lords of his Council to maintain the strictest silence on the subject. Search, said Ward, was to be made immediately in the vaults of Parliament Place, particularly in the passages and chambers beneath the throne, and everything they had done would now be found.

Winter repaired to White Webbs with this bad news; but Catesby, though he listened to every word in fever, could not stoop to personal fear. No doubt —he reasoned—the letter would lead to search being made; but search was not discovery; and, if Fawkes were on the spot, the heap of wood and coal might pass for what it seemed. While they were whispering to each other, Percy came to White Webbs, and this man's scorn of flight and failure overcame all previous doubts.

Percy had just arrived in town, where he hoped to hide himself at Rokewood's lodgings, in St. Giles's Fields. He had with him a large sum of money, belonging to the Earl, his kinsman, for which he had immediate use; but, feeling that to be in town without reporting himself at Sion was a dangerous thing, he sent Kit Wright to Isleworth, to mix with the grooms and pages and to learn from them whether his arrival in London was known in the household. Late in the night, Kit brought him word to Mrs. More's lodgings that his presence in London was known at Sion, in consequence of which it was resolved that he should go up the river next day and see the Earl.

Breaking up their conference at White Webbs, the conspirators rode back to town on Sunday evening,—Fawkes to go down at once to Vinegar House, where he noticed that the mine was still untouched, the rest to steal about the streets, from Parliament Place to Whitehall Gardens, where they found, to their amazement, everything dull and quiet as on ordinary winter nights. No stir at the gate, no torches in the court, no tramp of men in Parliament Place! Relieved in mind by what they saw, they crept at last to their lodgings in St. Giles's Fields, and waited for the dawn.

On Monday morning (November 4) they heard from Fawkes that all was well at Vinegar House. Who could now say their secret was known at court? To-day was the King's; to-morrow would be theirs. If Winter was a little down, Catesby and Percy were elate and proud. What cause had they for drooping of the spirit? Their mine was perfect, and their man resolved. In less than thirty hours their fate would be accomplished,—the House of Lords a wreck, the King a cinder, the city stunned, the country helpless, and the crown their prize. Percy ran out and bought a watch, which he set in true time and sent to Fawkes, so that the watcher in the vault would be able to count the very seconds which their enemies had now to live. Greenway and Oldcorne had left for the country, with good news,—the first for Goathurst and Coughton, the second for Hendlip Hall. Robarts was at Vinegar House. The final words were now passed from each man to his fellow, and the plotters parted for the day, each going to his post of duty, confident that the mine would now be sprung. Percy went off to Sion, where the Earl detained him to dine and sup. Tom Winter returned to Montagu Close. Rokewood and Kay remained in St. Giles's Fields, near stables in which Rokewood's horses stood with the harness ready on their backs. Catesby and Jack Wright rode out quietly to Enfield Chase, where they proposed to sleep, and trot on early next day toward Dunchurch, in the hope of reaching their rendezvous that night.

The plotters were hardly separated before a strange event occurred in Parliament Place. Lord Suffolk and Lord Monteagle came to Vinegar House, attended by a page, and passed into the vaults under the Prince's Chamber and the House of Lords. Suffolk was the Lord Chamberlain, and both the peers were members of the persecuted Church. No guards came with them, and they seemed to be light of mood, as though they were going through an idle form of search. Fawkes was in the vault, and watched their faces well. As they walked along the passages, they laughed and chatted with each other, and when Suffolk noticed Fawkes in the vault he asked him in a light tone who he was, and whose was the heap of wood and coal. Fawkes answered that he was Mr. Percy's man, and that the fuel was laid up for his master's use. Lord Suffolk made some joke about his merry preparation for the Christmas fires, and then the two lords went their way. The search being over, Fawkes came out to let Percy know of the event, which had at once confirmed and removed his fears. Percy had not come back from Sion; but the upshot of this official search was so important that Fawkes took horse and followed him to Isleworth, where he was sitting at table with the Earl. Percy came out into the yard, and, having heard the news, went in again, made some excuse to Northumberland, and rode with Fawkes to town.

The two men parted for the last time near Tothill Fields,—Fawkes going down into the vault, to draw on his jack-boots, to wind up his watch, and to light his lantern, Percy riding to Rokewood's lodging, where he had a room, to persuade his comrades who were still in town that all was now going well.

About ten o'clock in the murky November night, Rokewood, Kay, and Percy crept from St. Giles's Fields into King Street, near the palace-gates, to see and hear the news. Nothing they could see and hear alarmed them. The palace-gates were open, and the court was free. Parliament Place was silent. In the streets of Westminster not a sound of watch and guard was heard. In the palace a light burned faintly here and there, as if some page were rather late; but the windows in the King's apartments were dark, and the lords who had supped with him appeared to have gone to bed. Looking at the blank walls and silent courts of the royal quarter, could any man believe that James was conscious of what the morrow had in store?

When the clocks struck twelve, and yet no sign was made, the three night-watchers crawled past Charing Cross, up St. Martin's Lane, toward their lodgings in the lonely St. Giles's Fields, convinced in their hearts that long before noon next day the deed would be done that was to shake the world.

But, while they were creeping through the darkness to their den, the spring had been made, and Fawkes was a prisoner to the law.

The train being laid and the lantern lit, Fawkes was coming up the stairs of his vault into the small inclosed court behind the Prince's Chamber, when he was suddenly seized by strong men, bound hands and feet, and searched. Sir Thomas Knyvet was earning his reward. The watch which he had just wound up, a packet of slow matches, a quantity of touch-wood, were taken from his person; and a dark lantern, with the wick alight, was found behind the cellar-door. "What are you doing here?" asked Knyvet. "Had you but taken me inside," said Fawkes, who saw with a soldier's quickness that all was lost, "I should have blown you up, the house, myself, and all." Securing his prisoner, Knyvet proceeded to search the vault. The casks of powder were soon laid bare, and a rough account of them set down. From the cellars he went into Vinegar House, where he arrested Gibbins the porter and Robarts the priest.

In a few minutes Knyvet was in the King's presence at Whitehall; and in a few months he was a member of that House of Lords the frame of which he had so boldly saved.

CHAPTER XVIII.

HUNTED DOWN.

Betimes on Tuesday morning, Catesby and Jack Wright were in the saddle, winding through Enfield Chase toward Ashby St. Leger, which they meant to reach that night by easy stages, unaware that Knyvet had got possession of their mine, and that Fawkes was lying on his wisp of straw in the darkest dungeon of the Tower.

The plotters in St. Giles's Fields were roused in the night by news that Fawkes had been seized in the vault; and some of them crept into the streets to learn whether this report was true. Kit Wright ran off to Montagu Close, expecting to find Tom Winter, who had gone away to his lodgings near the Strand. But in the Close he heard a cry and parley which turned him sick with fear. A noble lord was calling under Monteagle's window, "Rise, and come with me to Essex House! I am going to call up my Lord of Northumberland!" Kit listened to what was said, and from the hasty words then dropped he learned that all was known. At five o'clock he found Winter in his lodgings near the Strand, and told him what he had heard under Monteagle's window. Tom leaped out of bed. "Go back, Mr. Wright," he begged, "and learn what you can about Essex Gate." In a short time Kit returned, saying surely all was known; for the lords were then with the Earl in council, and one Leyton had just ridden at full speed from the door. The business seemed high and pressing, for the lords came out to see him off. He had dashed up Fleet Street. "Go you then to Mr. Percy," whispered Tom; "for sure it is for him they seek. Bid him be gone. I will stay and see the uttermost." They parted at the door. Kit found his comrade Percy in the street; a word sufficed to warn him; and the two men leaped to horse, and rode away through Highgate, with the cry of mounting messengers in their track.

Percy had arranged his plans for leaving town, in case of failure, with such cunning art that for many hours the government were uncertain in what direction he had fled. A messenger was sent to Ware, as Cecil inferred that he would take the great north road; but the postmaster replied that he had not passed since Saturday, when he came up to town. The first news heard by Cecil was from Archbishop Bancroft, who reported that Percy had been met that morning near Croydon, where he cried, as he rode along, that all London was up in arms. The next news came from the Lord Chief Justice Popham, who reported that Percy was at Gravesend, where measures had been taken for his arrest. Later in the day, Sir William Waad, Lieutenant of the Tower, sent word to Whitehall that Sir Edward Yorke, in coming up to town that day, had seen him riding northward in disguise.

Winter passed down the Strand into Whitehall Yard, where he found the gates were closed and guarded; and thence down King Street, on his way to Parliament Place. The street was stopped, and soldiers were drawn across the road. No one was allowed to pass. Mixing with the crowd, he heard that a plot had been discovered for blowing up the King and Queen next day, and that the ruffian who was to have fired the train had been captured with his lantern and his match. Why need he wait for more?

Stealing swiftly to the stables where his gelding lay, Tom jumped into the saddle, and quitted London by the nearest lanes,—not for the rendezvous at Ashby St. Leger, but for what he hoped would be the safer asylum of his brother's house.

Kay hung about town until ten o'clock, and then took horse.

Young Rokewood was the last to fly. Proud of his great stud and his greater prowess, the Suffolk squire had placed relays of horses on the road from London to Dunchurch, so that when he rode down to the hunting-party he could devour the distance with amazing speed. Mounting his horse at eleven o'clock, he soon came up with his comrades in the road. At Finchley Common he overtook Kay, whence they tore on together until Kay, getting tired of his pace, fell off. Near Brickhill he overtook Catesby and Jack Wright, who had not yet heard the news; and a piece beyond Fenny Stratford they met with Percy and Kit Wright. From this village they held on together, pushing past Stony Stratford and Towcester at their utmost speed. Percy and Jack Wright, less nobly mounted than their fellows, had to cast away their cloaks in that furious race for life.

In two hours Rokewood rode thirty miles on a single horse, and made the whole distance of eighty-one miles in less than seven hours.

Unconscious of the fate then speeding toward them through the dark November night, two companies of country squires were waiting at Ashby St. Leger and Dunchurch in a riotous mood of mind. News having come down that the mine was safe and all going well at Westminster, Digby left his wife, his priest, and the two ladies, on Sunday morning, safe at Coughton, and came to Dunchurch with various gentlemen ready for the chase. The word was passed round the shires, and men were hurrying from every side toward the rendezvous. Robert Winter left his house near Worcester, and, trotting hard all day, arrived in Grafton, —where his wife's father, John Talbot, a rich old Catholic squire, then lived. The Littletons, leaving Hagley at the same moment, met Winter on Monday night in Coventry, where they slept at an inn. Next day, the 5th of November, they pricked forward to Dunchurch, where they found Sir Robert Digby of Coleshill and a strong muster of Catholic squires and their men, mounted on strong horses and armed with guns and pikes. The Littletons put up their horses and joined their friends in the village, while Winter rode on to Ashby, where he expected in a few hours to see his chief and receive the word to march. Ashby was full of guests, and Lady Catesby was just sitting down with them to supper at six o'clock, when a clatter of hoofs was heard in the court, and a moment later her son himself dashed in among them, white with passion and begrimed with dirt.

One word told all that there was left to tell.

Snatching down sword and lance from the baronial hall, the gentlemen rushed toward the stables, mounted their geldings in the dark, and made for Dunchurch, to see their comrades and resolve on what should now be done. The coming of Catesby in such a style threw everything ajar; and when the country gentlemen saw Digby and Catesby talking apart, in eager, tremulous tones, they felt sure that the scheme had failed, that government was master, and that the time had come for them to fly. Sir Robert Digby left. Humphrey Littleton also left. By twos and threes the company thinned, as the minutes waned, until, about nine o'clock, the army of Dunchurch was found to consist of few beyond those who had been sworn accomplices in the plot.

Fierce was the speech, insane the counsel, offered at Dunchurch that night; but Catesby's overpowering spirit at length compelled them to decide. Fawkes being taken prisoner, they had to count on his telling —under torture—what he knew. Their lives were forfeit to the law; and none but madmen could expect the King to overlook their crime. If they wished to live, they must strike for life. One chance was left them; an appeal to the Catholic people! Let the cry be raised. In Warwickshire they could not hold their ground; but Wales, in which they had recently invoked a powerful saint, lay open to their arms. Wales was sternly Catholic in creed. The country was difficult, the population warlike; and a religious war would feed itself on every passion of the Cymric heart.

Catesby's counsel being adopted, the meeting broke up about ten o'clock, and the company got on the road for Norbrook, which they reached in the dead of night, and rested their geldings for an hour. Digby snatched a pen and wrote a line to tell Garnet that the mine had failed, to ask his advice, and to beg that he would meet them at Robert Winter's house. Bates was sent with this note to Coughton, that he, as one sworn to the secret, might urge the good Father not to abandon them in their hour of need. Then, mounting once more, the band pushed forward in the early dawn toward Alcaster and Huddington, which they reached about two o'clock in the afternoon. Tom Winter had just come in. They were weaker in force than when they left Norbrook, for no one joined them on the road, and some of their stragglers had dropped behind. The country was rising round them on every side. In every stable from which they stole a horse, in every shop from which they snatched a gun, they raised up swarms of enemies. Men of all classes were on their track, the sheriffs of Worcester and Warwick being well prepared for such a chase by the recent musters and their admirable drill. How were they to turn, unless the Jesuits came?

A scene occurred at Coughton Hall. When Bates dashed up to the door, he found the Prefect in the hall, and gave him hastily his note. As Garnet opened the paper, Greenway came in, and asked him what the matter was. Garnet read the letter aloud, on which Greenway exclaimed, "Here is no tarrying for you and me." Bates begged that one of the Fathers at least would ride across to Huddington and comfort his young master. "I would go to him," said Greenway, "though it were to a thousand deaths; but my going would destroy the Society." Bates begged that they would come, and come at once. Then the two Jesuits stood apart, consulting in whispers for half an hour, at the end of which Greenway came out into the open air, attired in a suit of rich-colored satin covered with gold lace, and, a horse being brought round from the stable, he got on his back and accompanied Bates to Robert Winter's house.

The interview between Greenway and Catesby was in private. When it was over, Greenway took horse and rode away to Hendlip Hall. When the priest was gone away from them, Catesby called his companions, Rokewood, Percy, Morgan, and the rest, and begged of them to confess their sins and make up their souls for death. Father Hart, a Jesuit living in Winter's house, received them one by one in his closet, and, having heard the story of their crime, absolved them without a word.

The thing had to be done in haste; for Catesby was convinced that the hour was nigh when they must either die like soldiers or hang like dogs.

The confession over, and the absolution given, they took to horse once more, going straight up north through Stourbridge, to Stephen Littleton's house at Holbeach, in Staffordshire; where Catesby had a mind to make his stand and die, as he had lived, in conflict with the law.

Having crossed the borders of a county, he supposed that his friends were safe from pursuit for a few hours, while the next sheriff and his bands were getting ready; and, as much of their powder had been soaked in crossing a river, he asked Morgan, Grant, and Rokewood to assist him in the dangerous task of drying it before the kitchen fire. An accident ensued. A live coal fell into the platter on which the powder was spread, an explosion took place, and the four conspirators were blown off their seats, and their faces blackened and burnt. A bag of powder, big enough to have burst a castle, was carried through the roof unsinged. Yet the four men were so scorched and burnt that, when their comrades came into the kitchen, they shrank from the black and ghastly figures as from so many imps. A weak and superstitious fellow, Littleton stole away from his house in the night; and when morning dawned, the servants saw that Sir Everard and Robert Winter were also gone. Bates followed them; and then the bolder spirits of the plot were left alone. Tom Winter, stirring early, met Stephen Littleton, who told him Catesby was dead, and urged him to save his life by flight. "First I will go and bury the body of our friend," said Tom; on hearing which, Littleton slipped from the yard and left his house. When Winter found the specters, he asked them what they would do. "We mean to die here," they answered, in their pain. "What you do, I do," said the faithful Tom.

About eleven o'clock, Sir Richard Walsh and his company beset the house, and began to fire into the court. Tom Winter was the first to fall, though his wound was not mortal. Jack Wright was then shot dead; and after him fell Kit his brother. Then the assailants broke into the court, and Rokewood, shot already in the arm, was pierced in the body by a lance. "Stand by me, Mr. Tom," cried Catesby, "and we will die together." Tom was too much hurt to stand. "Sir," he said, respectful to the last, "I have lost the use of my right arm, and I fear that will cause me to be taken." One shot struck Percy and Catesby down, —a shot that won a pension from King James,—and then the fight was over, and the house secured.

Rokewood and Winter, Morgan and Grant, were taken prisoners. Catesby and Percy stood in sore need of help; but the only aid they could get from man was such as added to the pangs of death; for, while the sheriff was securing his prisoners and searching the house, the boors of the Black country swarmed into the court, and, finding the wounded men lying on the ground, they stripped them stark naked, stole their clothes and ornaments, exposed their gashes to the air, and caused them to expire in the accumulating agonies of bleeding, thirst, and frost.

CHAPTER XIX.

IN THE TOWER.

In less than a week from the assault of Holbeach House, the laymen of the plot were either dead or in the Tower. Catesby, Percy, Jack and Kit Wright were buried near the spot where they had fallen; but, by Northampton's orders, they were dug up from the earth and hung. Fawkes, Rokewood, Kay, Tom Winter, Stephen Littleton, Digby, Tresham, Bates, and Robert Winter were dispersed in the several prisons under charge of Waad, who brought them one by one before Northampton and the Lords Commissioners sitting in the Powder-Plot Room.

Their lives were clearly forfeit to the law, and Cecil knew that he could hang them all without incurring the reproach of dealing hardly with their Church.

The news of this plot was heard by the old English Catholics with more astonishment than rage, though the expression of their anger was both loud and deep. The priests were still more prompt to denounce it than their flocks. The venerable Archpriest, George Blackwell, took up his pen before a single man had yet been killed or captured in the shires, and in a brief address to the Catholic clergy stigmatized the plot as a detestable contrivance, in which no true Catholic could have a share,—as an abominable thing, contrary to Holy Writ, to the decrees of Councils, and to the instructions of their spiritual guides. Blackwell told his clergy to exhort their flocks to peace and obedience, and to avoid falling into snares.

While Blackwell was composing his letter, Ben Jonson, the poet, was standing in the Council chamber of Whitehall, denouncing the plot on behalf of his fellow-laymen, and offering his personal service in pursuing the gangs who had brought destruction on his Church. The poet was then about thirty years of age; for seven years he had been a Catholic; but he was a Catholic of the old English school, a pupil of St. Edward, not of St. Ignatius; and the part which he proposed to play in this drama was in keeping with his character and his creed. In his youth he had fought against Philip in the Low Countries, and after his conversion to Rome he had remained an enemy of the Jesuits and of Spain. A crime like that proposed by Catesby was one to fire his turbulent and generous veins with fury; crime in the name of religion, murder in the cause of God! He went down to Whitehall, had a talk with Cecil, and, on a blank form being given to him, he undertook to find an honest priest who could help in running the conspirators to earth. A form being placed in his hands, he went off to the Venetian embassy, where he reckoned on finding the Catholic chaplain eager to assist him in his search; and he was right in his belief; for that chaplain told him he had come on a good service,—one in which a man of conscience, who loved his country, must heartily engage. The chaplain, a foreigner, said he would seek out an English priest who knew the Jesuits and their haunts and would bring him to Cecil's chamber at Whitehall. But the poet's project led to nothing; for the priests, alarmed by the popular rage, which took no note of the difference between the children of St. Edward and the pupils of St. Ignatius, dared not come forth into the light. Ben's indignation was extreme; and he wrote to tell Cecil that the shame was so deep among the Catholics, that five hundred gentlemen would abandon their religion in a week.

The Council could hang the prisoners without reproach, and great would be the gains accruing from their death. The Puritan towns would be delighted, and the Puritan burgesses more pliant to the crown. The King could get his name into the calendar and the service-books. But Cecil and Northampton had other purposes in mind. They wished not only to discredit and destroy the Jesuit agency in England, but to cripple still more the partisans of war, by ruining the powerful Earl who was now their chief.

Week after week passed by, and the prisoners were not tried for their offense. In fact, they were undergoing a course of daily trial by Northampton in the Tower. Here they underwent a thousand interrogatories from Coke, a thousand hostilities from Waad, and a thousand treacheries from Forsett. This Forsett was one of Northampton's spies, a useful and despicable wretch, whom his master employed in overhearing and reporting the private conversations of prisoners with each other. Cecil's object in allowing these proceedings was, not to obtain a knowledge of Jesuit complicity in the plot, but evidence which could be adduced in a court of law.

The prisoners had a conscience in the matter, of a curious kind; for long after they had taken to accusing each other in their confessions, they continued to screen their priests. Both Fawkes and Winter affirmed that, when they took that oath on the Primer in Butcher Row, Father Gerard, who gave them the sacrament, was ignorant of the purpose of their oath. The names of Garnet, Greenway, Oldcorne, never passed their lips. But the object of their lying words and lying silence was to screen their persons, not to clear their fame. Of Father Owen they spoke quite freely; for Owen was beyond the reach of English law.

Though Cecil was an artist in deceit, he was amazed by the complexity of lying which he had now to study. Sir Everard Digby seemed on the whole, apart from his share in the plot, a man of honorable mind; yet Digby, while a prisoner in the Tower, considered himself free to say and unsay, from hour to hour. He told his questioners that he was not sworn; that he went to Dunchurch for the hunt and nothing more; that he was only with the band two days in all; that he quitted them of his own free will. Next day, on Fawkes being set before him, face to face, the poor young fellow told some part of the truth, and justified his former course of lies. He wrote to his wife a flood of letters and a stock of doggerel rhymes. "If I had thought there had been the least sin in it" (the scheme of wholesale murder), "I would not have been in it for all the world." Digby had been taught that assassination, in a certain cause, was not a sin ; that a false statement, in a certain cause, was not a lie.

Fawkes was pressed more closely for confessions against the Catholic peers; and, mainly on his avowals, the Earl of Northumberland, Lord Montagu, Lord Stourton, and Lord Mordaunt were brought into the Tower.

Tresham was the greatest mystery of all. For many days after Catesby's flight, Cousin Frank remained in London, going about the streets as usual, and even offering to assist the Council in seeking out the fugitives. Fawkes mentioned him as one of the sworn confederates; yet for one whole week he was left at large; and it is evident from his ways of life that he felt no fear of being arrested. At length he was committed to the Tower; and Sir Thomas Lake, the King's private secretary, considering him as a lost man, applied for a grant of Pipewell Manor, one of his estates, which James assured him he should have when it was forfeited to the crown. He made a cautious statement, saying he had seen Catesby and Winter, and had given them money, but was not a member of the plot, and had only paid the money in order to tempt his cousin to cross the seas. He seemed to know that the Council were bent on saving Lord Monteagle, and he fancied that Monteagle could not be saved unless he himself were spared. Monteagle's name appeared in all the chief confessions; but a tiny slip of paper was pasted over this name in every document that would have to be produced in court.

Tom Winter, in the ample declarations which he made in the Tower, described his mission into Spain, and mentioned the names of Tresham, Catesby, Lord Monteagle, and Father Greenway, as the men who sent him to Madrid. Greenway was known to have escaped, and Tom had therefore no concern to hide his share in the plots conducted from Enfield Chase; but he manfully refrained from saying one word that could have clouded Garnet's fame. Tresham was much more frank. He said that Father Garnet, as well as Father Greenway, had been present at their meetings in Enfield Chase, and was only too well acquainted with the mission into Spain.

The art of lying was a favorite subject of study to Cousin Frank, in whose house were found two treatises on the art: one, in favor of equivocation, by Father Garnet; the other, against equivocation, by Father Blackwell. The Jesuit's convert, following the Jesuit's rule, betrayed, without a kiss, the master from whom he had learned his art.

A few days after Frank gave his evidence against the Prefect, he was reported sick; on which his wife, Ann Tresham, applied for leave to attend him in his cell, along with her old servant, William Vavasour, an admirable scribe, who could write in many differing styles. Mrs. Tresham, a woman of the Dacre mint, procured from the sick man a paper purporting to be a full denial of his former charge against the Jesuit. A singular production was this paper. It began by saying that the man who signed it had been guilty of an infamous falsehood; it went on to say that he was now about to tell the truth,—on his salvation; it then asserted that Frank Tresham had not seen Father Garnet for sixteen years, had never heard from him in all these years, and had no knowledge of his being privy to the mission into Spain! The form was no less curious than the contents. Not being written in Tresham's hand, some evidence was wanting to prove it his. Mrs. Tresham said it was in her hand, and copied down by her from her husband's lips. A marginal note, in another hand, and signed with the name of W. Vavasour, affirmed that such was the truth.

On the morrow Frank was dead: in fact, he died the very night on which the document was signed.

Every word in that paper was a lie, and both Mrs. Tresham and her servant knew it to be a lie. During those sixteen years Mrs. Tresham had constantly received Father Garnet in her house. Nor was the paper in Mr. Tresham's hand. As both the lady and the scribe confessed later on, it was written by Vavasour himself.

As yet the evidence of guilt which Cecil could produce in court was far too slight to warrant him in arresting the Jesuit chief. A course was taken with the servant Bates, as one less likely to be cunning in his fence. The man, led on from point to point, and hardly seeing the drift of what he said, not only spoke of his confession to Greenway, but of his ride from Norbrook to Coughton, of his scene with Garnet in the hall, and of his night journey to Huddington in company with the gentleman in colored satin and golden lace. When asked where Greenway could be found, he answered that he thought he was living at Hendlip Hall.

Feeling that the tools of Philip were in his grasp, the Secretary of State proclaimed the three Jesuits, under the style of John Gerard, Henry Garnet, and Oswald Tesmond. The very same day he wrote a curious note to Anne, Lady Markham, of Beskwood Park.

This starless creature had been suffered to reside at Beskwood after her husband's liberation from the Tower on condition of his going to live abroad. But life was misery to her while Sir Griffin ate the bread of exile, and, by force of brooding on her grief, which she attributed, not unfairly, to the Jesuits, she fell into such obliquity of moral view as to think herself justified in doing them every sort of wrong. She had written a note to Cecil, hinting that her place among the Catholics, as one who had suffered in their cause, was such as enabled her to hear and see many things which it behoved the King to learn. Encouraged to speak out, she answered that certain persons then in custody could tell where the missing Jesuits could be found. From Hurleston, then in the Marshalsea, he might hear of Father Gerard; from Digby, then in the Tower, he might hear of Garnet. Cecil, while leading her on by the hope of a pardon for her husband, told her that Gerard, the priest who had sworn the confederates in Butcher Row, was wanted the first and most. To this communication she replied that, while she must be wary in her steps, lest the Catholics should suspect her of playing them false, she was eager to do his bidding and to win his favor. Garnet and Gerard, she could tell him, had been hiding in the house of Mrs. Vaux at Harrowden, and a stricter watch for two days longer would have forced them to come out. Garnet was gone, but Gerard was in the shires; and she offered to inveigle him to Beskwood Park and then deliver him up a prisoner to the King.

Cecil was free in promises. In letters dated from Whitehall, he told her he was loath to prosecute the Jesuits, but, on finding that they had been principals in the plot, he had no choice. Accepting gladly her proposal to ensnare Father Gerard, he sent her down a blank form of warrant, so that her people could arrest him the moment he set foot within her gates.

Lady Markham failed in her treacherous scheme, through the zeal of one Rutland Molyneux, a Nottingham squire, who, suspecting her purpose, met Father Gerard on the skirts of Sherwood Forest and warned him of the peril into which he was about to run. The Father made for Harwich, where he was lucky enough to find a boat.

Greenway came back to London, where, in a new disguise, he hoped to escape pursuit. One day he mixed with a crowd of people in the street, who were reading a proclamation for his arrest. One man in the crowd began to eye him sharply; and on his moving off uneasily this fellow followed him, and, seizing him by the arm, exclaimed, "You are known; I arrest you in the King's name; you must go with me before the Council at Whitehall." Very quietly saying there was some mistake, the Jesuit offered to go with him; and they walked on together, chatting, until they came to a deserted street, when Greenway sprang upon the fellow, threw him down, and got away. He hid himself for a few days in Essex, and then took boat for Flanders, which he safely reached.

Short shrift was given to the prisoners. Digby, Robert Winter, Grant, and Bates were taken from the Tower and hung near Paul's Cross; while Fawkes, Kay, Rokewood, and Tom Winter were drawn on hurdles, hung, and boweled in Palace Yard.

The Powder Plot was over; but the Jesuit agents of Spain were still to seek.

CHAPTER XX.

SEARCH FOR GARNET.

If Garnet and Oldcorne had chosen to escape beyond sea, they could easily have found the means. The Council would have been glad to see them go; for the flight of Garnet, as a broken and ruined man, would have been more than evidence of his guilt; it would have been a public confession that his mission from the King of Spain had failed.

Cecil drew a clear distinction between Garnet as a Spanish agent and Garnet as a Catholic priest. In the first of these characters he was an outcast; in the second he was a citizen, bound to obey the law. Cecil and Northampton were eager to prove that the old Spanish policy was a failure; and such a proof the Prefect was determined not to give.

Hence, when Greenway, dressed in his satin suit, rode off with Bates from Coughton, Garnet and the ladies kept in their rooms, avoiding strangers, and being served by their faithful people, until the news arrived that Digby was overtaken by the hue and cry near Dudley. Digby, who was weak of tongue, would be forced to speak, and the Prefect felt that Coughton was no longer a place in which he could safely hide. The country was up in arms, and every house suspected of having a Catholic mistress was certain to be searched. Where could he and his females hide until the uproar passed? While he was scheming, Oldcorne arrived from Hendlip Hall with an invitation for himself and train; when he moved, together with Ann Vaux and his servant Little John, to Mrs. Abington's friendly house.

Hendlip Hall, a Tudor house of vast extent, which stood on high ground and swept the country for many miles, had been recently built by Thomas Abington, on plans supplied by Little John, as a hiding-place for priests. Almost every room in the pile had a recess, a passage, a trap-door, and a secret stair. The walls were hollow, the ceilings false. The chimneys had double flues,—a passage for the fire, and a second for the priest. One hollow in the wall was covered with most cunning art,—a narrow crevice, next to the fire-place, into which a reed was laid from Mrs. Abington's bedroom, so that soup and wine could be passed by her into the recess, without the fact being noticed from any other room. Except the builders and the Jesuits, no one had a key to the whole maze of secrets; but the local gentry were aware that the Hall had been contrived for the concealment of priests; and when the proclamation against the Jesuits came out, Sir Henry Bromley, of Holt Castle, an active justice of the peace, was not surprised to receive an order from the Council to search the house. His orders were minute. He was to surround the Hall with his men, to set a guard at every door, to suffer no one to come in, no one to go out, until the priests were found. The servants were to be watched by day and night, to see that they carried no food into strange places. The dining-room was to be carefully examined, and the wainscot pulled down to see if any passage lay beyond. The cellar-floors were to be broached. Every room in the house was to be measured, so as to see whether the lower apartments corresponded with the upper in length and breadth. Even the chimney-stacks were to be pierced and probed.

The searchers came upon Mrs. Abington with so much secrecy and suddenness that the priests and their servants had to run like rats into their holes. Garnet and Oldcorne crept into the crevice near the fireplace, from which the reed for passing soups and wine conducted into Mrs. Abington's room. Chambers and Little John, their servants, hid themselves in a kind of cupboard. No preparation for their stay in these hiding-places had been made. The priests' recess was nearly filled with books and lumber, and the only food which it contained was some pots of marmalade. The servants had no food at all, and their den was stuffed with what Bromley calls "Popish trash."

When the justice showed his warrant from the Council, Mrs. Abington assured him that no one was in hiding at Hendlip. Abington, her husband, was then from home; but, on his coming to the Hall, he confirmed the statement of his wife, adding that he knew nothing of Father Garnet personally, and had not seen Father Gerard for several years. Bromley was surprised; but, his orders being strict, he proceeded to search the house, to measure the rooms, and to count the beds. With a list of the family in his hand, he passed through every chamber, noticing which was occupied and which was not. He found more beds in the rooms than guests; and, on carefully testing the condition of these beds, he found that some of those which were said to be unused were *warm.*

Mrs. Abington kept her room, in anger at the search being made. Bromley would have had her quit the Hall while his troops were there; but she refused to go, and he dared not turn a lady of her quality—the sister of so great a man as Lord Monteagle—out of doors. He could not guess her reason for so obstinately shutting herself up in a single room,—eating there, drinking there, sleeping there, day and night.

But after some days of careful watch had been kept in every room—except the one in which Mrs. Abington lay—a panel in the wainscot opened, and two specters stepped into the hall. The ghosts were Chambers and Little John, whom Bromley took to be the Jesuit and his man. Mrs. Abington pretended not to know them; but the facts were soon discovered; and the search was then continued for their masters with a warmer hope.

The crevice in which Garnet and Oldcorne lay was low and strait; and, being filled with books and furniture, the Fathers could neither stand on their feet nor lie down at length. Their flesh began to swell and their bones to ache; they could hear the searchers tapping at the walls; and, from their talk and laughter as they called to each other, they learned that Chambers and Little John were caught. "We were very merry and content within," said Garnet afterward, when describing the scene to Ann Vaux, "and heard the searchers every day most curious over us, which made me think the place would be found."

But, as day after day slid past without result, the magistrate, after setting a watch in every room and corridor, rode home to Holt Castle on his own affairs, for the sake of a little rest; and while he was absent from Hendlip, more precise and positive news of Oldcorne being hid in Mrs. Abington's house was received from Worcester jail.

Humphrey Littleton was being tried for his life in that city; and this poor fellow, whose only crime had been a desire to command a troop of horse against the Dutch, was highly sore against his old confessor. On quitting the gangs at Dunchurch, Humphrey sent a pressing prayer for Oldcorne to join him at once and tell him what he should now do; but the Jesuit, feeling safe at Hendlip, and hearing that the shires were up in arms, declined to come; on which Humphrey whimpered that his confessor had drawn him into rebellion and then left him to his fate. So long, however, as a chance of life remained to him, he held his tongue; but when the day for hanging him at Worcester had been fixed, he sent his keeper to tell the sheriff and justices that if his sentence were respited he could render much service to the King. Of course the respite was given, and a magistrate went to his cell, where he heard from the prisoner's lips that Oldcorne was concealed in a recess at Hendlip, and that one of the servants then in the jail could take a pursuivant to the spot.

Elated by this news, Sir Henry rode back to Hendlip, and, renewing his search, soon found the hollow in the wall. The soldier who slid the panel, seeing two men darkly in the hole, ran back in fear, expecting them to fire. A crowd was soon at the door, to whom Garnet spoke, bidding them be quiet, and saying they would yield themselves in peace. Bromley recognized Garnet from the proclamation. But the Father would not give his name. "You are a learned man?" said Bromley. "Let me be taken before my Lord of Salisbury," answered Garnet: "he will know me." Cecil's cunning courtesies had so far told upon the Prefect, that he thought himself an object of the Secretary's grace.

Abington, arrested with the lie on his lips, was driven, with the four Jesuits whom he had feloniously concealed, to Worcester in Bromley's coach. "I hoped to have lodged you in a citizen's house," said Bromley to the Father; "but I cannot, and you must lie in the jail." Garnet started at the word: "A God's name, I hope you will provide we have not irons, for we are lame already, and shall not be able to ride after it to London." Bromley said he would see to it. He put Garnet into a private room, and left him for a time. On his return, he placed the prisoners in his coach once more, and drove them to Holt Castle, where they remained as guests in his house, well lodged, and sitting at table with Lady Bromley and her people, until Candlemas, to recruit their strength. A banquet was then given, and in the midst of dinner Sir Henry called for wine, and, standing up, bareheaded, drank to the King. The Prefect rose to his feet, and pledged the health, as he says, "in a reasonable glass."

Ann Vaux and Mrs. Abington were left at Hendlip Hall.

At length the cavalcade set out from Holt Castle. "I parted from the gentlewomen, who were very kind to me," wrote the Jesuit, "as also all the house." The journey was made by easy stages, and a treacherous kindness met them at every turn. From Bromley, Garnet heard that it was by Cecil's express command that he was used so well. He rode the best horse in the company. He traveled at the King's expense. He halted when he pleased, and ate and drank of the best. On the road he met, as it seemed by chance, Dean Abbott and Dean Barlow, two of the court divines. They had a long talk together at an inn, and Garnet was struck by the air of respect which the two Deans put on. Yet these divines were the bitterest enemies of his Order and his Church. When Bromley arrived in London with his charge, he lodged the Prefect in the Gate house, near Whitehall, Abington in the Fleet, Little John and Chambers in the Tower.

On St. Valentine's eve Garnet was marched through a crowd of people to the Council chamber of Whitehall, where Cecil and Northampton received him with the treacherous courtesy that had already thrown him off his guard. When he knelt, they bade him stand up. When he began by protesting his innocence of Catesby's plot, "I wish," said Cecil, mildly, "you would not protest so earnestly, since we have certain proof." With smiling courtesy Cecil inquired his opinion about equivocation, about the doctrine of excommunication, and about the Pope's dispensing power. "You see, Mr. Garnet," he insinuated, "we deal not with you in matters of religion, as of your priesthood, or of the real presence." He only asked a question about the oath. Garnet was pleased, as he wrote to Ann Vaux, "to be accounted a traitor without, and not within, the plot." But he was cautious in what he said. To Cecil's question, whether it was held by Catholics to be lawful to take up arms against the King, he answered that no one could rise against his prince unless that prince were excommunicated by the Pope. He thought King James was not excommunicate; and, even if he were so, he declared that no one could proceed against him without the Pope's express command. A Catholic could only rise against heretics. Being pressed to say whether the English were not held to be heretics, he answered, "The religion is heretical: of the persons I cannot judge." Cecil put the question, "May the Pope excommunicate our King?" Garnet replied by the evasion, "The Pope is successor to St. Peter, to whom Christ said, *Pasce oves meas*, and so he may excommunicate Kings." Cecil urged him to say "our King;" but he refused to do so, as he alleged, "out of reverence." "Could the Pope release subjects from their obedience?" "There is a canon, *Nos Sanctorum*, wherein is such a rule, which lies beyond my power to abridge." The questioning by Cecil and Northampton lasted two hours, after which Coke attacked him for one hour more. Garnet refused to name his partners in the mission, and even to admit the names by which he was known to his penitents.

Next day, St. Valentine's day, he was committed to the Tower,—to a "horrible dungeon," probably the Keep; but, after suffering two bad nights in his miserable den, he was removed, for a reason which he could not guess, into Leslie's old chamber, on the lower tier of the Bloody tower.

"I am allowed every meal," he wrote to Ann Vaux, who had followed him to London, "a good draught of excellent claret wine; and I am liberal with myself and neighbors for good respects, to allow also of my purse some sack; and this is the greatest charge I shall be at."

Contrary to their nature, Coke and Waad, both acting on a hint from court, were civil to the prisoner. Even Popham's awful brow unbent when Garnet came into the Powder-Plot Room. During one of his examinations, Garnet said he did not fear to die, for he should die innocently, and death would be welcome. "That were a pity," said Coke; "for you are a man to serve your King and country." One day, when Coke was talking of the time at Hendlip, Garnet said, "If I had a calendar I could tell, for I think it was St. Sebastian's day." "You have saints for every day?" "We have for the most part," answered Garnet. "Well," quoth Coke, "you shall have no place in the calendar." "I am not worthy of a place in the calendar," said Garnet; "but I hope to have a place in heaven." Waad rallied him about Mrs. Brooksby's child, born at White Webbs; but Popham came to his defense by saying that Brooksby, her husband, lived in the house. Brooksby was bald, and Coke could not resist the opportunity of saying that the baby was seen with a shaven crown.

Once, indeed, Garnet was drawn by these treacherous pleasantries into making what he thought a serious offer to the King. Waad was saying, what he knew to be in Cecil's mind, "The Jesuits' Order shall be dissolved upon this as the Templars' was;" to which the Prefect answered, "Private faults do not prejudice the whole." "The Jesuits shall now all out of England," added Sir William. Garnet then made his offer: "If the King would grant free liberty to other Papists, I will presently send away all Jesuits." Popham started. "That is more than you can do?" he urged. "I will try," said the Prefect, making to his judge a most dangerous confession of his power over that band of outlaws.

Well lodged, well fed, with plenty of sack and claret, with civil judges and obsequious keepers, Garnet was highly pleased with what was going on. If he could have his "morning delight," he wrote to tell Ann Vaux, he should be happy. What his "morning delight" was, we can only guess: the lady knew, no doubt.

An obliging keeper carried his letter to Ann; and in less than a week after it was sent, Ann Vaux was herself a prisoner in the Tower.

CHAPTER XXI.

END OF THE ENGLISH JESUITS.

THE whole group of English Jesuits were now in charge of Sir William Waad.

Father Fisher was in the Keep, on the walls of which he inscribed his name. Garnet and Oldcorne, after passing some fifty hours in a dark hole, had been placed in adjoining rooms under Raleigh's lodgings in the Bloody tower. George and Little John were thrown into separate dungeons, dismal and far apart. Abington alone was in the Fleet.

But where was Father Robarts all this while? This Father, the companion of Fawkes in Vinegar House, was taken, as it were, in the fact. His guilt was evident. No jury could have doubted for a moment that he knew of the mine being laid. Near him, in his room, a quantity of Popish books and papers had been seized. These papers were of moment, and in the first hours of their seizure they had been freely used by Coke. Yet from the night of Fawkes's arrest the Father and his papers disappear from view. Robarts was afterward seen at large; but what became of him during those five months in which Cecil and Northampton were routing and destroying the Jesuit conspirators, no soul can tell. This sudden disappearance of a man who had come direct from Rome to stand by the side of Fawkes, is one of the darkest mysteries of that mysterious time.

One day, a keeper, of whom Garnet thought he had made a friend by giving him a little sack and a little coin, told the Prefect as a secret that his comrade, Father Oldcorne, lay in the adjoining room. Garnet listened to his words, and then the man, encouraged to go on, pointed to a slide in the wall, and told him that on pushing it back he might converse with his friend. But the thing must be done with care, as keepers might be about who were unfriendly to him, and then the panel would be nailed up. Garnet tried the panel, and found his keeper right. Oldcorne was there; and the two Jesuits, after a short prayer in Latin, made confessions to each other, beating their hands the while upon their hearts.

Two spies, named Forsett and Locherson, had been so placed by Waad that they could hear the two priests; and the main part of their conversation was taken down by these spies. "I had a note from Rokewood," they heard Garnet say (Thomas Rokewood was a brother of Ambrose), "and he telleth me Greenway is gone. . . . I had another from Gerard, that he meaneth to go over to Father Persons. . . . I think Mrs. Ann is in the town; if she be, I have writ a note, that my keeper may repair to her, and convey me anything unto her, who will let us hear from all our friends. I gave him an angel yesterday, . . . and he took it very well, with great thanks; and now and then at meals I make very much of him, and give him a cup of sack, and send his wife another, and that he taketh very kindly. . . . You should do well now and then to give him a shilling, and sometimes send his wife somewhat. . . . He did see me write to Mr. Rokewood." The talk was long and curious; for the two Jesuits had not seen each other since they arrived in town. "I must needs confess White Webbs," said Garnet, who had at first denied being there; "but I will answer it thus,—that I was there, but knew nothing of the matter." Oldcorne spoke in a lower tone, and the spies could not always catch his words. "Mr. Attorney," Garnet went on to say, "told me, very friendly, that he would make the best construction of my examination to the King, and do me good. If I can satisfy the King, it will be well; but I think it not convenient to deny that we were at White Webbs. . . . They pressed me to be there in October last, which I will by no means confess; but I will tell them I was not there since Bartholomew's tide; neither will I tell them of my knowledge of any of the servants there, for they may examine and perhaps torture some of them, and make them yield to some confession. . . . I am persuaded I shall wind myself out of this matter." Poor fellow! A noise was now heard in the passage, for the spies had learned enough for the day; and Garnet was heard to say in a whisper to Oldcorne, "Hark you—hark you—Mr. Lieutenant! Make a hawking and spitting while I shut the door."

Two days later, the keeper to whom Garnet had given his money and his wine made a motion that the coast was clear; on which Garnet slid back the panel and held a second confidential chat with Oldcorne. "They charge me," said Garnet, "with some advice in the Queen's time for blowing up the Parliament House with powder. . . . I told them at that time it was lawful, but wished them to save as many as they could that were innocent." Here was the evidence that Cecil and Northampton needed for his condemnation. "They pressed me," Garnet added, "what noblemen I knew that have written any letters to Rome. . . .

Well, I see they will justify my Lord Monteagle of all this matter." What he said next was doubtful; for a cock in the Lieutenant's garden under his window gave a lusty crow. The spies reported that he mentioned the names of Lord Northumberland, Lord Rutland, and one other, though in what connection he referred to these noblemen they could not tell.

The two Jesuits held a long debate as to how they should shape their confessions not to differ in the main. Garnet complained that Oldcorne was rather lax, not standing to the bargain they had made while hiding at Hendlip. "They went away last time unsatisfied," said Garnet, speaking of Northampton and the other commissioners, "and therefore we may expect the rack. . . . Mr. Attorney was about to write, but when he had written these lines he gave it over, and seemed to be angry, saying, 'I had lost my credit, for *he* had undertaken for me to the King.'" The spies reported that Garnet spoke much of a gentlewoman, and said that if he were charged with her he would excuse her coming with him; but how he was to do it they could not plainly hear him say. They made a noise, as if some one were coming, on which Garnet asked Oldcorne to take a shovel and rattle the coals while he closed the dividing door.

These secret conferences, overheard by spies, continued for a week. In one of his brief confessions to his fellow-priest, Garnet admitted having drunk so much that he had twice been obliged to be put to bed. Oldcorne mentioned that he had heard from some one that their servants were being questioned; when Garnet replied that his own man, Little John, would never confess to anything against him. While he was using these words, this faithful servant, broken by his fear of the rack, was dying in another cell.

Up to the previous day Little John's strength had not been tried. Being asked in the ordinary way how he came to Hendlip, he refused to say; he knew neither Garnet nor Oldcorne; and though he had known Chambers for some years, he could not tell them whether he was Oldcorne's man or not. But on his thumbs being tied together, and his body being raised by a beam, he instantly gave up his master's name. This clever architect could not bear the torture, and while his limbs were stretched he answered every question they chose to put. He had served Father Garnet from the date of the Essex rising. He had been with him often at White Webbs. He went with him down to Coughton, where he heard him say mass before the insurrection broke out, and afterward to Hendlip Hall, where Garnet and Oldcorne dined and supped with Mr. and Mrs. Abington every day until the search began. These were the confessions of which Oldcorne had heard some hints; but Waad, who thought he could tell much more, told the lay Jesuit that his next examination should be taken on the rack.

The threat sufficed. Next day Little John complained of sickness, when his keeper lent him a chair to sit on and a knife to cut his meat. The broth for his dinner, he said, was cold; and, feeling very faint, he begged the keeper to put it for a moment on the fire in an adjacent room. So soon as the man was gone he ripped himself open with his knife, and, gathering up the straw about his knees, sat still and bled until the keeper came. Seeing his prisoner covered with straw and dabbled with blood, the man ran off to the Lieutenant, whom he found at table with his guests, and gave the alarm; on which Waad and the gentlemen who were dining with him rushed to the suicide's cell. The Jesuit was gone past hope, and the only speech they could draw from him was that he had killed himself in fear of the rack, lest in his weakness and his agony he might be tempted to betray the lives of men who had always been his friends.

A brave man, worthy of a nobler fate!

Ann Vaux was no less brave. In following Garnet to London and taking lodgings near the Tower, she knew the dangers into which she ran. About the time of her arrival, her house at White Webbs was searched, and her servant, James, was seized. Tied on the rack, this servant told the story of her life in Enfield Chase, —her false names, her priestly guests, her dangerous visitors; yet for two or three weeks the Council allowed her to remain at large, and to correspond with her confessor in the Bloody tower. She sent in parcels of linen and boxes of marmalade. Garnet asked her for money to pay his fees, and he told her she must come to his keeper's mother for instructions how to act. If she came to the Lieutenant's garden, near his window, she could see him, though she must not try to speak. He told her to get some of the Society's money if she could, as he wanted to buy beds "for James, John, and Harry, who have been tortured." This note—and much that followed it—was sent by a private hand; but the Lieutenant seems to have seen it before it passed the gate.

Ann Vaux, arrested and committed to the Tower, was sharply questioned as to her residence at White Webbs, and the gathering of conspirators beneath her roof. She answered boldly, confessing that Catesby, Winter, and Tresham had been her guests, and frequently at her table; that she had gone with Lady Digby to St. Winifred's Well; that she was at Coughton on the 1st of November last. But not one word could be drawn from her against the Jesuits. She would not say what priests were at the Well. She had heard no prayer, no mass, at Coughton. Told that Garnet had confessed the plot, she expressed her sorrow and surprise, as he had made to her many protests to the contrary. When they found her useless as a witness, they remembered her noble birth and set her free.

Nine days later, Ann sent to the Tower a pair of spectacles, wrapped in a bit of paper, on which were written, in plain black ink, these harmless words, "I pray you prove whether these spectacles do fit your sight;" but, when this piece of paper was held before a fire, the text of a letter, written in orange-juice, came out. She told the prisoner that Coke, at supper-time on Saturday night, had spoken of him. He had said that Garnet, feigning to be sick, had gone to his chamber, where his keeper saw him take a letter from a box of marmalade, just then come in, and burn it. He had also said that Garnet had confessed to his knowledge of the powder, though he still denied any practice in it. She told him that the box and paper were from her hands. She was glad they reached him. The spectacles and scrap were from her; and if they came to him safely, then other of his friends would write, and steps could be taken to supply his room. She added, "For myself, I am forced to seek new friends; my old are wearied of me. I beseech you, for God's sake, advise me what course to take. My hope is you will continue your care of me, and commit me to some that will for your sake help me. To live without you is not life, but death. Now I see my loss, I am and ever will be yours; and so I humbly beseech you to account me. Oh that I might see you!"

On this letter being read by Coke, the writer was again arrested, and her house examined, when a heap of relics, altar-stuff, and priestly trappings was discovered. She said they belonged to her sister and herself. She confessed that Father Garnet had lived with her at White Webbs; that her cousin, Frank Tresham, had often come to see them; but she declared that the Jesuit had always counseled him to be patient in his griefs. The notes of this second examination were sent by Coke to Cecil.

As nothing could be learned from Ann Vaux, the government were forced to make use of the conversations which had been overheard by their spies in the Bloody tower.

Oldcorne was carried into the Powder-Plot Room and charged by the commissioners with having held a clandestine conversation with Garnet in the Bloody tower. Startled by the announcement, Oldcorne confessed that he had spoken with his friend through the door, and, being pressed by Coke, admitted details which were fatal to his comrade and himself. He was often at White Webbs, where he had met with Garnet, Gerard, and many more; but Garnet had told him in the Tower that he would never confess to being at White Webbs. Garnet had also told him, in the Tower, that he had taken the lead in those prayers at Coughton, which in public he had strenuously denied.

Garnet was now brought in and questioned. Secret conference with Oldcorne! Never. He had not seen his fellow-prisoner; had never exchanged a word with him. When shown the paper signed by Oldcorne, he said it was all a lie; that Oldcorne might accuse him, but he would never accuse himself. On being threatened with the rack, however, he confessed to the main facts; and then he was sent to trial under a special commission, consisting of Sir Leonard Halliday, Lord Mayor, the four Catholic Earls to whom Cecil had read Monteagle's letter (Nottingham, Northampton,

Suffolk, and Worcester), Sir John Popham, and some others. The trial took place in Westminster Hall; the King was present behind a curtain, and the Lady Arabella looked on the scene from a private box.

Oldcorne had been already tried, condemned, and executed.

Garnet's trial (March, 1606) was a form only, for he had been already tried in secret and condemned to die. The trial lasted some hours; Garnet defended himself with subtilty and spirit; and Northampton made a long and scurrilous attack on the Jesuits in a speech, which he afterward printed in London and explained away in Rome.

From the Tower gates the Jesuit was carried to Ludgate Hill, in front of St. Paul's Cathedral, where a gallows had been built for him. A multitude of people came to see him suffer, and, like many a worse man than himself, he made a devout end. The injury which he had done to Ann Vaux was on his mind to the last, and he spoke some words on the scaffold to clear her fame. "There is an honorable gentlewoman," he said, not aloud to the people, but in a low, sad voice, to those about him, "who hath been much wronged by report, for it is suspected and said that I should be married to her, *or worse.* I protest the contrary. She is a virtuous gentlewoman; and for me a perfect virgin." He prayed for the King and Queen. He said he had held out in denial, because he thought the Council had no proof against him. He now confessed his fault, and hoped that the Catholics would fare no worse for his sake. As he was saying his prayer, "Maria Mater gratiæ, Maria Mater misericordiæ," the cart was drawn from beneath his feet.

CHAPTER XXII.

THE CATHOLIC LORDS.

WHILE Cecil and Northampton were employed in driving and seizing the priestly members of the Plot, they were not unmindful of those Catholic peers who, from their name and faith, could not help being the most acceptable of Englishmen in the court of Spain. Such peers as Montagu, Mordaunt, Stourton, and Northumberland were counted in their several ways, by foreign princes, most of all by Philip the Third, as the living force of the Catholic cause,—the men by whom the country would be drawn at some future time into what they called the ancient family union of the Church. These peers might be out of favor; but men who had half the population of England at their back could never be out of power.

Cecil and Northampton had to show the Duke de Lerma that a foreign minister who counted on these Catholic lords was counting on a bundle of broken reeds.

The facts which came out in the earliest questioning of Fawkes and Winter in the Tower enabled them to take defensive measures against these lords without appearing to go beyond the stern necessities of the case. Fawkes had lived in the household of Lord Montagu, Kay in that of Lord Mordaunt. Stourton, who lived in Clerkenwell, was married to Frances Tresham, a sister of "Cousin Frank." Catesby was known to have warned Stourton and Mordaunt against coming to the House of Lords. Percy was not only a kinsman and servant of Northumberland, but was known to have supped with him at Sion on Monday night. Such facts, as they came out one by one, excited the public mind; but Cecil, in giving orders to restrain the four great Catholic peers, took every opportunity of hinting that he meant them well. At first they were confined to their several houses; then some of them were removed to the houses of aldermen and justices of the peace; but in less than eight weeks after the arrest of Guy Fawkes they were all committed to the Tower.

Anthony Maria Browne, second Viscount Montagu, of Cowdray in Sussex, was a youth of thirty-three, a master of many manors, colleges, and farms, and the husband of Lady Jane, a daughter of Thomas Sackville, Earl of Dorset, the eminent poet and Lord High Treasurer of England. He lived in Montagu Close, the great Priory of St. Mary Overies, near London Bridge, a pile which had been given by Henry the Eighth to his grandsire, the first Lord Montagu of his line. The Priory was Church property, and when the Brownes became Catholic under Mary it was hoped they would cease to hold an estate which belonged to God. In fact, the old Viscount had become strict in his principles; he had married Maud Dacre; he had called his grandson and heir "Maria;" but he stuck to Montagu Close as firmly as though he had been the laxest heretic in the realm.

The case against Anthony Maria, Viscount Montagu, was ugly enough under any explanation, and he had the misfortune to give more than one explanation of the leading facts. The points which told most against him were that Guy Fawkes had been one of the servants near his person, that Catesby had given him some hint of what would occur when the King was seated on his throne, and that he had proposed to be absent from his place in Parliament on the opening day.

To the first point he answered that Fawkes was placed by his grandfather in his household when he married, that he was then a boy under nineteen, and that Fawkes was in his service only about four months. But he could not say that he had never seen him since that time. On pressure, he confessed that Fawkes, after the first Viscount's death, had slept in his house and served at his table. The explanation was that his steward, one Spencer, a kinsman of "the miserable fellow," had given him a few days' lodging in Montagu Close, and, while he was staying there, had turned his service to account. All this took place twelve years ago, and since that time he had scarcely ever seen or thought of him.

To the second point he answered that he met with Catesby in the Strand by accident on the Tuesday before All Saints' Day, as he was going to the Savoy to dine; that the conspirator gave him no warning to absent himself from Parliament; that their speech was only general, as to the cause of his being absent in the country. But the very next day he corrected the date on which these dangerous speeches had been held in the Strand into the Tuesday fortnight before All Saints' Day,—a date which he could fix, he said, from the fact that he was dining in the Savoy with his aunt, Lady Southampton.

To the third point he answered that he proposed to be absent from London on the opening day by the King's good leave, and not otherwise,—a leave which he hoped to procure through the Earl of Dorset, his father-in-law. If this leave could not be obtained for him, he meant to be in his place. The old Viscountess

Montagu (poor Maud Dacre) knew about it; for on telling her of his plan for going down into the country she had begged him not to go, unless he could first get leave of absence from Parliament, as the hard riding would be too much for his health.

From Sir Thomas Bennet's house he was carried to the Tower; but for the sake of Lady Jane, if not for his own, the Council dealt with his inconsistencies in a tender spirit. Brought before the Star Chamber, he was condemned to a fine of four thousand pounds and imprisonment during his Majesty's pleasure. In the end he compounded for his fine, and lay in the Tower about forty weeks.

Henry Mordaunt, fourth Baron Mordaunt of Drayton Manor in county Northants, and of Turvey in county Beds, was descended on his mother's side from the old Catholic family of Darcy, one of whose members had forfeited his honors by the Pilgrimage of Grace. Mordaunt was a close friend of Catesby, but, being a Catholic of the old English school, he could not be intrusted with the secrets of his plot. He was a weak and pliant creature, whom the haughty Catesby had to manage and despise. Some one had proposed to swear him. "Not for a church full of diamonds!" cried the man who knew him best. If Mordaunt were told the secret, even on the Primer, Catesby was of opinion that he could not keep it. Easy and yielding, he was used, like the two Littletons, by that mastering spirit, who induced him to permit his servants to be employed in raising men, under cover of a design to fight in the Archduke's cause. Two Irish fellows, named O'Ferrall, who had been tempted to enlist, gave evidence against Mordaunt's man. More than one of the prisoners confessed that Catesby had given some hints to his friend; and Mordaunt had made excuses for not being present with his peers, on the ground that his conscience would not allow him to attend the King at church.

Turvey, his ancient seat in Beds, was a notorious nest of Jesuits. Kay had lived in his house, and Kay's wife was the teacher of his children. All these things were against him. Brought before the Star Chamber, Mordaunt was sentenced to a heavy fine, with imprisonment during the King's pleasure; and, after six months of rather sharp privation in the Tower, he was liberated on conditions which left him a broken man. In succeeding reigns the Mordaunts rose again,—chiefly in the person of Henry's grandson, the meteoric Earl of Peterborough; but for twenty years to come his utmost care was needed to preserve in his family that lordship of Turvey which had been their own since the reign of Henry the First.

Edward Stourton, ninth Baron Stourton of Stourton, in county Wilts, was the second son of that wretched Charles, Lord Stourton, who had been hung, in a silken cord on account of his quality, for the murder of his neighbors, the two Hargils, father and son. Edward, then a boy, was said, like his elder brother John, to have been privy to the crime; but the lads were spared on account of their youth; and, after eighteen years had passed over the public memory, the two brothers were restored in blood, in order that John might sit, as one of the old Catholic peers, on the bench which was to condemn Mary, Queen of Scots, to death. This John, eighth Lord Stourton, died without issue; and Edward, his partner in suspicion, came into the honors of his race.

A dark and gloomy fanatic, with hands not free from blood, and weighted with the curse of his father's shame, this Edward, ninth Lord Stourton, had lived a lonely life, the companion and the victim of monks and priests. Lady Stourton was Frances, a daughter of Sir Thomas Tresham, and therefore a sister of "Cousin Frank." Their London house was in Clerkenwell,—a part of the famous priory of that place; for the Stourtons, like the Brownes, had no objection to receive Church lands

Brought before the Star Chamber, Stourton, who could neither deny his intimacy with Catesby and "Cousin Frank" nor explain to the court his reason for absenting himself on the opening day, was sentenced to a thousand pounds fine and imprisonment during pleasure in the Tower. This fine was compounded, and the prisoner released; compounded, not paid; for two years after his release from the Tower the fine was returned in a draft of outstanding public debts. What was due to private persons had been paid to the uttermost coin.

Compounding for fines was a curious and immoral traffic, and, being conducted with the utmost secrecy, was understood by few. Lord Stourton happened to be one of those few, his wife being a Tresham, and one of a family which had been driven by their misfortunes into studying the mysteries of this immoral trade.

When Cousin Frank went out with Essex into the Strand, he fell into so much danger that every one expected him to share the fate of Cuffe and Lea. But the Treshams were rich, and some great ladies in the court were poor. A communication was made to Sir Thomas, in a roundabout way, on behalf of a young lady who might be able to help his son. This young lady, the daughter of no less a person than Lord Howard of Walden, Constable of the Tower (afterward Earl of Suffolk,—the same who went into the vault and jested about the coal and wood), was represented as being willing to plead for Frank, on certain trusts being executed in her favor by the master of Rushton Hall. Catherine Howard was then a child, too young to speak with her Majesty on any subject more serious than a toy; but her mother, Lady Howard, the sharpest intriguer living, had arranged with her lover, Sir Robert Cecil, that this girl should some day be the wife of his eldest son; and therefore it seemed right in the Secretary's eyes that Catherine should be provided with a dowry out of traitors' lands. Sir Thomas, knowing that the life of his son was in their power, consented to lodge with a third party, not to be named in the writings, certain bonds of large amount, on the understanding that these bonds were to be handed over to certain "honorable persons" when a "matter" not set forth in words was performed, and to be returned to Sir Thomas in case that "matter" was not performed. How much money was paid to the young lady by Sir Thomas remains a secret: one of the bonds was drawn for twenty-one hundred pounds, and several were for a thousand pounds apiece. The bribe was so large that Sir Thomas always said the payment crippled him for life.

Through some such channel as Lady Suffolk's daughter, Stourton compounded for his fine.

But the ruin of these three barons was of less importance to Cecil and Northampton than that of the great northern Earl, the friend of Raleigh, the mainspring of the war party, the future hope of the Catholics, and the most powerful personage living beyond the Trent.

CHAPTER XXIII.

HARRY PERCY.

Harry Percy, ninth earl and twenty-first baron of his line, had won his spurs of knighthood in the Low-Country war and in the Armada fight,—in which, though a good Catholic, he had fought with heroic fire against the King of Spain. But his hope of achieving a great career in arms had been quenched by the many and unseemly quarrels into which his violence of temper led him.

Even when the flush of youth was gone, he had no control over his tongue and pen, and at thirty he behaved like an overgrown boy in a public school. For two years he had fought in the lines of Ostend with credit, when his mutinous passions entrapped him into an indecent broil with his commander, the illustrious Vere, whom he wished to call out and fight. He quarreled with his comrades, and separated from his Countess. This lady, a sister of Lord Essex and of Lady Rich, was of a temper heated and unruly like his own; and when they bickered in their golden halls, Northumberland rode away from her, engaged a mistress to live with him in open shame, and hired a lodging for her near the court in order to provoke his wife.

Apart from an infirmity which he shared with his ancestor and namesake, Harry Hotspur, Percy was a gallant soldier and a princely friend. Raleigh respected him as a companion-in-arms. Neither Pembroke nor Southampton rivaled him in his sympathy for science and the liberal arts. Peele and Heriot were his constant companions. Spenser sent him a sonnet, and a copy of the Faery Queen. Peele composed for him his poem called "The Honor of the Garter;" and Heriot owed to his bounty that leisure for investigation which led to his discoveries in solar and stellar science. It was said in Percy's praise that no scholar ever turned disheartened from his door. Himself a student of art and nature, he toyed with every subject in its turn,—with numbers, with music, with the starry heavens, with alchemy, with the elixir of life. Bacon looked to him as a patron of the new learning: "Your great capacity and love toward studies and contemplations of a higher and nobler nature than popular (a nature rare in this world, and in a person of your lordship's quality almost singular) is to me," wrote Bacon, "a great and chief motive to draw my affection and admiration toward you." In person, he was the soul of honor; and, if he could only have curbed his petulant tongue, he would have been one of the most perfect paladins in the English court.

The name, the valor, and the possessions of Percy had pointed him out as Lord Protector in case the kingdom should require such an officer on the Queen's demise. The whole north country would have rallied to his flag; and the known wishes of the great Earl, as to the coming in of James, had done more to make his entry pleasant than those of any other man.

The King, too well aware of his service, had hardly crossed the border before he called him to his Council by a special act. Yet the lines were drawn between Cecil and Percy from the opening day of the new reign; and every slight that could be made to gall and wound a spirit only too quick to see offense was put on Percy by his smiling and respectful adversary. Percy, who had thought of finding great employments under

James, was sore at heart, and, being sore at heart, was certain to be loud of tongue. He talked to Bethune. He inspired Watson with hope. Even if he had been careful of his words, he could not have failed to be the subject of conversation in taverns like the Hart's Horn, in slums like Butcher Row; and he was far from careful of his words. The circle at White Webbs made many inquiries about him. Once, indeed, they thought of making him their general, in place of Stanley; but his fanatical kinsman, who had come to think of godliness as a thing of fasting, whip-cord, and a horsehair shirt, reported that the Earl had given up religion for science and the worldly arts. When Raleigh was arrested, Percy went down to Windsor Castle to defend his chief; and, but for Cecil's fear of trying too much at once, he would have been wrecked in the Arabella Plot instead of in the Powder Plot.

So great a man could not be readily set aside, and Percy was associated with the court in many offices of grace. He was made Captain of the Band of Gentlemen Pensioners; he was chosen as witness when Prince Charles was created Duke of York; he bore the basin when Princess Mary was christened. The Countess of Northumberland was one of Mary's godmothers,—the King's cousin, Lady Arabella, being the other. Sion House, which Percy had previously rented from the crown, was now settled on him by grant.

Still, he had little actual power; and after Raleigh's trial and reprieve at Winchester he retired in weariness of spirit from a world in which he could find no peace, and tried to console himself with the intellectual delights of study, building, gardening, and the like. The Lord of Wressil in Yorkshire, of Petworth in Sussex, of Alnwick in Northumberland, of thirty other manors, parks, and castles, he had scope enough for the indulgence of princely tastes. The Earl spent much of his time at Sion, where he transformed the dull monastic garden into a laughing lea of flowers, among which he played with his four little ones,—Algernon and Henry, Dorothy and Lucy; boys and girls who were, each and all, to live remarkable lives,—Algernon as tenth Earl of Northumberland, one of the heroes of the Civil War; Henry as Lord Percy of Alnwick, the favorite cavalier of Queen Henrietta Maria; Dorothy as Countess of Leicester, and mother of Algernon Sydney; Lucy as Countess of Carlisle, the friend of Strafford and of Pym, and the subject of a thousand rapturous songs.

Northumberland was clever, popular, and rich. Some envied his reputation; many coveted his lands. Even while he was training his plants and sporting with his children on the lawns at Sion, his fate was drawing him toward that dungeon which had been the dwelling of so many of his race.

Most of the old fighting Percies had been prisoners in the Tower. More than one had been murdered in its chambers; and many of them had passed through the Bye-ward gate to the block on Tower Hill. The Beauchamp tower and the Bloody tower were dark with the traditions of his house; and now another tower on the Ballium wall was waiting to receive her guest and grow into sudden fame as the prison of Percy the Wizard Earl.

Incapable of prudence, Northumberland had been more than usually imprudent in his dealings with his kinsman, Thomas Percy, the conspirator; for he had not only given him a place in the Band of Gentlemen Pensioners, but had suffered him to enter on his duties without taking the customary oaths. There he was wrong, and wrong beyond excuse. Percy knew that his kinsman disliked the King; he ought to have known that he was a convert and a tool of the Jesuits. Such a man was unfit for a post so near the King, and, even if he had been fit for such a post, he ought never to have been admitted without the usual forms. The great sum of money which Thomas Percy had brought to London was the Earl's property, and Northumberland seems to have been careless in exacting from him his vouchers and returns of rent. But the circumstance of darkest note was that supper on Monday night, when Fawkes rode down to report the official searching of the vault. Fawkes had no sooner confessed to having found his master at Sion, than the Earl was commanded by the Council to keep his house. In vain he pleaded in defense his secluded ways, his absence from court, his devotion to his books, his plants, his children, and the innocent pleasures of a country life. Taken from Sion, he was given in custody to Richard Bancroft, Archbishop of Canterbury, and remained at Lambeth Palace for twenty days, when he was carried down to the Tower, in which he lay five months without being either accused or heard.

At the end of June (1606) he was brought before the Star Chamber, and accused (1) of wishing to put himself at the head of the Papists and to procure their toleration; (2) of admitting Thomas Percy to be a Gentleman Pensioner without taking the oaths. Four additional articles were drawn, but they were only variations of these two. The sentence was, that the Earl of Northumberland should be fined in thirty thousand pounds; that he should be deposed from the Council, and removed from his Captaincy of the Pensioners; that he should cease to be Lord Lieutenant of any shire; that he should be kept a prisoner in the Tower for life. He raised a passionate cry against the justice of such a sentence; but the lords were deaf to his wrongs, and Sir William Waad conducted him once again to that gloomy fortress in which his father had been shot to death.

CHAPTER XXIV.

THE WIZARD EARL.

A SPACIOUS and secluded house was found for Percy in the Martin tower, on the northeast angle of the Ballium wall,—a house which had been occupied before his time by Lord Rochfort and other gentlemen connected with Anne Boleyn; which was occupied after his time by Archbishop Sancroft and his fellow-sufferers in the Church. The vaults of this mural tower, which are exceedingly strong, were used during many reigns as the royal jewel-house; and here occurred the desperate attempt of Colonel Blood to steal the crown. Here also occurred the comicalities of the Tower ghost. But the ghost which haunts the stairs and terraces around the Martin tower is that of Harry Percy, who lay in it for sixteen years, and whose quaint garb, unusual studies, and strange companionship caused him to be known as "The Wizard Earl."

The terrace on the wall connecting his lodging with the Brick tower and the Constable's tower is called the Earl of Northumberland's Walk. Heriot's sun-dial, fixed by that famous astronomer, is still to be seen on the southern face of the Martin tower.

Percy's wild youth continued into his middle age,

and his character was a puzzle to the wisest men. Nobody could dispute his courage, his attainments, his munificence; though every one could see that his temper was bad, his learning fantastic, his conduct suspicious. He was a student, a swordsman, a sorcerer; a man given equally to cards, to science, and to pleasure; as prompt with his blade as he was saucy with his tongue. But the scornful habit, which had wrought him so much evil in his younger time, soon softened when he came to reside in the Martin tower. Injustice acted on his mind in an unusual way; for he who could hardly bear a prosperous fortune like a man of sense, bore the miseries of a harsh and undeserved imprisonment with noble pride. The wife who could not live under his roof at Sion and Petworth came to share his cell in the Martin tower, where her pretty children became the spoiled darlings, not of their father only, but of every person in the Tower.

The Countess was but too familiar with her new and dismal home,—the Tower. Stout Sir John Perrot, the father of her first husband, died in one of its vaults. The dust of her brother Robert, Earl of Essex, lay in the dark little church under Develin tower. Many of her brother's old friends and rivals—Raleigh, Cobham, Grey—were daily seen in the garden and on the wall. Her second husband was now a prisoner,—not to come forth, though happily she could not know so much, until long after she had worn out her life with care and watching.

No man then lying in the Tower was kept a prisoner on more flimsy pretexts than the Earl. His real offense was being too great; his pretended crime was being a kinsman of Thomas Percy. He had no more to do with the Gunpowder Plot than with the Arabella Plot; but, having a hot temper and a vast estate, his fellows of the Council-board were anxious to stop his tongue and to get his land. Such a fine as thirty thousand pounds, he said, was never laid before on any subject in any realm. It was a king's ransom,—equal to one hundred and fifty thousand pounds in our present coin.

When Percy urged that such a sum could not be wrung from a private estate, the King was advised to take his affairs in hand and try his skill in collecting rents. It was bad advice,—bad in law, and bad in business; for the Star-Chamber sentence had left the Earl's property intact, and the crown had no legal right to levy the fine by seizure and distress. But what was law to men like Cecil, Suffolk, and Northampton, the three great peers who now ruled the King? The manors were seized, the farms were let on lease, and the rents were collected by agents for the crown. In vain the Earl protested. "This method is not used," he wrote: "my lands are spoiled, my houses ruinated, my suits in law prejudiced, my officers imprisoned, my debts unsatisfied." All this was true. The King's receivers grew fat; but the King himself got little of the spoil. These receivers were allowed two shillings in every pound of rent, and, as they paid their receipts into the county courts only once a year, they had the use of his money for many months. To get the place of a receiver of Northumberland's rents was to get a good thing. "In all this provision for them," cried the Earl, "I find not a thought of one penny for either wife, child, or myself. There wants nothing but strewing the land with salt."

The Countess came to court, and threw herself at James's feet, as Lady Raleigh was then doing daily, though with gentler passion and livelier hope; praying that his Majesty would not suffer the bread to be taken from her children's mouths. James told her, with far more kindness than his wont, that he would never hurt her and her children. She was his old friend's sister, dear to his heart for that old friend's sake. She must rely upon him. Lady Northumberland flew to the Martin tower with these gracious words; and Percy, who thought his time had come, drew up a statement and petition to the King, in which he asked no more than leave to go home to his house in Petworth. "Hum," said James, in answer; "I must take my own time."

While waiting on the King's leisure, which was long in coming, Percy made the best of his crowded rooms. He hired from Lord Carew, Master of the Ordnance, the adjoining house—the Brick tower—as an occasional residence for his son Algernon, in whose young face he loved to recall the heroes of his line. Lady Dorothy was often with him. Lady Lucy came and went, like a summer bird, bringing gleams of light from the outer world into his cell. In that cell he made a collection of books, globes, astrolabes, and drew to himself a society of learned and ingenious men. Thomas Heriot came to live with him in the Martin tower, and in the midst of his many embarrassments Percy never allowed the poor student's pension to go unpaid. Walter Warner and Robert Hues were also his constant visitors; and these three men of science were known in the Tower wards as the Earl of Northumberland's Magi. John Dee, the astrologer, came also to the Martin tower; where he met with a host of scholars, such as Thomas Allen, Nathaniel Torperley, and Nicholas Hill. To all these servants of science the Wizard Earl was a bountiful patron and enduring friend.

One comfort in a confinement which was long without being always strict, lay in the occasional freedom of his intercourse with Raleigh, in whose experiments of the still-house he felt a warm and mystical interest; hoping that the phials which held the Great Cordial would one day hold the Elixir of Life.

All his wife's appeals to James were fruitless. Solomon told the Countess he should like her husband to prove that Thomas Percy had *not* given him notice of the plot. "Your Majesty, that is so great a scholar," answered Northumberland, with biting sarcasm, "cannot but know how impossible it is to prove a negative."

At length, some change came over his affairs at court, in a way which he had neither expected nor desired. As his children grew up, they fell into love with other young people of their age and rank. Of course they fell into love with persons whom their father scorned as unworthy of alliance with the Percy blood. Algernon was kneeling at the feet of Lady Anne Cecil, grandchild of Lady Suffolk; but, on a match between the youth and maid being proposed to the recluse in the Martin tower, the Earl proudly exclaimed against it, crying, "The blood of Percy would not mix with the blood of Cecil, if you poured them into a dish." In time, though not with Percy's consent and blessing, that match of Algernon with Lady Anne took place.

The love-affairs of his daughter Lucy crossed him even more than those of his son. This girl, whose incomparable beauty as a woman was the theme of a dozen poets, from Waller to Carew, and the snare of eminent men, from Strafford to Pym, was fluttering into a first young love with the favorite, James Hay, afterward Earl of Carlisle. The Wizard raved and stormed at her folly. What could a Percy have to do with upstart curs like Hay? Believing in his heart that Hay was following Lady Lucy for her money,—as he heard, right truly, that Lady Suffolk was courting Algernon for his money,—he sent the Scotch favorite word that if she married any man without his leave she should never get a penny from his purse. But Hay, in love with a pair of bright eyes, and never troubling himself to count the cost of his love, ran off with this message to the girl, caught her up in his arms, obtained her consent, and married her in a trice. The King, who was present at their nuptials, which took place at court, with a thousand gayeties and fooleries,—eating the wine posset, throwing the left shoe, and running at the ring,—made a bridal present to Lady Lucy Hay of a promise for her father's enlargement from the Tower.

But Lady Lucy found it an easier task to get a pardon from the King than to induce her father to accept it. Percy would not owe his liberty to Hay; and when the order for his release was read to him, the venerable Wizard, swearing he would not owe thanks to Hay, went back to his books, his globes, and his magi in the Martin tower. That tower had come to be his home. Lady Northumberland was dead; his son was married; his health was failing; and he cared no longer for the glory and greatness of the world. His comrade Heriot was in correspondence with Kepler on things of higher moment than the intrigues of a court: on the laws of vision; on the cause of rainbows; on the sun-spots, which he noticed before they had been seen by Galileo; on the satellites of Jupiter, which he was the first in England, perhaps in Europe, to observe. He was busy with the theory of numbers, to which Percy had given a good deal of his time. In the face of such studies, what to the Wizard Earl were the rivalries of Buckingham and Hay?

The doors were open; but he would not go. The Lieutenant informed him that he had orders to use him with honor and to announce his departure with saluting guns. Lord Percy and Lady Lucy, whom he received in sorrow, as children who had lowered his family pride, persuaded him that he ought to go down to Bath for the benefit of his health. But he was long in making up his mind to go. At length he allowed himself to be put into a coach, and carried away from his nightly lodging and his daily walk, under a joyous salute of guns. But the old Adam was not dead in his veins. On reaching his house, he heard that the new Duke of Buckingham was driving about town in a coach with six horses. Six horses! Who was this Villiers, that he should outbrave a Percy in magnificence? With a cry of contempt, the Earl commanded his servants never to drive him through London with less than eight horses to his coach.

On his return from Bath, he lived mainly at Petworth, with Heriot constantly at his side, laying up in the library of that baronial seat the letters and papers which in a new generation added so much to the glory of English science.

CHAPTER XXV.

A REAL ARABELLA PLOT.

At length the young lady, in whose name so many gallant men had been accused of treason and committed to the Tower, was herself an offender against the King, and a prisoner in the dungeon of her race.

For Lady Arabella Stuart had the presumption to fall in love, and marry her lover, without the King's consent,—an act of disobedience, in one so near the throne, to bring her within the penalties of that law which had been passed to punish her starless grandmother, Margaret Douglas, the sister of James the Fourth.

No passage in the story of our royal house has a more pathetic comedy than the tale of Arabella Stuart's love for her young and graceless kinsman, William Seymour; of her secret marriage to that cold and calculating paladin; of her sudden arrest and long imprisonment; of her romantic efforts to escape from London; of her final separation from her lord, and the train of evils which that escape and separation brought upon the adoring wife.

This pair of lovers were descended from Henry the Seventh, and had the turbulent Tudor blood careering in their veins. Seymour was a grandson of Catharine Grey, whose grandmother was Mary Tudor, Queen of France; Arabella was a granddaughter of Margaret Douglas, whose mother, Margaret Tudor, was the Queen of Scots. Each of these personages stood too near the throne for safety; and many of the keenest critics of the court imagined that the young lady would be one day Queen. "Some time," Elizabeth had been heard to say, when speaking with the French ambassador's wife, "this child will be lady-mistress here, even as I am."

When James the First came in, his cousin, a fair young woman of twenty-eight summers, with round blue eyes, soft oval face, arched brows, and ripples of curling hair, was the Rosalind of a dull court,—tender in spirit, young in wit, lightsome in manner, full of prank and jest. Without being much of a beauty, she had not the less been thought, in her younger time, a most engaging and attractive girl. A good talker, a fine musician, she was the delight of every house in which she lived. As a princess of the royal blood, she had been pursued by adorers. Princes had sought her from north and south: the King of Poland, the Duke of Parma, nay, Henri the Great, had dreamed of her blue eyes and ripples of curling hair. "I should not refuse the Princess Arabella of England," he remarked to Sully, "if she were once declared heiress-presumptive." The stern necessities of the crown had doomed this royal lady to live an unwedded life.

Arabella had always been an object of speculation in foreign courts. She was a favorite in Rome and Madrid; and her religious views were thought to be rather Catholic in their bent. Philip regarded her as a friend of Spain.

This tendency on the part of foreign kings to busy themselves with her affairs was one chief cause of her being watched with unsleeping care by Cecil; and, now that Cecil was growing faint, by Suffolk and Northampton, with increasing fear. Lady Suffolk was anxious to have no rival in Philip's cabinet, which a royal princess, married and having issue, could not fail to be, whether she wished it to be so or not. A king's cousin, growing old in her single state, might be a person of the court, but she would not be a public power.

Enriched by the gold of Spain, Lady Suffolk had nearly as strong an interest as the King himself in compelling the Lady Arabella to live and die in her unwedded bliss.

When Arabella had passed her thirty-fifth year, the King, who had come to regard her settlement as a standing jest, was rude enough to tell her she was now free to marry anybody who would have her. She took him at his word. Rosalind had seen Orlando in the person of her young kinsman, William,—a youth of twenty-three, a man of books and theorems,—cold, sedate, and clever, given overmuch to pondering on his birth, his poverty, and his family wrongs. For the Seymours, grandsons of Catharine Grey, sister and heiress of Queen Jane, inherited all the rights of that popular idol; so that after the King's issue and the Lady Arabella, William and his brother Edward, Lord Beauchamp, were the nearest claimants to the crown.

That Seymour could be moved by noble passion his after-life in the Civil War, through which, as Marquis of Hertford, he fought on the side of Charles the First, abundantly made known. His offer to be put to death instead of the King has covered his name with such romantic light and color that the harsh and calculating lover of Arabella Stuart appears in the story like a different man. But Seymour's childhood had been spent in a bitter school. His family, one of the proudest in England, was a wreck. His father was a child of the Tower. His grandmother, Lady Catharine, died under the brand of an illegal union. Nearly all his kinsmen for a hundred years had fallen by the axe. No man in the realm, not even of the Percy and the

Howard families, could claim so large a share in the noble dust of St. Peter's Church. Under the flags of that darksome pile lay the ashes of his kindred by the male and by the female lines; of Edward, Duke of Somerset, Lord Protector of England; of Thomas, Lord Seymour of Sudeley, Lord High Admiral; of Henry, Duke of Suffolk; of Lord Thomas Grey; of the Nine-days' Queen; to all of whom he and his brother Edward were immediate heirs. His grandfather, the aged Earl of Hertford, had been ruined by a monstrous fine. His father had been tainted in his birth, and been compelled to fight in the courts of law for more than thirty years in order to establish his mother's fame.

That father had passed away, worn out by rage and sorrow, leaving his sons to the care of a feeble old man, whose spirit had been broken more than forty years.

William, the younger son, with his fortunes all to seek, could not foresee that his brother would die without issue and leave him heir. He was poor, and wanted to be rich; obscure, and wanted to be great. He looked around him in the world, and saw no way in which a younger son could rise so quickly as by marrying a royal bride.

When the court was at Woodstock, Seymour was at Magdalen College, and in the leafy groves of that royal park Rosalind and Orlando rambled unobserved, their ages and their kinship covering them from the malice of prying eyes and whispering tongues. The lady thought she was free to love, and Seymour was sedate beyond the warrant of his years. At thirty-six a lively woman, who has lived among poets and adorers, is pretty sure to be quick in feeling and susceptible to fire. When Arabella rambled in the park of Woodstock, she was in the mood for love; and the youth of twenty-three summers, seeing where the woman of thirty-six was weak, found his way into her room, threw himself at her feet, and made her an offer of his heart. Such words had not been heard by her of late. The poets praised her beauty, the courtiers extolled her wit; but no one dared to speak to her of love, since it had been always said at court that James would never allow his cousin to enjoy the consolations of a wedded life. She bent her round blue eyes upon him, and raised the enamored youth into her arms.

Informed by spies of what was going on in Lady Arabella's room, Northampton caused her gentleman-usher and her lady-in-waiting to be seized and committed close prisoners (March, 1610), while he placed the lady herself in charge of Lord Knyvet, the man who had arrested Fawkes in Parliament Place. Nothing could be proved against her, for nothing illegal had as yet been done; and in some respects the rumors which had got abroad came back to her in grace. The King bethought him of her state; a woman debarred the privilege of her sex; a royal princess, with a scant provision and a load of debts. He sent her a box of plate, he gave her a thousand marks to pay her people, and he settled on her a pension of sixteen hundred pounds.

But she was now in love, and money would not stay the beatings of her heart. On Candlemas-day—seven weeks after her first arrest—she received William Seymour in her private room at court, and pledged him her troth in a way which, in her own opinion, made her his lawful wife.

When the news of what they had done came out, and Seymour was called before the Council to answer for the outrage of betrothing himself to the King's cousin without the King's consent, he treated the affair with cool and provoking scorn. He was poor, he said, and wanted means. He was a younger brother, he said, and wanted rank. He knew that the lady he loved was great, and from her style of living he thought she must be rich. As a young man, having his way in the world to make, he felt justified in trying to win her. But he did not mean to offend the King. He fancied that she had her sovereign's leave to marry: if his Majesty raised objections, he would proceed no farther in the match. No contract had been made between them, such as binds betrothed persons to each other; nor had either the lady or himself ever dreamed of proceeding to betrothal without the King's consent.

The King was pleased with words so frank and loyal; and, on Seymour promising to forego his suit, the scandal died away. When quizzed about her youthful adorer, the lady took the jest with a laughing grace, and seemed to be more intent on masques than marriage. On the creation of Henry as Prince of Wales, a gallant masque was offered by the Queen, in which Arabella, dressed in shells and corals, played a nymph of the Trent. She was an admirable artist, and the court was giddy with her praise. The young Prince loved her; the Queen was always at her side; and, but for Northampton and Lady Suffolk, the King himself would hardly have treated her like a brute. So far as money could soothe her grief, she had no reason to cry out, for, in addition to his previous gifts, the King made over to her a license to sell wines and usquebaugh in Ireland for a term of one-and-twenty years,—a privilege worth not less than a hundred thousand pounds.

The young dissembler held his tongue.

Three or four months slipped by without much trouble to the pair, when Seymour, who was vainly expecting the King to yield, took his sharp cousin,

Edward Rodney, into his confidence, telling him of his secret contract, and of his resolution to marry the King's cousin, cost her what it might. He made Rodney swear to keep his counsel, and to help him by his suit and service when the time of action should arrive.

A month after Lady Arabella had been tickling the court gossips by her garb of shells and corals, Seymour called on his cousin Rodney, to tell him of his plans and to seek his help. The two young men dropped down to Greenwich, where they found a poor priest, John Blague, who was willing to perform the rite; and early next day (July 9, 1610) the young fellows went up into the lady's chamber in the palace, where the nuptial knot was tied by Blague, in the presence of her two gentlemen, Hugh Crompton and Edward Reeves, beyond the power of kings and councils to untie.

Here then, at length, a genuine Arabella Plot had risen to perplex the court. When the secret came out, the King was furious with the Seymours, feeling that he had been cozened and deceived, as well as outraged and defied. The aged Earl, who had ruined himself by marrying Catharine Grey, was thought by James to have urged this new and more dangerous suit, so as to bring the family of Seymour one step nearer to the throne than they already stood. But the abject protests of the broken man appeased him. Orders were given to arrest the conspirators, of whom Rodney alone escaped pursuit and capture. Blague, the priest who had married them for a fee, was committed to the Gate house in Westminster; Crompton and Reeves, the gentlemen who stood by as witnesses, were sent to the Marshalsea in Southwark. The bride was given in custody to Sir Thomas Parry, who lodged her in a fine house on the Thames near Vauxhall; while Seymour was placed in the house of Sir William Waad, Lieutenant of the Tower, until fitting apartments could be got ready for a man of his rank and taste.

CHAPTER XXVI.

WILLIAM SEYMOUR.

THE bride and bridegroom, parted in the first hours of their honeymoon, took the blow in their several ways. Seymour lost his temper, and his partner broke her heart.

Seymour's chief trouble was the want of money, of which he had none, and his wife not much. Blue eyes would not pay his weekly bills, and Seymour's weekly bills were likely to be large. He wrote to his grandfather for an allowance; and, with the King's consent, Lord Hertford consented to allow him fifty pounds a quarter for his maintenance in the Tower. The rooms assigned to Seymour for his future home were the handsome chambers in St. Thomas's tower, in front of Raleigh's Walk; but Seymour thought these chambers were cold and bare, needing much arras, plate, and furniture to give them a cheery look; so that while Rosalind was crying in Parry's fine house, refusing to be comforted in her grief, Orlando was wrangling with Waad about hangings and cups, about presses and stools. Tapestries were bought for him, and the chambers opening on the Thames were brightened with serge, with silver, and with books. To Waad's surprise, however, this prince with a thousand wants had not a single pistole in his pouch to pay for the things he ordered; and, much to the Lieutenant's wonder when he came to think of it in after-times, this husband of a royal princess got into his debt. Sir William was not a man to pay for other people; and once he set his teeth, even in the tradesfolk's presence, against his haughty and exacting guest. Seymour, who wanted new tapestries for his sitting-room, induced Waad to order five pieces for him from Jenning the upholsterer, at ten pounds apiece. One of these pieces Seymour cut across, so as to make it fit his fire-place; by which he destroyed it as an article of furniture for use in any other room. Waad, who had pledged himself thus far, declared that he would give his name no more.

Seymour was not nice in the art of helping himself to what he needed. The princess, now his wife, had a villa of her own at Hackney; and to this villa he sent for such things as he could not get from Waad,—kitchen-stuff, linen, silver trenchers, candlesticks, drinking-cups; and when his rooms had been duly brightened up (on credit) he took jaunty leave of the Lieutenant's house, and went to live in his chambers over Traitors' gate.

Those comforts of the flesh which Seymour prized so much had no great hold upon his wife. The bride was not closely kept; she was served by her own people; she had a garden to walk in; and no restraint was put on her use of books and pens. Her servants could come and go; her table was well supplied; she was in correspondence with her friends. But she felt no comfort in her freedom, since her soul was in the chamber on the wharf, where her husband, as she dreamt, was pining out his soul for love. She wrote to him in tender and moving tones, to which the young bridegroom answered her not a word. In fact, he saw that his marriage was a mistake of means. His wife was not rich; nor could she help him to become great. He had vexed the King to please her; and—she was thirty-seven years old.

When Arabella heard from him at all, it was through Smith, a servant, who told her that he had been ill. Then Rosalind snatched a pen and wrote, with her delicate banter, to her bridegroom in the Tower:

"I am exceeding sorry to hear you have not been well. I pray you let me know truly how you do, and what was the cause of it, for I am not satisfied with the reason Smith gives for it. If it be a cold, I will impute it to some sympathy betwixt us, having myself gotten a swollen cheek at the same time with a cold. For God's sake let not your grief of mind work upon your body. . . . In what state soever you are, it sufficeth me you are mine. . . . You see, when I am troubled, I trouble you too with tedious kindness; for so I think you will account so long a letter, yourself not having written to me for this good while so much as how you do. But, sweet sir, I speak not this to trouble you with writing but when you please. Be well, and I shall account myself happy in being your faithful, loving wife."

Seymour was too busy for such tender and unprofitable humor; the winter passed and the summer came again without much writing to his wife. He was looking to himself, to his present comforts in the Tower, to his future rank and place at the royal court. He was writing to the lords of the Council, praying to be restored in grace, asserting that his health was ruined, and begging to be allowed the full liberties of his prison.

All the love, and nearly all the daring, were on the

lady's side. Growing bolder as the days went by, she got into a barge, dropped down the river, and paid a visit to her husband, with whom she may have spoken through his grated window on the wharf. Such facts were sure to become known at court; this daring visit was reported at Whitehall; when the King gave orders that a dozen counties should be put between his romantic cousin and his impudent prisoner in the Tower.

Arabella was to be placed in charge of William James, Bishop of Durham, with orders to repair forthwith into the north, and there await his Majesty's pleasure; while Seymour was to be watched in St. Thomas's tower with a sharper eye.

And now came a strife between Solomon's craft and Rosalind's wit,—a comedy in its course of deception and surprise, a tragedy in its conclusion of insanity and death.

Early in June (1611) the court was fluttered by a message from Sir William Monson, dated from a tavern at Blackwall This tough old sailor, taking boat for Billingsgate on his own affairs, was told by his watermen that a swift barge, having some of Seymour's friends on board, had dropped down the river on the previous night. The barge had been lying off St. Katherine's Wharf. A boat was in attendance at the Tower stairs; a bundle of clothes had been thrown into this boat; at nightfall a man in a black wig and a carter's dress had come alongside; a parley had taken place between the carter and a young gentleman in the boat; the carter had gone away, and the young gentleman had told the watermen to pull for the barge. Some of the men engaged in the business were known to be Seymour's kinsfolk. Who could say whether Seymour himself might not have been that carter in the black wig?

Monson, a friend of Lady Suffolk, a partisan of the house of Howard, suspected that an escape was being attempted from the Tower, the defeat of which would be likely to make his fortune. Instead, therefore, of landing at Billingsgate, as he had meant to do, he bade his men pull lustily for Blackwall, where he jumped on shore, ran into the river-side tavern, and learned from the man who kept it that a young gentleman, or one who by his dress and figure wished to pass for a young gentleman, had come on the previous evening to his house on horseback, in company with a lady of middle age, and, after staying in a private room for two or three hours, had at last taken oars for Gravesend. He also learned that Lady Grey, a daughter of the Earl of Shrewsbury, had come down to Blackwall, from which she was pulled across to Greenwich. This Lady Grey was a cousin of Lady Arabella. Every word he caught was full of mischief. Pressing his host still further, he learned that late on the previous evening two gentlemen, dressed in the same sort of clothes, from rosette to plume, had come to Blackwall, one of them by land, the second by water; that they seemed to be looking for some one who was not there; that the youth who came by water had mounted a horse and ridden away, while the one who came by land had taken oars and put off from the wharf, as though he were following the young gentleman and the lady of middle age.

While Monson was extracting this news from his landlord, men from a vessel in the river stepped on shore. They had come up the Thames that day, and, in reply to the Admiral's questions, they could tell him that a French bark, then lying in Leigh Roads, had taken a strange party on board and sailed at day-break on the course for Calais. Sure that an escape was being made, and also pretty sure that Seymour was on board the French bark, he saw what a golden chance was thrown into his path. Of late he had been falling back. A reign of peace was not a reign in which men of his trade could thrive; and Monson had been vainly striving to obtain at court the prizes he could no longer obtain at sea. If Seymour had broken prison, the man who captured and brought him back would do a striking service, not only to the Howards, but to the King.

Familiar with the winds and currents of the Straits, he knew that the French bark, sailing from Leigh Roads at dawn, could not have passed the Foreland. The wind was high, and the water rough. The bark would then be rolling in the chops beyond Margate Sands. If the wind should keep in the same quarter, that bark would not be able to make the port of Calais before set of sun.

Quick in action as though he were on his quarter-deck, the brisk old sailor took his course. Throwing a few men into an oyster-boat, he pushed them down the Thames. Mounting a good rider, he sent off a message to the admiral commanding in the Downs. Writing a letter to Cecil, he informed the Secretary of his news, and then pulled over to Greenwich, where he asked for the use of a royal ship.

His high rank in the navy made his wish in these matters a command; so that in less than an hour after his coming to the inn-door at Blackwall he had opened the chase of his unknown fugitive by water and by land.

CHAPTER XXVII.

THE ESCAPE.

Arabella had done her part, as women always do, with singular and successful art. Before she was carried away from Lambeth she had procured the liberation of her servant, Hugh Crompton, from the Marshalsea. Among her many merits, this royal lady had the grace of making all her people love her. By nature soft and kind, she made companions of her attendants, from whom she could not bear to part, still less to see them suffer on her account. When Reeves and Crompton were in prison, she sent to the Marshalsea almost every day to learn how they were doing, and wrote most pressing letters for them to the Council and to the Queen. She seemed to suffer more pain for her people than for herself.

The Council was hard of heart, for the Howard party was anxious that the King's cousin should never more regain her old ascendency at court; but when plague broke out in the Marshalsea her prayers became so urgent that they could not be denied; and when she was ordered into the north country, Crompton, as the man most used to her ways, was suffered to share what was understood by Lady Suffolk as her banishment from the English court.

Before going north, the lady made one last appeal to the Lord Chief Justice of the King's Bench and the Lord Chief Justice of the Common Pleas. In marrying, as every woman was free to do, she conceived that she had done no wrong; but, if others thought so, she demanded to be tried for her offense and punished according to the law. "If your lordships," she wrote, "may not, or will not, of yourselves grant me the ordinary relief of a distressed subject, then I beseech you to become humble intercessors to his Majesty that I may receive such benefit of justice as both his Majesty by his oath (those of his blood not excepted) hath promised and the laws of this realm afford to all others." She added, with equal modesty and dignity, "And though, unfortunate woman that I am, I should obtain neither, yet I beseech your lordships retain me in your good opinion, and judge me charitably, till I be proved to have committed any offense either against God or his Majesty, deserving so long restraint or separation from my lawful husband."

The Lord Chief Justices to whom she wrote were Sir Thomas Fleming and Sir Edward Coke, courtiers and creatures of the Howards. Her prayer remained unheard; and warrants were issued by the Council for Sir Thomas Parry to bring her "person" to Whitehall.

She protested against this seizure, and had to be removed by force.

Rightly or wrongly, the lady conceived the idea that she, a free woman of the blood royal, was being treated with lawless violence by a faction in her cousin's court, against whom it would be fair in her to use whatever stratagems her wit could devise.

The courtiers, reading her prayers and protests, and fearing to place her at the Council-table, where some sudden burst of feeling might touch the King and cause him to change their plans, requested the Bishop of Durham to go in person to Vauxhall and there receive her into charge. The lady was in no mood to submit in silence to this change. The Bishop produced his letters. She refused to stir. With tender art, for the Bishop was a godly man, he tried to soothe her rage, by telling her the story of patient saints, and of prisoners far less happy than herself. She wept, she raved, she fainted on the floor. At length they picked her up, placed her in a coach, and carried her to the Thames, and so through the town to Highgate Hill. Scant preparation had been made for her reception on the road. A cold March wind was blowing in her teeth. The inns were mean and full of people, and her escort was instructed to hurry her along. She had to be carried in a litter, in which she fainted thrice before they reached the Hill. Moundford, her physician, gave her cordials to restore her strength; but late in the afternoon he began to fear she would not live, and in a fainting state she was put to bed. A rider was sent back to court, where Suffolk, suspecting that her sickness was put on, sent Sir James Croft, a court physician, to see her. Sir James reported that her sickness was not feigned. Still force was tried to make her go. Sergeant Mynors, one of her escort, lifted her out of bed into the coach, and bore her to Barnet, where Moundford declared that she could not travel, and to carry her farther would be murder. Mynors himself was frightened when he saw her lying on the floor, her face like death, and her tunic stained with blood.

The good Bishop wrote from Barnet to the lords, describing her sickness, and asking for orders what to do. The doctors and parsons who came to see her told but one story. She was unfit to travel; and when the King perceived that he could not drive her on without the risk of killing her on the road, he gave an order for her to rest a month and then go forward toward the north.

A cottage was hired for her from Thomas Conyers, at East Barnet, near Hampstead Heath, in the fresh air of which her spirits suddenly revived. She kept her counsel well, so that only her trusty maid and her faithful Crompton knew how she really was in health. The Bishop went north to prepare her chamber, leaving her in the charge of Croft. Moundford rode backward and forward between the Heath and Charing Cross, where the Council pressed him to compel her to go on. He begged for another month, but the lords refused her another day. As Croft and Moundford seemed to them too yielding, they sent for Mynors, who told them the lady was not fit to travel; but they cut the keeper short by saying it was the King's absolute will that she should go at once to Durham, even if she rode no more than a mile a day.

She wrote to the King and Queen. She made a friend of Mrs. Adams, the wife of a clergyman who came to see her. She wrote to her aunt Mary, Countess of Shrewsbury, who espoused her cause, to the peril of her freedom and estate. Her uncle Shrewsbury was a member of the Council; but his brain was too weak for influence on a board at which Cecil and Northampton sat. In her distress of mind for her niece, Lady Shrewsbury appealed to the new favorite, Robert Carr, now Viscount Rochester; but the young minion of royal grace was in love—in most disloyal love—with Suffolk's beautiful daughter, Lady Essex, and therefore was a slave to that powerful peer. Taking his cue from Northampton, the Nestor of his Lady's house, Carr answered the Countess of Shrewsbury that he could not solicit the King in a matter which was unfit for her to ask and for the King to grant. Northampton wrote an account of this "faithful and sound refusal" to the King.

But Mary, Countess of Shrewsbury, was not a woman to yield at once. She knew how near the throne her kinswoman stood, and she hoped that Seymour and Arabella would leave a son to inherit their claim and perhaps to wear the crown. By fair means if it might be, by foul means if it must be, she resolved that the young man and his wife should come together in some country beyond the reach of James.

Sending for Hugh Crompton, she told him of her hopes, her means, and her designs. She hoped to unite the husband to his wife. She had plenty of money; and she fancied that on spending gold enough she could buy the means for their escape into France. Crompton listened to her speech. With wit and money, anything might be done,—servants corrupted, disguises bought, confederates paid, and vessels hired for flight. Crompton went to East Barnet, and told his mistress all that Lady Shrewsbury had opened her mind to say. The lady leaped to her offer, and with ready wit suggested the particulars of a plan for their joint escape into France,—she from her keepers at Conyers's house, and Seymour from his lodgings in the Tower. Her servant, seeing the way laid out, engaged to prepare disguises, to arrange for horses, and to hire a skipper in the Thames. They only wanted money; and money the Countess undertook to find. Great sums—not less than twenty thousand pounds in all—were quickly raised and poured into Arabella's lap, "to pay her debts." Jewels were bought; a cloak and hat, a rapier, and a pair of cavalier's boots, were carried in secret to Conyers's house. In her private room, the faithful Hugh instructed his lady how to wear her hat and sword.

Money was sent to Seymour in the Tower, with details of a plan for his own escape. Young Rodney entered with all his soul into Crompton's scheme. Two suits of clothes, exactly alike from rosette to plume, were made; for the cousins were of an age and size to match; and these two suits were to be used on the day of flight. A second disguise was got for Seymour, in the shape of a carter's frock and whip. Batten, his barber, made him a great black wig. One Monsieur Corvé, a French skipper, was hired to lie in the Leigh Roads and wait for certain parties who would give him a pass-word and come on board his bark.

Croft now told his patient she must resume her journey toward the north, where the Bishop of Durham was waiting to receive her into his charge. Every one about Conyers's cottage pitied her, even those who had to answer for her; and, on the physician's plea, a second month was given her to recruit her strength. That month was May; a month of rare delight on the breezy Hampstead heights. She seemed to be winning back her health. At once playful and meek, she lulled suspicion; and Croft, believing that his patient wisdom had prevailed over her fretful spirit, advised the Council that she was now resigned to the King. When, late in May, he pressed her, in the King's name, to resume her journey toward the north, she named Monday, the 3d of June, as the day on which she would be ready to set forth.

About four o'clock on Sunday afternoon, dressing herself in cloak and hat, drawing on a pair of cavalier's boots, slinging a sword by her side, and putting her jewels into her pocket, Rosalind came out of Conyers's cottage with Mrs. Bradshawe, the daughter of a gentleman of East Barnet, followed by William Markham, one of the gentlemen of her suite. A walk of half an hour brought them to a lonely inn, where Crompton was waiting with horses ready saddled for their flight.

Sick with hope and fear, poor Rosalind gave her hand to a groom, who helped her to mount; and, as the party pricked away toward London, this lad turned round to his fellow-groom and said, "Poor young gentleman! he will hardly reach London alive." A quick ride brought the blood into her cheek; but on reaching the inn by the river at Blackwall, where she expected to find her husband safe and well, she almost fainted from her horse. It was six o'clock, and Seymour was not come. Boats were hired for Woolwich; the luggage was put on board; the men got ready to start; but Rosalind would not stir from the Blackwall inn until Orlando came. A precious hour was lost; the village clock struck seven. Mrs. Bradshawe urged her to go on board, as the pursuers would be soon upon her track. The oarsmen grew impatient, for night was coming on. Still she would not stir from the little parlor of the water-side inn. What to her was liberty unless her husband was at her side? A few minutes more might give him his only chance.

When the church-clock chimed eight, the watermen told her she must either go at once or wait until another day. They could hardly now make Woolwich Reach before dark, and they did not care to be out on the Thames all night. With a heavy heart she stepped on board, and the boat pushed off from the Blackwall stair.

CHAPTER XXVIII.

PURSUIT.

Lady Arabella and Mrs. Bradshawe were in the leading boat; Crompton and Markham, her gentlemen-in-waiting, in the second. They had with them a heap of diamonds, pearls, and rubies, and a sum of three thousand pounds in gold. Five minutes after they left Blackwall stair the sun went down; but they had still an hour of light; and when they were fairly in the stream she asked the men to carry her past Woolwich and put her on shore at Gravesend, which they were willing enough to do for a purse of gold. At the second port she found a skipper, who agreed, for a high fee, to take her down the river to Leigh Roads, where Corvê's bark was to take them all on board. In the dark summer night they passed the bark without seeing her, and in Leigh Roads found a ship at anchor, which they hailed. The master of this ship, John Bright, bound for Berwick, refused Arabella's offer of a large sum of money to carry her into France. Bright told her that a ship was lying in the Roads about two miles up the river, which ship she fancied must be Captain Corvé's bark. Turning back in her search, she hailed the strange vessel; and, finding her to be French, she made herself known to Corvé by the pass, and in a few seconds her party was taken up on board.

The wind was cross. For four days past it had been blowing east by south; the sea was running high, and, with the best of fortune, the bark could hardly have passed the Foreland and got her tack. But Corvé made no haste; for his royal passenger begged him to hang below the Nore, in the hope of picking up Seymour from some craft. Their plans were so well arranged that she was sure her husband had left the Tower. Some accident had spoiled their meeting at the Blackwall tavern; but she felt no doubt that he was somewhere tossing in his boat at sea. She lost some hours in reaching the Narrows, and long before they got into open water in front of Calais their happy chance was gone.

A swift war-ship, the Adventure, had been sent from the Downs on Monson's order, to sweep the Straits. The Adventure appeared in sight. The French coast was near, and the bark threw out her sails; but a boat was lowered from the Adventure to give chase. The princess wept; the captain fought his best; but, after thirteen shots had been fired into him, Corvé struck his flag and gave up his freight.

Seymour had taken care of himself. By the help of Rodney, he procured his black wig and his yellow frock. Feigning sickness, he kept his room in the Water gate. The Lieutenant had no conception that Seymour was such a deep and wily youth; and, even when the bird had flown away from his cage, he was chiefly vexed at finding that the fellow had cheated him of his perquisites by secretly sending away from his lodgings the best of Arabella's plate!

On the Saturday night, when everything was ready at East Barnet for the lady's flight, Rodney went to a house near St. Catharine's Hospital, kept by a woman with whom he had formerly lodged, and hired a room, on the pretense that he felt himself a little unwell and wanted a change of air. He sent his man to this woman's house with a great bundle of clothes, which were laid in his room. Early on Sunday morning the man came again, with a fresh bundle, and asked whether his master had yet arrived. Two strange persons called during the day, one of them a female, who stayed in the house until all the stuff brought in by Rodney's man was carried to a boat at St. Catharine's wharf.

All that day poor Seymour was thought to be lying ill in bed. Just at sundown, a cart drove up to the Water gate, when Seymour, leaping out of bed, put on his carter's frock and wig, snatched up a whip, stepped out into the street, and drove the horses along Water Lane through the Byeward gate.

Rodney was waiting for him with a horse and boat near Tower stair. Seymour mounted the horse and rode away, while Rodney stepped on board and pulled for Blackwall; where the two men met again about nine o'clock. Seymour had changed his dress, and the landlord of the inn observed that the cousins were dressed alike from head to foot. Seymour soon learned that his wife had come and gone. The young men parted company, Rodney riding away to baffle pursuit, while his friend and cousin dropped down to Leigh. The French bark having sailed, Seymour made no effort to follow his wife, but, finding a collier beating about the Narrows, he bribed the master to take him on board and land him in Ostend.

When the crew from the Adventure leaped on board Corvé's bark, Arabella came forward, made known her rank, and yielded herself a prisoner to the King. They asked her where Seymour was; to which she answered, smiling, that she had not seen him, and could not tell them; but she hoped he had got across into France, and said that her joy at his escape consoled her for her own mishap.

Passengers and crew being taken on board the Adventure and brought into the Downs, Sir William Monson dispatched a messenger with his news to court. The King was cross, and Northampton inflamed his passions; but Cecil, an advocate always for the middle term, prevailed with James to adopt a more moderate course than Northampton would have had him take. Northampton tried to make the King believe that Arabella's flight was a deep political plot, and he drew a fanciful picture of a series "of plots that were to follow" her escape into France. Cecil laughed this nonsense out of court; yet the proceedings taken against the suspected persons were sharp enough. Even before Monson had brought his prisoners up the Thames, a number of men and women had been committed to the various jails: the Countess of Shrewsbury to the Tower, Sir James Croft to the Fleet, Mr. Adams and Dr. Moundford to the Gate house, the barber Batten to the Keep. When the captives arrived in town, the King gave orders that his fugitive cousin should be lodged in the Tower, and the apartments chosen for her were the chambers occupied by Margaret Douglas, the common grandmother of Arabella and the King. William Markham was sent to the Marshalsea, Hugh Crompton to the Fleet. Corvé was lodged in Newgate, then much used as a sailors' prison. Edward Rodney, seized near London, was put in the Gate house, questioned by Northampton, and committed to the Tower. Gilbert, Earl of Shrewsbury, and Edward, Earl of Hertford, were restrained to their several homes.

The proceedings lasted long, and wore out many lives. One by one the minor agents in the escape either died in prison or gained their liberty by telling what they knew. Croft, who knew nothing, was discharged from the Fleet; while Dr. Moundford and

Mr. Adams, who knew little more than Croft, were liberated from the Gate house. As nothing could be learned from Rodney, he was suffered to go abroad, where he joined his cousin Seymour at the court of France.

Crompton and Markham, the companions of Arabella's flight, were brought from the Fleet and Marshalsea to the Tower, and pressed by questions in the torture-chamber, until they told some part of what they knew.

When niece and aunt were brought before the lords and questioned as to the escape, Arabella was gentle and yielding, while her aunt was haughty in manner and hot in speech. Why, asked the Countess of Shrewsbury, was she brought before that secret and unjust tribunal? Northampton bade her answer the questions put to her. She would not answer. She would not be tried in private. She appealed to the law. If they had evidence against her, let them produce it in open court. Northampton stormed upon her. Was that the way to deal with the King's Council? Still prouder and more scornful, she demanded to know whether that was the way to treat a lady of her rank.

Lady Shrewsbury bound herself by a great oath never to reveal the particulars of her niece's flight.

CHAPTER XXIX.

DEAD IN THE TOWER.

WHEN Lady Arabella was taken on board the French bark, she had three thousand pounds in gold, and a great wealth of rings and bracelets in her trunks and on her person. This money, and these jewels, the property of Lady Shrewsbury, had been seized by the King, and the money had been used for paying the cost of Arabella's capture. But a heap of gold and a case of jewels were the smallest parts of Lady Shrewsbury's loss. This wealth was Arabella's force; and the raising of so large a sum of money was proof of Lady Shrewsbury's share in her flight. But neither niece nor aunt could be drawn into confessing each other's guilt; and, after many of Northampton's attempts to snare them had been foiled, the two ladies were sent back to the care of Sir William Waad.

Rich enough to buy herself every indulgence, Lady Shrewsbury procured a suite of rooms in the royal quarter, consisting of the Queen's old lodgings,—three or four chambers in which she could live and walk about, but worn by time, and bare of hangings, furniture, and wainscots, the windows being broken, the doors unhung, the ceilings open to the sky. Not a single servant of her own was suffered to be with her. Gilbert, her husband, wrote to Cecil, who obtained for her some relaxation of the rules. But the lady would not help her friends; her stomach was said to be too high for a private person, even of her exalted birth. A servant was allowed, as an especial grace, to wait upon her. The ceiling of her room was mended, so as to keep out wind and rain. But the Countess was tormented in her prison by Northampton, who came to the Tower in the interest of his new tool and dupe, Sir Robert Carr, now hungering for escheats and fines. Carr was eager to get Sherborne Castle from Raleigh; a part of the thirty thousand pounds from Percy; a case of Arabella's diamonds; a lump of Lady Shrewsbury's vast estate; and the hoary pander to this young man's passions came down to see the prisoners, one by one, to pry into their ways of life and find some pretext for proceedings yet more harsh. Every one in the Tower had cause to regret his coming. Raleigh and Percy were confined to their cells; Lady Shrewsbury was insulted in her apartments; and the Lady Arabella suffered from the incivilities of Waad, an officer only too anxious to please his patrons at the court.

The darkening crimes and breaking strength of that bad old man were hurrying him to an end; but whether that end would be a felon's dungeon or a councilor's grave, the nimblest wit in London could not tell.

Lady Shrewsbury, saucy and silent with the lords, was brought before a Select Committee of the Privy Council, at York House, the residence of Ellesmere, to answer for not answering; an offense which Northampton said amounted to a contempt of the King. They told her that Crompton had confessed to all she had done in the marriage and escape of her niece, and they wished her to supply information on certain points. She would not speak to these points. She pleaded her vow; she pleaded her peerage. If she were charged with an offense, she claimed to be tried by her peers, according to the law, and in open court, not by a Committee of the Council, sitting in a private room.

Four of the judges, consulted on her case, subscribed to a view of the actual law which, on a sentence being passed in the Star Chamber, would have laid her open to a fine of twenty thousand pounds, and imprisonment during the King's pleasure. That a verdict could be gained against her in the Star Chamber, if promoted by the Council, who could doubt? Yet the Countess was not frightened into speech. Sent back to the Tower, she lived on, year by year, in her old defiant mood, until her enemy Northampton died and the "Friends of Spain" were broken and dispersed.

Seymour amused himself in Brussels and Paris, wrote abject letters to King James, and squabbled with Waad about the plate and hangings he had left behind him in St. Thomas's tower. In less than six months he forgot his wife, and almost forgot his debts. Waad wrote to Cecil that the flown bird had left nothing behind him of his own, since the best things in his rooms had been either fetched from the Lady Arabella's house or taken from the Lieutenant's store. A few things he had bought from tradesmen, but for these things he had never paid.

In the chamber which her grandmother Margaret had occupied in the Tower, poor Rosalind, having lost her all for love, remained a prisoner to her cousin five years. Some of her letters, written from the Tower to the King, have been preserved,—tender and winsome letters, full of sad humor and wife-like grace. Her pleas were simple. When the King had told her to marry whom she pleased, she thought herself free. She allowed her heart to become engaged. Her lover pressed her, and she plighted him her troth. That act of plighting made them, in her conscience, man and wife. Before she learned that the King objected to her match, the deed was done. If she had given offense, it was because she had been driven to choose between the law of God and the law of man. "Most humbly I beseech your Majesty," she wrote, "to consider in what miserable state I should have been, if I had taken any other course; for, my own conscience witnessing before God that I was then the wife of him that now I am, I could never have matched with any other man." She signed her letters "A. S.," which luckily answered to either Arabella Stuart or Arabella Seymour. But the King was dead to her sorrow. Trying him on every side, by turns gay and cheerful, sad and submissive, she appealed to his pity, to his pride, to his affection; and she tried him on every side in vain. When the "Queen of Hearts" was married to the Palsgraf of the Rhine, poor Rosalind hoped that her cousin's heart would open to her woes. "Mercy, mercy! for God's sake, mercy!" was the burden of her daily prayer. The King was deaf.

In her lonely chamber she plied her needle on a canvas which she meant to send as a remembrance to the King; a dainty piece of labor, to have touched a kinsman's heart. But James would not accept her present. Then she fell sick, and pined in her room, and wandered in her thoughts.

The rules under which she lived in the Lieutenant's house were harsh, and even in her days of sickness they were not relaxed. Waad knew his masters, and guessed their minds. No news, he felt assured, could reach Northampton's ear so welcome as that of Arabella's death; and hence, when his functions gave him power to trouble his unpardoned captive, he pressed against her with all his weight. He refused to let her servants wait upon her. He compelled her to eat the ordinary prison fare. She asked for posset, and for clothes befitting a sick-room and a lady who kept her bed; but she asked for these indulgences in vain. In her search for help, she turned to her bitterest foe at court, and in a plaintive letter told Northampton of her misery in the Tower. "I have been sick," she wrote, "even unto the death; from which it hath pleased God miraculously to deliver me; but find myself so weak, by reason I have wanted those ordinary helps whereby most others in my case, be they never so poor, are preserved alive —at least for charity." She had little hope from Northampton, and her note was more a menace than a prayer. In words direct enough, she told him that the privations under which she lay in prison would be not only "the certain" but "the apparent" cause of her death. She warned him that if either he, or his nephew Suffolk, had "possessed the King with such opinions of her as should cause her to be restrained until help came too late," she knew her course. "I dare die," she added, "and oppress others with my ruin, if there be no other way."

The strain was now too great for her feeble strength to bear. Her tender musings passed into fierce convulsions; and when her doctors had chased the agony away, her mind was found to be a wreck. Rosalind was become Ophelia!

Days, months, went by in hopeless waste of love and life. She lost all sense of passing things, and prattled in her madness like a child. The Lieutenancy of the Tower was changed, a more unscrupulous tool of Lord Northampton coming to rule over her; but she took no heed of what was going on. Some friends she found, in the Tower and beyond the Tower,—men who pitied her, and would have given their lives to help her; but these were not the great ones of the earth. Palmer, a divine of the English Church, and Crompton, her faithful servant, put their heads together and, in the summer of 1614, in the third year of her imprisonment, contrived a plan for her escape. It was a wild design, which led to nothing, except their own arrest and imprisonment, a letter of congratulation from Northampton to Carr, and a resolution on the part of James to guard her better in the time to come.

The rumors of her proposed escape were useful to Northampton in drawing people's eyes and thoughts away from a frightful drama which had just been closed in the Bloody tower.

She lived a year after Crompton's attempt had failed; tenderly drooping day by day; always gentle, sometimes playful, never morose; now plying her needle through the flowers, now touching her well-worn lute, and humming her evening song, until at length the weary woman fell asleep.

In the dead hours of an autumn night her ashes were taken from the Tower and laid in that Abbey which was the tomb of all her race,—laid beside all that remained of her grandmother, Margaret Douglas, and her great-aunt, Mary Queen of Scots, with neither line nor stone to mark the spot in which she sleeps.

Seymour lived abroad, keeping his eye on events, and hoping to come back, which he was now convinced he could never do while his consort was alive. He never wrote to her, never sent her token of his love. He heard that she was sick, he heard that she was crazed; but Paris was gay, and nothing in her fortunes seemed to touch his young and calculating heart. When he heard that she was gone, he threw himself upon James's mercy, implored his pardon, and obtained permission to return. Attaching himself to Charles, he became that prince's councilor and friend, fighting at his side through the Civil War, and making at its close that theatrical offer of being put to death for his King, which is the best-remembered of his feats. But, to make things safe whichever side should win, he took a second wife from the popular side; marrying Lady Frances Devereux, sister of Lord Essex, the great Parliamentary general. Seymour kept his head and his estate, and when Charles the Second came back to London he received the reward of his many virtues in his elevation to the rank of Duke.

It is not known that Seymour ever paid for the hangings supplied by Jenning at ten pounds apiece for his comfort in St. Thomas's tower.

Yet before the royal lady passed into her rest in the great Abbey, she heard that the hoary and wicked Earl, who had wrought her so much evil, was no more; that in his later time he was a loathsome object in all men's eyes; and that he was gone to his grave suspected of a hideous crime, for which, on proof and judgment given against him, he would probably have been hung.

CHAPTER XXX.

LADY FRANCES HOWARD.

The last and latest of the many tools by which Northampton worked his will at court was the beauty of his nephew's daughter, Lady Frances, the young wife of his ally, Robert Earl of Essex.

In the long line of our female criminals there is hardly one more fascinating and more odious than Lady Frances Howard, the daughter of Lady Suffolk. When she was yet a child of thirteen springs, she appeared at court in one of the parts of Ben Jonson's Masque of Hymen. A daughter of the house of Howard, she was chosen by Cecil and Northampton as the first victim in a series of matches by means of which they hoped to fuse into one great party four rival houses; the other victims of their policy being her elder sister, Lady Elizabeth, and her tiny sister, Lady Catharine. These girls were given in marriage by plotting graybeards to two boys and one old man; Lady Frances to Robert, Earl of Essex, Lady Catharine to William, Lord Cranborne,—boys no bigger than themselves, whom they could neither love nor hate in that tender age,—and Lady Elizabeth to William, Lord Knollys of Greys, a kinsman of the great Queen. The prize of this union of the four great houses of Cecil, Howard, Devereux, and Knollys was to be the control of king, court, and government for a dozen years.

The King was thought to have made the match between Earl Robert and Lady Frances, and the wedding came off in a scene which was gay with all the gayety of a court. The King and Queen were present. James, who gave away the bride, and heard Montagu bless the children, ran with them from the chapel to the masque, where they were dazed by the lights and company, by the ripple of Jonson's verse, by the surprise of Inigo Jones's sceneries, by the masquers' white plumes and the ladies' ropes of pearl. When the feast was eaten and the romps were danced, the boy and girl, now man and wife according to the Church, were sent away to school. Lord Essex went abroad with his tutor, while his child-like bride went home to her mother's house.

Reared in the court of France, living much in Huguenot homes, the Earl grew up into a grave and religious youth; while the Countess, his bride, being trained under her mother's eye, grew up into a woman unspeakably venal and impure. A youth of parts and figure, soft in his ways, especially with the gentler sex, quick with fire and manhood, proud of his great name, inclined, like the old warriors of his house, to cleave his way not by his wit but by his sword, Earl Robert grew up into a perfect knight, armed at all points with the courtier's grace no less than with the soldier's art. During the five years which he spent abroad, he does not seem to have thought very much of that festive scene at the English court, and of that fair young face which had filled the galleries of Whitehall with light; and when he returned to London, after a long absence, to claim his wife, now grown into a lovely woman, he heard with equal surprise and pity that the fair young girl whom he had kissed and promised to love was thought by some of his family to have been led by her kinsmen into unwife-like ways.

The girl was cursed with the rarest gifts of person. Tall and lithe, with oval face, small pouting lips, straight nose, and masses of shining hair, she would have taken captive every heart without the aid of her brilliant eyes. If those said sooth who knew her best, those eyes were fired with a wondrous and wicked glow. They set the poets raving, drove the painters to despair, and, even when they shone in eclogues only, furnished critics with the theory of what Johnson calls the poetic propagation of light.

Living with her mother Lady Suffolk, with her sister Lady Knollys, both of whom made wreck of their repute, she learned, while yet a child, to see the value of such gifts. A husband far away, of whom she heard as poring over strange books, as crossing swords with unknown sparks, was not the man on whom her fancy loved to dwell. Though young and noble, she heard that he was grave and proud, averse to courts, contemptuous of pomp and show, a soldier more like Grey than a cavalier like Carr. Unhappily for the girl, no friend was at her side in those perilous years who could have shown her a better way. Her mother had for many years been lost to all sense of shame. Of her elder sister, now the wife of a man old enough to be her grandfather, it is enough to say that she was (afterward) that Countess of Banbury whose married life has been the subject of judicial inquiry ever since she died. From her father, and from the old man who was more to her than father, she had little more than venal counsels to expect.

During the dozen years of the new reign, the Howards had driven a thriving trade in honors and estates, though the ducal coronet of their house had not yet been won.

Henry, the Nestor of his family, was Baron Marnhill, Earl of Northampton, Constable of Dover Castle, Lord Warden of the Cinque Ports, Lord Privy Seal, High Steward of Oxford, Knight of the Garter, a Commissioner for the Office of Earl Marshal, and Keeper of Greenwich Park. Among manors and castles which he had begged from James were Castle Rising in Norfolk, the lordship of Ash in Suffolk, the manor of Buckland in Dorset, the manor of Clare in Salop, Wark Castle and the manor of Tyndale in Northumberland, the Chase of Baggeridge and White's-wood in Stafford. Besides his official salaries, he got a personal pension of two hundred pounds a year for life, one hundred pounds a year of the surrendered pension of Lady Walsingham, and a royalty on all the starch either made in England or imported from abroad. He had built a great palace at Charing Cross, which he called Northampton House, and a second great palace in the country, which he called Audley End.

Thomas, his nephew and favorite, was Baron Howard of Walden, Earl of Suffolk, and Lord Chamberlain, with nearly as many pensions and perquisites as his uncle.

Since Cecil's death, no single courtier had been able to stand his ground against the Howards, whose high connections and unscrupulous talents had made them every year more dangerous to the King. James loved them little, but he feared them much. He liked their supple knees and slimy tongues, but trembled when he thought of their riches, their experience, their ambition, and their greed. One thing about them gave him comfort: they were hated by his people; so that he had little doubt, if ever he should have to turn against them, that he could do so with the nation at his back. Northampton asked for the White Staff, the wand then borne by the Lord High Treasurer; and the King, not daring to give him that staff, on account of his religion and his unpopularity, put the Treasury in commission for six months. Then commenced a new series of intrigues, through which the hoary and wasting Earl expected to win his place. He threw out lures and hints, and played a most curious game of give-and-take. He favored the reduction of Northumberland's fine, in order to catch the support of Lady Lucy's lover, and actively pursued his young crony, Lord Vaux, the nephew of Ann and Helen, until that pupil of Garnet was condemned to the loss of his estate and to imprisonment in the Fleet for life. He gratified the London mob by hanging Father Richards and Father Sahagun, two priests who returned to England without license; at the same time taking some pains to soften the surprise in Rome by sending his nephew Arundel to weep at the foot of the gallows on which the priests were hung. So well was his game played out, that the world began to talk of Northampton's "Protestant zeal," and for this outbreak of English virtue he was rewarded by the Dons of Cambridge, who added to his many offices and honors that of Chancellor of the University,—a step which brought him sensibly nearer to the Staff.

Northampton, gazing on Lady Essex's lustrous eyes, began to dream of an alliance with the royal house; and this old man, who should have been her guide and stay in the path of honor, taught the poor child how to beam on the young prince, and blessed his stars when he observed how the warm boy flushed and trembled beneath her gaze. But Henry, though he liked to toy with the siren, never dreamt of asking her to be his wife. Too soon and easily he clipped her chains. Once, when she dropped her glove at his feet, a courtier drew his eye to the sign of favor; but he passed it by, saying, "No: it has been stretched by another."

The tale of Prince Henry and Lady Essex having been locked in a room may not be true; but Lady Suffolk and Lord Northampton had the sort of fame in the city which left them open to suspicion of the vilest acts. In that dozen years during which they reigned at court, the tone of life in the upper ranks had undergone a change. To those who had seen the stately and decent court of Gloriana, that of her successor on the throne appeared like a cock-pit and a bear-garden. Fulk Greville, in a ripe old age, which was certainly not penitential and severe, described for the amusement of after-times the vices of great lords and ladies as he saw them,—a picture of courtly manners to be mated only in the annals of some Cæsar in ancient Rome, some Regent in modern France. Lady Suffolk was no solitary queen of vice, nor was Northampton the only broker in his country's shame. All ranks seemed rotten; the finest ladies to wear their prices, so to speak, upon their sleeves. A royal closet, unclean with the litter and language of a kennel; galleries besieged by gamesters, pensioners, and jades; ante-chambers choked by sorcerers, poisoners, and pimps; a garden walked by bravos, ready for any service, however foul and dark, that stood beyond the hangman's reach; with a bald and febrile man of middle age presiding over the dice and drink, the sale and cozenage; scenes which were varied and disturbed by Lake's reports, by Montagu's divinity, and by Archie's broad grins,—such was the court in which the hoary and dying Northampton was seeking to obtain the Staff.

Having failed in his hope of catching the Prince of Wales, he turned his face elsewhere, and, having made his calculations, taught his pupil how to bend her beautiful, burning eyes on Carr.

CHAPTER XXXI.

ROBERT CARR.

Robert Carr was a Scottish lad of handsome person, for whom James had conceived a sudden and ridiculous whim.

The King, who could not live without having some youth about him whom he could pat and pinch, tickle and slobber, had cast his eyes in turn on Herbert and Hay, young fellows with flowing beards, pink cheeks, and empty skulls, who rarely troubled their brains with anything worse than a masque and a saraband. He kept his darling for a time, and then dethroned him for some newer and fairer face; but the darling of a day was seldom so unlucky as not to retire ennobled and enriched. Hume, Herbert, Hay, were all created Earls.

The Countess of Suffolk, knowing that the King was blind to the beauty of women, laid herself out to supply him with removes of handsome boys. She spent her days in seeking for arch eyes, pink flesh, and graceful forms; and, when she had found her Ganymede of an hour, she curled his locks and sweetened his breath to the royal taste. She taught these youths to leave politics alone, and to devote their talents to the service of beauty, as imaginary Knights of the Fortunate Isles, and to fight for such golden truths as—

Beauty supplies the world with valor;
None but lovers can be happy;
No fair lady ever yet was false.

Carr was the youngest of these curled and silken favorites. A page of Hume, he had spent some months in Paris, where he learned to dress and dance, to ride and run the ring. Coming to court, he put on his best attire, and walked into the Tilt-yard, when the King was present, in a scarlet frock, a foam of lace, and an embroidered shirt. Contriving to be knocked over in the game, he caught the King's eye by his fall; and when James was told that the pretty boy was one of Hume's old pages, he carried him up into his room, put him into bed, and nursed him with his own hands, until the strength of a roe returned to his feet and the bloom of an apple to his cheek. Thus began his fortunes. In a few months the King dubbed him Sir Robert, paid his debts, put jewels in his ears, swore him of the bed-chamber, and promised him the Lady Ann Clifford for a wife.

Left to his own devices, Carr would have risen like Herbert and Hay, to set like Montgomery and Carlisle. A coronet, a rich wife, a house in town, a chase in the country, would have quenched his appetite for favor; but by the side of Carr stood a young man, poor as himself in purse, but richer in the gifts of wit, of policy, and of speech. This youth was Thomas Overbury, a member of the House of Commons, a Puritan in morals and in thought, if not in opinion, a poet, a prose writer, a politician of consummate power. These lads had come to court in company. Something in Carr had taken the fancy of his more intellectual mate, who, measuring James from head to heel, had seen his way to making use of Carr in his attempt to rise. Swearing a league of friendship, the two young men had come to Whitehall with an understanding that, in seeking a fortune which they were to share and share alike, Carr was to find beauty of person, while Overbury was to find strength of brain. They meant to make a figure in the world.

In their first five years at court they rose very high; for Carr, who was to enjoy the pleasures while Overbury was to exercise the powers of the high station they might win, was lifted from the position of a private page to the state of an adviser and the rank of a viscount. Overbury, careless of show, was satisfied with being dubbed a knight and consulted in every affair of State. A man of subtle and commanding genius, equal to many kinds of work, with powers of mind which made him easy master of every craft, Overbury had raised Carr to the height on which he stood; but neither King nor court as yet knew the strength of Overbury and the emptiness of Carr. While the new Viscount reigned at court, Overbury was the actual minister of the crown. "There was a time," said Bacon on the trial, "when Overbury knew more of the secrets of State than the whole Council." What Bacon said afterward other people knew at the time. In the City taverns it was a pasquil that Carr ruled the King, and that Overbury ruled Carr.

To the outside world, the rise of this favorite was that of a shooting star. Who could tell where his flight would stop? He was now Viscount Rochester; he had the promise of an earldom; nay, a Marquisate of Orkney was likely to be his next birthday-gift. In those years we had neither duke nor marquis in the country, and a Marquis of Orkney would be the highest person in James's court. There were hints of the King adopting him as a son. Here, then, was no passing favorite, such as the world had seen in Herbert and Hay. These men were liked; but Rochester was all in all. After the death of Cecil, who had kept him in his fitting place as a gentleman of the bed-chamber,

Carr seemed to be the only man of whose presence and advice the King was never tired. Acting on Overbury's lessons, and speaking the words set down for him, the raw Scottish lad achieved a certain popularity, not only in the closet but in the street. He had the name of a stanch Protestant, and the reputation of an enemy of Spain. If his life was not lovely, he was not more lax in morals than many who had less than half his tempters to resist. No man's name, no woman's fame, had yet been smirched by Carr. If men could say that his rise had been swift, his accumulation of riches sudden, they could add, with truth, that he had shown many of the virtues as well as some of the vices of a royal favorite. Even in temper, gracious in bearing, bountiful in disposition, he had gained admirers even where he had not secured friends. A man of Overbury's gifts could not have worked with a fool. To the poets Carr was uniformly kind; both Jonson and Donne have written in his praise. Even Bacon, though he owed him nothing, was not unwilling to grace him with a masque. For the rest, his power to go wrong was checked by a feeble will.

For two or three years this favorite had been watched and thwarted by Northampton, Knollys, and Suffolk, who saw that he was not as they were; though they crossed him less for his own sake than for that of Overbury, whose principles and talents they equally feared and shunned. On Cecil's death, a scramble had taken place at court, not only for the White Staff, but for the important post of Secretary of State. The place of Secretary, though of less dignity than that of Treasurer, was of more importance, since the holder of it was in daily intercourse with the King; and a man of active genius would be sure to make it the center of every movement in the realm. The inner circle of the Council was now composed of three great peers, allied in blood and marriage,—Northampton, his nephew Suffolk, and that nephew's son-in-law, Knollys; and these great peers, in seeking to gain these offices for their party, had the advantage of voting with a single voice. Northampton spoke, and the younger men obeyed. When they had got the Staff put into commission, as the only thing that could then be done, they fought for the minor and nearer post of Secretary. Winwood, Wotton, Bacon, Lake, were mentioned, as men who could serve their country; but the King, though he did not like to say so in the outset, was resolved to have no other Secretary than Carr.

Now, Carr in the King's closet, writing letters on public business, was, as Northampton felt, but another form of having Overbury for a master. Carr was Overbury's voice; and Overbury was an enemy of Spain. If Overbury were to shape the policy of James, Northampton and Suffolk would hardly be worth their salt.

Lady Suffolk had already tried her arts on Carr; but Overbury, whose morals were austere, though he hungered after power even more than his ally after flattery and female smiles, repelled her. Overbury had a difficult game to play; for Carr, though popular at court, was far from popular in the town. The qualities which took the King—his dainty face, his splendid garb, and his Lowland Scotch—provoked the people into scorn. The London crowd could not endure a Scot. Poor in purse and quick in speech, his bold eye, his ready hand, his saucy tongue, disgusted men who either would not or could not see his nobler side. To them, his courage was the merit of a mastiff, his abstinence the virtue of a fox, his loyalty the cringing of a slave. Even his religious ardor pained them, as a passion in excess; and no reproach appeared to them severe enough for the roaring, rieving callant who aped the fashion of a court in the midst of filth and rags. Now, Carr, though handsome, civil, and well dressed, was still a Scot; and Northampton made the King believe that to give him Cecil's post in the closet would provoke a rising in the streets.

Unable to have his way, the King declared that in the future he would act as Secretary of State himself.

Northampton was not deceived by James's move. He saw that Carr was rising in the world; and, hungering after posts which none but Carr could give him, he was base enough not only to dream of gaining him over to their party through his lovely niece, but shameless enough to teach that girl how to lay her beauty in his path.

The young lady did not need much training to go wrong. She knew the way too well. Only too early in her life she had found a priestess of indulgence in Ann Turner, the famous White Witch. Ann, who had been a lovely girl, was still a winsome woman, white, graceful, slender, looking like a lady of birth, a little faded from her prime. Even when she stood, years later, at the bar of justice, the poets could only sing,—

"The roses on her lovely cheeks were dead."

Now, this White Witch professed, among other arts, to understand how to preserve youth, to kindle love, and to chill desire. In the task which Northampton set her, Lady Essex had need of all her charms. From Ann Turner the fair Countess got one philter to chill the man she called her husband, another to warm the man she wished to call her lover. When these philters failed to work her ends, at least on Essex, who truly loved his wife, Ann took her noble pupil to a great magician living in a lonely house in Lambeth Fields. This sorcerer was Simon Forman, a fellow known to be driving a brisk and profitable trade in potions, horoscopes, and charms. Forman had more to do with great ladies than Mayerne himself; and, as he impudently set down in his diaries, he took his payment from these dupes in various ways. This knave supplied the young Countess of Essex with enchanted papers, a few wax puppets, a scarf full of white crosses, and a piece of human skin. Later on, he adopted her as his "daughter" in the black art, permitting her to call him "father," and giving her a scroll on which he had noted for her use a list of the principal imps in hell.

Lady Essex had scant need for magic. Carr was only too soon in love with her bright eyes, and asking no aid from Forman's scrolls and fiends. Northampton played Old Pandarus to this guilty pair, just as he had done when Cecil was the Troilus, Lady Suffolk the Cressida, of his play. He put the young wife in the young favorite's way, and even lent them his house to meet in. Often beneath the roof, sometimes in the sight, of that old man, they kissed and swore to each other to be true.

Suffolk, younger and less base than his uncle, forced his daughter to live in her husband's house. Essex, though grieving to see that his wife's heart was gone from him, never dreamt that her honor was also gone; and, kind in temper as he was princely in gifts, he set himself to win once more the love which for the moment he saw that he had lost. She pouted, raved, and mocked him, hoping he would flash into anger and turn her out of doors. Her husband bore with these humors, thinking they were but the ways of young married girls. His wife was dark to him as night. Nor could two such natures as his and hers come nearer than they stood. He, pious and severe, rode to sermon; she, profligate and superstitious, went to mass. He loved the country, while she adored the town. Masques, balls, processions, priests, dress, sports, and triumphs, all the things to which her heart lay open, he would have shunned for himself and for the woman whom he loved. Early hours, long rides through the summer woods, attention to the poor and sick, the duties of a country household, all that round of love and usefulness which Essex craved as the purest work that he could find on earth, his Countess flung at his feet in anger and contempt.

Ann Turner's service to her mistress did not end in the magician's study. She hired a house for her in the medical quarter of St. Paul's, near Amen Corner, in which she might meet her lover, unseen by watchful critics of the court. Carr was young and she was fair. No devil on Forman's list found more delight in doing wrong than Lady Essex. Yet, in the midst of all her profligacy, she was careful to make her game. Lord Rochester being the most powerful man at Whitehall, she made up her mind to share his power,—not for a season only, but for life.

The obstacles in her path were vast. She had a husband to get rid of; Rochester, a friend to put away; and with these two men she was only too well aware that she would have to conduct a duel to the death.

CHAPTER XXXII.

THE POWDER POISONING.

ESSEX, a man of high rank, was proud of his name, and quick to avenge affronts. How could she get rid of such a man? She thought of poison; she thought of steel; she thought of Holy Church. A divorce would be the best of all; but how could a divorce be got? The only plea to be set up in such a case as hers—that of nullity from the first—was one which no man likes to admit and few women like to urge.

Listening, now to Northampton, now to Ann Turner, she conceived a triple scheme for getting rid of the husband whose name she bore. She egged on her brother Henry to send him a challenge; she paid the Lambeth wizard to waste his strength by magic; she gave a diamond ring, with the promise of a thousand pounds, to Mary Wood, a Norfolk hag, renowned for ridding ladies of their inconvenient lords, for a philter warranted to kill in three days. But all these efforts failed her. The King forbade the duel; the wizard's dolls and scarfs were powerless; and the Norfolk hag deceived her with a philter which would not kill. When magic, steel, and poison failed her, she fell back on her idea of divorce.

While the Countess was poring through the ways and means for getting a divorce from Essex, the White Witch and some lesser agents of evil were employed in removing Overbury from her path. In spite of his high talents, Overbury lay open to such arts as Northampton's corrupt nature and Italian education had taught him to abuse. Pride of genius led him into unwise scorn of men who had been schooled to rise by paths more devious than his own. The very frankness of his opposition to Spain armed Northampton against him, while his nobleness of soul prevented him from seeing to what desperate shifts a man of such high rank could stoop. He overrated Carr; not his power of resisting money and favor,—for there his friend was strong,—but his power of resisting the more perilous trial of liquid eyes and a wanton tongue. A sense of original force, which, often as it was tried, had never yet failed him, gave to Overbury's native haughtiness an austerity and emphasis very hard to bear. The Queen complained of him; the King resented his scornful tone; and citizens wagered their golden angels as to which was the proudest, Raleigh, Overbury, or Lucifer. The prize was given to Overbury. None of the courtiers loved him, for he took no pains to please them. Weak on every side except that of his intellect, he invited and defied Northampton's arts.

So long as Overbury thought his friend's intrigue with Lady Essex was the fancy of a day, he let it pass in silence, smiling grimly at the old man's baseness in selling the honor of his house for a mess of pottage; but he felt that it would never do for him to let this fancy of a moment sink into a permanent madness of the heart; and when he saw that Carr was running after the siren day and night, he warned him gravely against her vicious wiles. He spoke too late. Calypso had sung her slave to sleep. A fact came out by accident to have startled him from his dream of enduring happiness with such a woman. Mary Wood, the Norfolk hag, was arrested for petty theft, and, in her rage at being abandoned by her noble patrons, confessed her name, her trade, and her employers. The story of the poisonous drug and the diamond ring was told;

and the truth of her tale was confirmed by Richard Grimston, the pursuivant, on a very important point. This story was referred to the Council, in which her kinsmen sat; but the secret inquiry came to Overbury's ears and roused him to take a decided course. With consummate art,—for Carr was proud and hasty, not to be schooled too openly,—he warned him against her alluring smiles, now tickling him with easy banter, now stinging him with grave advice. To show what sort of woman a man should seek in wedlock, he wrote his poem called The Wife; that gracious picture of holy love in contrast with unholy lust. A wise man, said the poet, first seeks in a wife—not beauty, rank, and wealth; fools seek for such things first; but —the higher virtues of the soul. First, he hopes to find her good—then wise—then fit—and last of all comely. All that Lady Essex was, he urged his friend to shun. But Carr slept soundly in Calypso's lap, as deaf to the poet's verse as he had been to the Witch's charge.

Lady Essex and her Nestor now resolved that he must die. Their plans required his death. That he could stop their suit for a divorce, they knew; that he would use his power, they also knew. Less than his blood would neither serve their ambition nor appease their wrath. At first they thought of hiring an assassin. Unlike Essex, the poet was not a master of his sword; and Lady Essex sent to Greenwich for Sir David Wood, a soldier of fortune, who had been crossed by Overbury in a job. "I am told you have grievous wrongs against Sir Thomas Overbury," she began at once: "I am also told you are a brave gentleman. He who has wronged you has wronged me. I should be glad to hear he is no more." Wood hung fire. They were alone in her chamber, and she quickly explained her hints. She told him that she wished him to kill Sir Thomas; she promised him a thousand pounds, and offered him the friendship of Carr and the protection of all her kin. Wood was willing, but only on condition that Carr should come forward in person and assure him before a witness of his safety when the deed was done. She promised that Carr should give that pledge. But she dared not ask her lover for such a promise; and, sending for Wood once more, she told him she would pledge her own life for his safety, come what might. Wood answered, bluntly, that he was not such a fool as to go to Tyburn on a lady's word. "Why," urged the Countess, "the thing is easily done: he sups every night at Sir Charles Wilmot's house; stop his coach; drag him out and run him through." The bravo shook his head and left her in despair.

Northampton hit upon a safer plan.

The King was not fond of Overbury; and the pages who were near him, taking Northampton's cue, began to fret his ear by telling him that the people who met in fairs and taverns made jests against him, saying that he could not rule his realm without Overbury, since Overbury found all the wit for Carr, and Carr found all the wit for him. James swore a big oath that Overbury should be sent abroad,—as far as Moscow,—if only to let folk see whether the King could not rule without his aid. Overbury declined to go. They had taken care beforehand that he should decline, and so offend the King; but he had only refused the task on Rochester begging him not to go, since the proposal was a trick of their enemies to put the seas between them. Thus, he declined; when James, incensed at his refusal of so high a trust, gave orders for his instant arrest.

Overbury was lodged in the Bloody tower.

Out of sight, the poet soon fell out of Carr's remembrance. How far Rochester consented to his murder is uncertain; though it is clear that many of the steps which led to it were taken by him in person. Lady Essex and the White Witch had resolved to poison Overbury long before he was committed to the Tower. When they had locked him fast, they fell to work, like artists knowing what they meant to do.

The first step was to change the Lieutenant; for Waad, though insolent and slavish, was not the man to put his neck into a coil of rope by murdering one of his prisoners in open day. Who could assure him that his deed would never come to light? Murder will out; and when murder comes out, it is hard for any man to cheat the gallows of its due. Northampton had his agent ready; and when he sent for Waad to his mansion at Charing Cross, that agent was waiting in a room below. The Earl accused Waad of being too lenient with his new prisoner, and told him bluntly that he should not go back to his post. Waad was surprised; but on Northampton hinting that much of Lady Arabella's plate was missing, and that the Lieutenant was supposed to know what had become of it, he was so much frightened that he gave up his commission on the spot. He left Northampton House with fourteen hundred pounds in his pocket, and a promise of six hundred pounds more if he would only hold his tongue. A ruined gambler, one Sir Gervase Helwyss, was then brought in. What passed between the proud peer and the obscure knight we shall never learn; but that very night, without a warrant, without an oath, this ruffian was installed as Lieutenant of the Tower. The note of his appointment was scrawled at Northampton House, and the record of it afterward inserted in a blank corner of the Council-book. All his instructions, as to the treatment of his prisoner, Helwyss received directly from the Lord Privy Seal.

The second step was to change the keeper; for in such a business they could not trust an ordinary fellow to do their will. In Ann Turner's house there lived a servant worthy of such a mistress,—one Richard Weston, a tailor, with a soul too big for a yard and goose. Having tried his skill in sorcery and coining, he had run through a round of jails before adopting the more profitable trade of pimp. As Mrs. Turner's man, he had been employed to carry notes from the Countess to Carr, to arrange their guilty pleasures in Paternoster Row, to watch over their secret meetings at the Brentford farm. He knew his masters, and they knew their tool. A bag of gold would buy him, body and soul; and the Countess never paused to count the cost of what she had a mind to buy. She asked Sir Thomas Monson to get this fellow appointed keeper in the Bloody tower; but Monson, though eager to oblige so great a lady, thought it well to consult the Privy Seal, —an act of prudence to which he afterward owed his life. Northampton told him not only that Weston's appointment to wait on Overbury would be right, but that the King himself wished Weston to be placed in charge. Monson took him to the Tower and put him in the poet's room.

From that night Overbury's strength began to fail. Though his offense was only a contempt, he was confined more strictly than men who had been condemned to die. A secret order from Northampton closed up every avenue to the Bloody tower. Sir Nicholas, his father, and Lady Lydcot, his sister, were turned away from his door. Lydcot moved the court for leave to visit him, but he was only allowed to see him at his grated window. Davis, one of his men, proposed to be locked up with his master, day and night; and he was kicked away from the Tower. Sir Robert Killigrew, the physician, was clapped in the Fleet for trying to speak with him. Even Rochester's messages were stopped. Northampton was resolved that he should die, and he took pains that none save creatures of his own should enter into Overbury's cell. Yet the poet's strong stomach caused much delay; and letters got in and out, in spite of the Lieutenant's care. Monson told the Lieutenant that notes might pass under his eye in tarts and jellies, if he were not sharp; and when Simon Marson, the King's musician, brought to the Tower a present of jellies, which Lady Essex wished to be given to Overbury in the name of Carr, the Lieutenant, poking into them for correspondence, found that they were poisoned, and refused to let them pass. Weston sneered at such scruples; but Helwyss could not tell how far his employers wished him to go, and he had a strong desire to escape a murderer's doom.

On Tower Hill, in a small shop, lived one James Franklin, an apothecary, less honest in his trade than he who put poison into Romeo's hands. Like all the agents employed by Lady Essex, Franklin was a Papist; and this fellow, though he professed to keep a devil, and was said to have poisoned his wife, was brought to assist in committing murder, not only by the payment of a hundred and twenty pounds in gold, but by the hope of doing good service to his Church. From Franklin, Weston received a phial of stuff like water, which Mrs. Turner instructed him how to mix with his prisoner's drink. But Helwyss, still in doubt, detained the phial, and poured the drug upon the ground, even while he was suffering Weston to lay the tarts and jellies from Lady Essex on the prisoner's dish.

These poisons crept into the poet's veins. His cheek began to pale, and his voice to drop. On Overbury begging in his misery that a friend and a physician might come to see him, Rochester appeared in person before the Council, and procured a warrant for Lydcot and Killigrew to enter his cell; but when the favorite was gone away from the Council-board, Northampton and Suffolk revoked their pass. The prisoner, they wrote to Helwyss, must be closely kept; and, if he needed a physician, *they* would send one to him.

To draw his mind from thoughts of their foul play, Suffolk caused Overbury to be told that Rochester and he were on bad terms; and, on Northampton's hints, he even went so far in this deceit as to ask for Overbury's good offices with Rochester, in return for his own in Overbury's favor with the King. Northampton took these messages to the Tower; and, when the poet was thought to be off his guard, the French adventurer, Mayerne, rode down to the Bloody tower and marked his prisoner with a poisoner's eye. Lobel, a French apothecary, and Reeve, his English boy, were appointed to do the deed.

The poet knew that he was being poisoned. Helwyss told him that Lord Rochester had sent him an emetic, as his lordship wished him to look sick, in order that the King's compassionate feelings might be touched. The poet was annoyed at such feeble tricks; and Northampton schooled his Lieutenant into exciting Overbury to use the language of reproach toward Rochester, while he himself pressed on the work of drugging him to death. When all was ready, Lobel made the glister, which his apprentice Reeve applied.

The poet was no more.

CHAPTER XXXIII.

THE END.

Carr heard of the poet's death without a sigh. The courtiers who watched him closely saw, or afterward thought they saw, a gleam of unusual brightness pass across his face when he heard the news. He flew to his enchantress, told her the story of his death, and sealed her rapture with a lover's kiss.

Northampton, fearing that men's tongues would wag against him in the city, requested Helwyss to send for Lydcot to the Tower, but to take care that the corpse should be buried before he came. The poet was put under ground before his flesh was cold.

The wedding-day was fixed, the feast of St. Stephen, 1613. Rochester was made an Earl, so that Lady Essex would not have to descend from her former rank by marrying him. Sherborne Castle was torn from Raleigh to provide them with a country-seat. Lady Raleigh put up her hands to heaven; and then the splendid nuptials of the Earl and Countess of Somerset were celebrated in the royal chapel at Whitehall, with a splendid ceremony, a round of dances, and a gorgeous masque.

Just eight years earlier, on the same day, in the same chapel, before the same King and Queen, in presence of nearly all the same lords and ladies, with the same officiating bishop, the young lady, then a fair and innocent child, had been married to the young and handsome Earl of Essex. Two years later, that brilliant throng was scattered to the winds. The hero and heroine of that day, now man and wife, with their passions chilled, their spirits broken, their lives forfeited, were lying in the Tower, a bickering and unhappy pair, conscious of their fall, and eager to impute their ruin to each other's crimes. Lady Somerset now contemned her low-born husband; Lord Somerset now abhorred his wicked wife.

Northampton never got the White Staff for which he had done so much, for nature could not wait, and when the surgeons who were called to Northampton House had cut the putrid sore in his side, he fell at once. A priest, who waited in his chamber, gave him the host, laid pall and cross on his bed, and set tapers burning for him night and day. He died with yells of accusation ringing in his ears, which all his power as a Privy Councilor could not silence. Peers, burgesses, and citizens accused him of being not only a Papist and a pensioner of Spain, but the secret soul of all the Catholic plots. In vain he raved and stormed; in vain he threw himself at the favorite's feet; in vain he pointed out what he had done against Fawkes and Garnet. The mask was falling from his face, and men began to see him for what he was. He died in a gorgeous chamber of Northampton House (June, 1614),—in time, but only just in time, to save himself from a cell in the Bloody tower.

For the poet in his grave had begun to make war on the peer in his palace. Friends of Overbury, who were also friends of virtue, had printed his poem The Wife, and the public snapped up five editions of that noble satire in as many months. The reader of the poem talked of the poet, and then old tales were told once more about the manner of his death. An accident gave to these rumors a sudden, ominous shape; for Reeve, the French apothecary's lad, fell sick in

Flanders, and in his agony of conscience spread the news of what his master had been hired to do. Trumball, the English Resident in Flanders, hastened home with this report, not daring to write such words as Reeve had spoken in his fear and pain. Winwood, the new Secretary of State, a Puritan, who hated the Howards with a good deal of secret energy, received Trumball's news with a grim delight, and sent him back to Flanders, with orders to keep an eye upon the lad.

Winwood moved with a wary step, for the boy's confession touched the fame of some of the highest persons in the realm. He dropped some hints that Helwyss was unfit for such a post as Lieutenant of the Tower; and when that officer, in trying to excuse himself, had half confessed his guilt, the Secretary of State rode down to Royston and laid his proofs before the King.

James read the confessions, and sent them on to Coke, by whom a swift and secret search was made for further facts. The injured Waad came forward; and his evidence touched not only the more active agents in the crime, but Monson, Northampton, Lady Somerset, and Carr. After he had arrested Mrs. Turner, her man Weston, and the apothecary Franklin, Coke applied for powers to examine Helwyss, Mayerne, and Sir Thomas Monson. The facts which came to light suggested that the murder of Overbury, daring and open as it was, had been no more than a single act in a great drama of public crime. Ann Turner spoke of Prince Henry as having been poisoned with a bunch of grapes; and Weston talked of wizards and druggists going over to Heidelberg with orders to cut off Frederick and Elizabeth. Carr began to tremble; and, thinking it might be well to cover his past life by a general pardon, he sent for Sir Robert Cotton to his room, and begged that antiquary to seek among his papers for the largest pardon ever granted by a sovereign prince. Cotton found a pardon issued by a Pope for the crimes of treason, murder, felony, and rape, and on the model of this grant the Earl of Somerset drew a pardon for himself and got the document signed by James. But Ellesmere refused to pass it, saying that to put the Great Seal of England to such a paper would subject the Lord Chancellor to a premunire.

Coke was so far ready with his proofs, that the King was forced to appoint a commission of inquiry into the poet's death; Ellesmere, Lennox, Zouch, and Coke were the commissioners; and their meetings were held in the Lord Chancellor's residence, York House, to which they summoned Helwyss and Monson, as well as Weston, Franklin, and Mrs. Turner. Weston told them the story of his crime, the love-affairs of Lady Essex and Carr, the secret meetings in Paternoster Row and at the Brentford farm, the original prompting of Lady Essex to the murder, the promises given in her name by Mrs. Turner, the appointment made through Monson for him to wait in the Bloody tower, the failure of his philters, the altercation with Helwyss, the receipt of the poisoned tarts and jellies, the impatience of Lady Essex to have the thing done, the visit of Mayerne, the employment of Lobel, and the glisters which caused the prisoner's death. Ere long, Mrs. Turner and Franklin confessed their guilt; the first giving up the implements of magic received by her from Forman,—the roll of devils, the scarf of white crosses, the bundle of waxen dolls, and the scrap of human skin; the second raving against his imp and his employer,—one for not warning him in time, the other for bewitching him to his ruin and then leaving him to perish.

The day of Lord and Lady Somerset was come. In raking up evidence against Mrs. Turner, the Commissioners found that on the day of her arrest Lady Somerset had not only sent her secret messages to fear nothing, but had got her husband to sign a warrant for John Poulton, a pursuivant, to search the Beaver Hat, a house near Temple Bar, and to bring away all the papers which he found there in a certain trunk and bag. The Beaver Hat was kept by Weston's son, and Poulton was accompanied in his search by Lady Somerset's maid. The contents of these papers could be guessed, and, when the Commissioners learned that Poulton had taken them to Somerset's house, they dispatched their messenger with orders for the Earl to keep his lodging near the Cockpit, and for the Countess to remain either in her own house at Blackfriars, or with her elder sister, Lady Knollys, near the Tilt-yard. Husband and wife were not to see each other. A messenger bore a letter to Royston, where the King was hunting, signed by Egerton, Lennox, Zouch, and Coke, urging that the proofs against Somerset were now so strong that he ought to be stripped of the Seals and lodged for safety in the Tower.

James kissed his favorite and gave him up.

The tools of Lady Somerset were quickly put away. Helwyss was hanged in chains, and the gibbet on which he swung was left to stand for a warning on Tower Hill. Mrs. Turner was hung at Tyburn, in her yellow bands and powdered hair, in the presence of a mighty crowd, many of whom wept for the beautiful though faded creature who knew the secret ways to all female hearts. She stood on the gallows, raving at the world she was about to leave, and calling down fire from heaven to consume it in the midst of sin and shame. Franklin and Weston were strung up like dogs.

How was justice to deal with the greatest criminal of all? Could a lady of the race of Howard be hung for a private murder?

Somerset had burned the papers seized by Poulton at the Beaver Hat; but the confessions wrung from Weston, Franklin, Helwyss, and Mrs. Turner would have sufficed to hang the principals, had such been the King's desire. Taken from his lodgings near the Cockpit, Somerset was placed under charge of Sir Oliver St. John; and when the Privy Seal had been taken from him, he was carried, with a single servant, to the Tower. As he passed from Water Lane through the dark archway, Raleigh was coming out. "It is the case of Haman and Mordecai," said the great captive, then going out into freedom. James was told of this speech. "Raleigh," he observed, "may die in that deceit." The King was probably of Carr's opinion, that the storm would soon whirl by.

Sir George More, the new Lieutenant, conducted the Earl and Countess of Somerset to the Bloody tower, and bade them enter. "Put me not in there!" cried Lady Somerset, white with terror. She knew it was the room in which she had murdered her husband's friend. "I shall never sleep again!" she shrieked; "his ghost will haunt my bed! put me elsewhere!" Somerset went in; and the Lieutenant urged her to follow him. In fact, he had no other lodging ready for prisoners of such high rank. But she would not stir. "Put me elsewhere! put me elsewhere!" she sobbed. Sir George had to carry her back to his own apartments, until Raleigh's house in the garden could be got ready for her use.

Somerset raged and pouted in his prison, bullying the new Lieutenant, Sir George More,—sending for Lord Hay,—demanding to see the King. When told that Sir George must write any message which he wished to be forwarded to James, he refused to send at all. When the Commissioners offered to hear him, he turned on his heel with a gesture of contempt.

At court the conflict of opposing forces raged with fury, for the Howards and their kinsfolk were a party in the state, with nearly half the public offices in their hands. Suffolk had got the Staff for which his uncle pined. Among them the Howards had the Mint, the Treasury, the Admiralty, the Army, the Household, the Cinque Ports, and the Channel Fleet; and as Lord-Lieutenants they commanded the nine counties of Berks, Oxon, Cambridge, Norfolk, Suffolk, Surrey, Dorset, Herts, and Kent. Opposed to this great family were the Puritans and patriots of every shade,—men so various in opinion and accomplishment as Pembroke and Bacon, Winwood and Raleigh, Villiers and Southampton. Clever as the courtiers were in guessing, they could not say which side would prove the stronger. Writing his Golden Age for a Christmas masque, Ben Jonson trimmed his verse to the uncertain winds; but nobler poets than Jonson spoke the indignant passions of the time. Ford, with fearless chivalry, composed a history of Overbury's Life and Death. He also wrote some verses on The Wife,—as did a stronger and wiser pen than that of Ford. In the massive measure and volcanic heat of the lines by W. S. (prefixed to the seventh edition, and published in the exciting days between the arrest and trial) some critics see the last public service done by Shakspeare. It is certain that his patrons, Pembroke and Southampton, took a leading part in bringing the poet's murderers to account.

The King's heart melted toward his minion, but he dared not free him from the Tower until his innocence had been proved in an open court. The town was full of Overbury, and books of which he was the hero were on every stall in Cheape and Fleet Street. A ninth edition of The Wife appeared, and a companion poem, called The Husband, was brought out. Overbury was known to have been a Protestant, an enemy of Spain; so that patriotic passion entered deeply into the cry for justice on his murderers, and the King was borne upon a stream which he could neither stem nor turn.

When the Commissioners closed their labors, and fixed the day of Lady Somerset's trial (May 24, 1616), the arraignment was considered by the country as a national solemnity. All private business was suspended for a time. The shops were closed, the parks deserted. Every one who could afford to spend five double angels bought a seat in Westminster Hall; and the thousands who could not press inside the Hall choked up the avenues of Palace Yard, in order to catch the first news that the weak Earl and his bad Countess had been convicted of murder and condemned to die.

The Countess held up her hand in answer to her name. A warder stood beside her with the axe. Attired in a gown of black tammel, a cypress chaperon, and a large lawn ruff, looking as penitent as she was beautiful, she bent her pale face to her judges, pleading guilty to her crime. Bacon, as the Attorney-General, spoke without harshness to the fallen Countess; Ellesmere, as Lord Chancellor, pronounced her sentence; and the warder, as executioner of the court, turned toward her the gleaming steel. She shed abundant tears, and begged the Lords to intercede for mercy with the King.

That night, Sir George More was alone with Somerset in his room. The prisoner was morose and threatening, though he knew that his wife had pleaded guilty and been condemned to die. He defied the judges and the peers. He said he would not answer to his name. More hinted that the King was anxious that he should confess his crime, accept a verdict, and trust his bounty for the rest. But Somerset would not yield. For six or seven days there had been much negotiation between the crown and the prisoner. Lord Hay had been chosen on the part of James. Sir George had been authorized to make Carr a specific promise that, on pleading guilty and evading proof, the life of Lady Somerset should be spared and his own honor as a peer should be saved. He rejected every offer. He said he would not plead. In look and tone, if not in words, he dared the court to bring him before his peers.

Late in the evening, More took horse for Greenwich, and, after a midnight interview with the King, rode back to the Tower.

Early in the May morning, More was at the door of Somerset's room. The Earl was already dressed,—in black, as if in mourning for his wife. He wore a plain black satin suit, laid with two satin laces in a seam; a gown of velvet lined with unshorn fleece; the sleeves trimmed with lace, and the gloves adorned with satin tops. He had the George about his neck. His hair was neatly curled, and his beard fell richly on his chest. More noticed that his eyes were sunk in his head, and that his face was very pale.

A moment before he stood up in court, the Lieutenant whispered in his ear that if he said one word against the King he should be dragged down, sentenced in his absence, and immediately put to death. To show his prisoner that he meant what he was saying, he placed two strong fellows close to him, each with a cloak on his arm, with orders to watch his lips, and, on a word being dropped about the King, to throw their cloaks over his face, pull him down, and hurry him away on the ground that he was mad.

Somerset denied the charge, and put his accusers to the proof. That part of the evidence which concerned Mayerne, Lobel, and his boy Reeve had been suppressed; and the court could not prove his guilt unless that evidence were produced. Bacon was very skillful; but his proofs were vague and incomplete. The long May day wore out in speeches which divided and perplexed the public; and when the torchmen entered with their lights, the darkness in the street was not more evident than the darkness in the hall of justice. Ellesmere asked for a verdict, and broke his staff; but, when Somerset went back to the Tower that night, no one could say that he was guilty of the murder, though every one knew that he had been condemned to die.

The Earl and Countess of Somerset came near together once again, but not as man and wife who love and trust each other. The doors of the Bloody tower and of the Garden house were left ajar, and they were sometimes overheard in angry talk. If Overbury's ghost could have visited them, either by day or night, the murdered man might have felt avenged by a misery so complete.

Their dream of state was gone; their hope of rest not come. The last years of their lives were to be spent in poverty, in loneliness, in mutual scorn. In time, on a pardon being vouchsafed them by the King, they left the Bloody tower and Garden house together, —going away, men said, to live in some country place, in a small house which had been left to them. There they dwelt under a common roof for a good many years to come; living apart; nursing a blue-eyed girl who had been born to them whilst they lay under the charge of murder; but otherwise groaning in a state of misery which was not untruly described as hell upon earth.

But out of evil comes, not seldom, by a higher law than men can fashion, a form of goodness to redeem it. Even as a lily feeds and grows out of dust and ashes, that blue-eyed girl, the child of so much sin, was to grow up in that secluded house, ignorant of her mother's shame, into one of the purest and proudest mothers in a land illustrious for her noble women. Lady Ann Carr was the only child of the guilty pair; and this daughter of a murderess lived to become the mother of that Lord William Russell who was to lay his head upon the block in the very same cause for which Raleigh died.

INDEX.

www.ingramcontent.com/pod-product-compliance
Lightning Source LLC
LaVergne TN
LVHW010241110826
845151LV00004B/1358

* 9 7 8 1 4 2 5 5 2 4 1 7 3 *